Kama Sutra

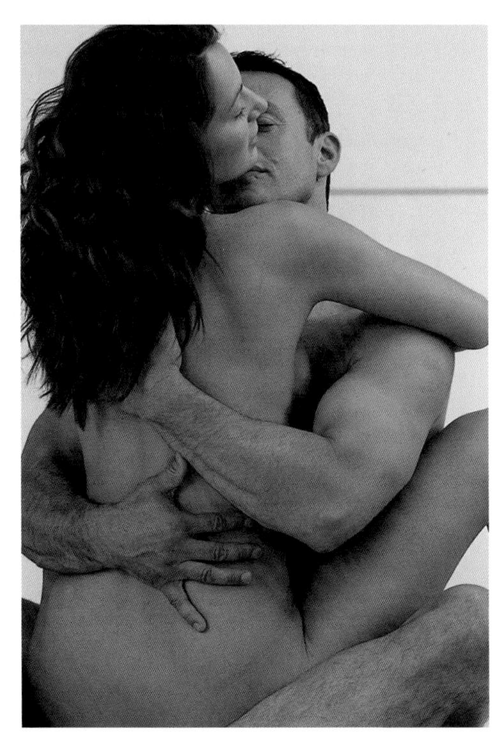

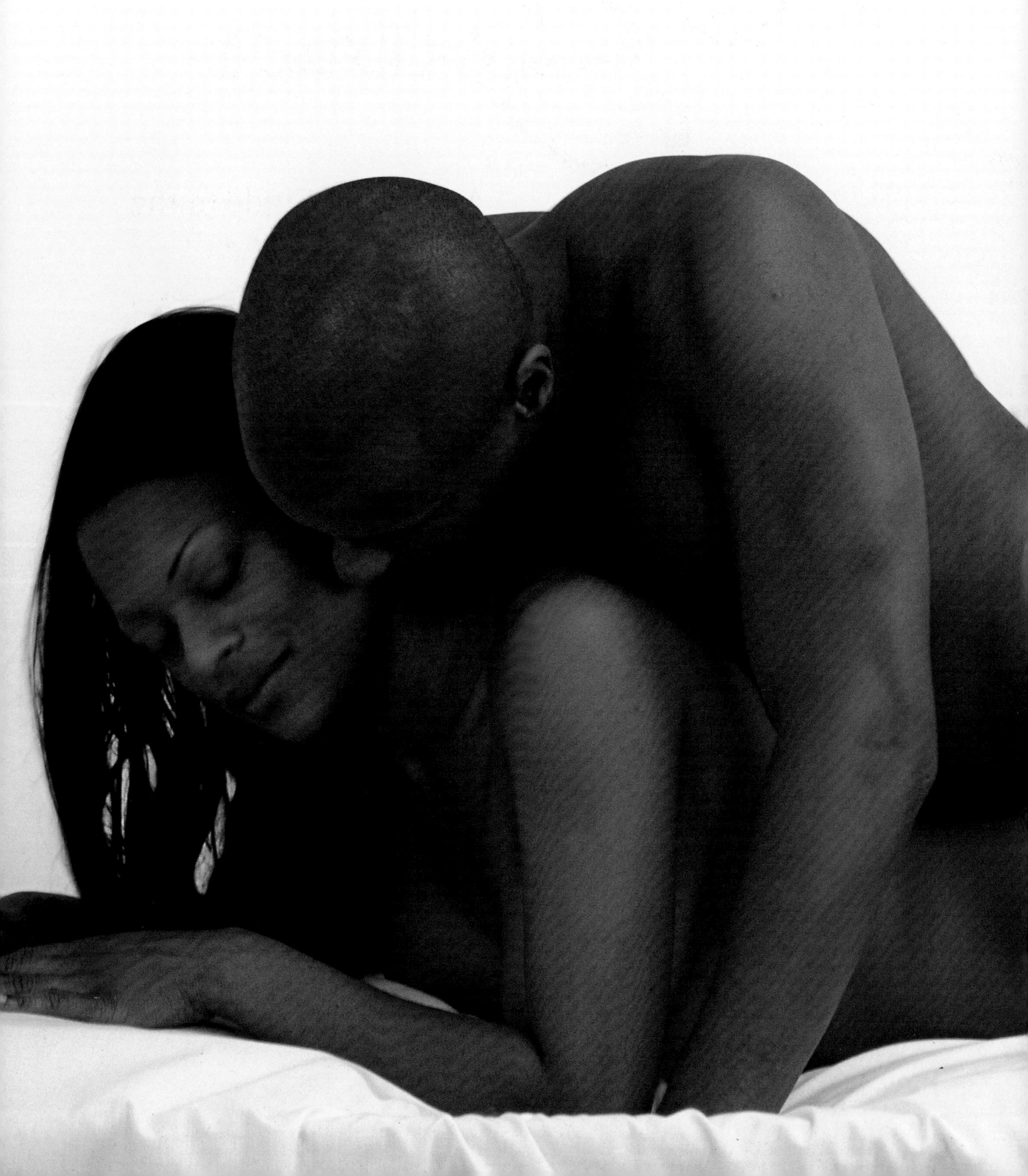

Kama Sutra

A Modern Guide to the Ancient Art of Sex

Nitya Lacroix

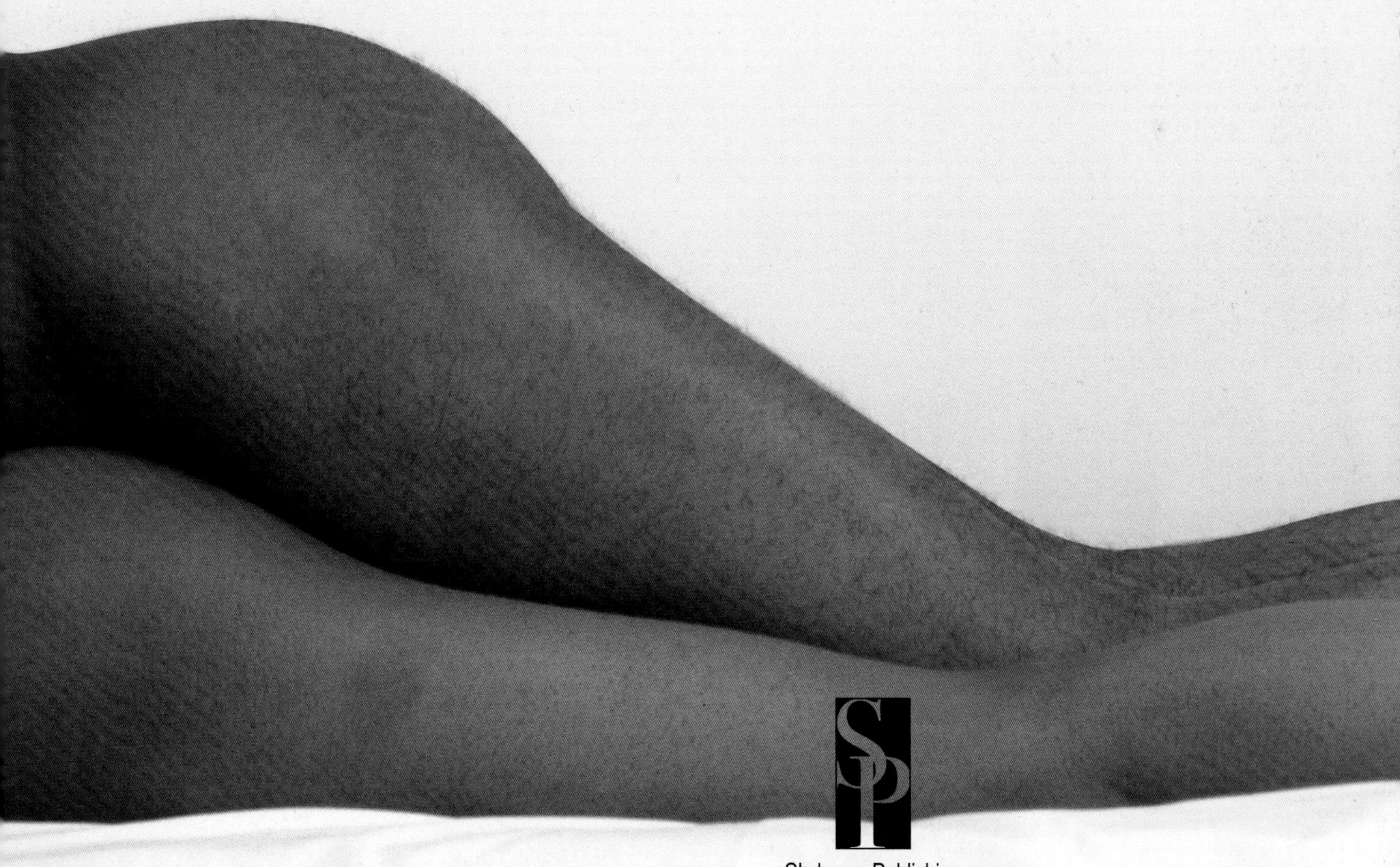

Skyhorse Publishing

First published as *Kama Sutra* by Nitya Lacroix in 2003 by Hylas Publishing

Skyhorse Publishing books may be purchased in bulk at special discounts for sales promotion, corporate gifts, fund-raising, or educational purposes. Special editions can also be created to specifications. For details, contact the Special Sales Department, Skyhorse Publishing, 307 West 36th Street, 11th Floor, New York, NY 10018 or info@skyhorsepublishing.com.

www.skyhorsepublishing.com

10 9 8 7 6 5

Library of Congress Cataloging-in-Publication Data is available on file.

ISBN: 978-1-62914-207-4

Printed in China

Contents

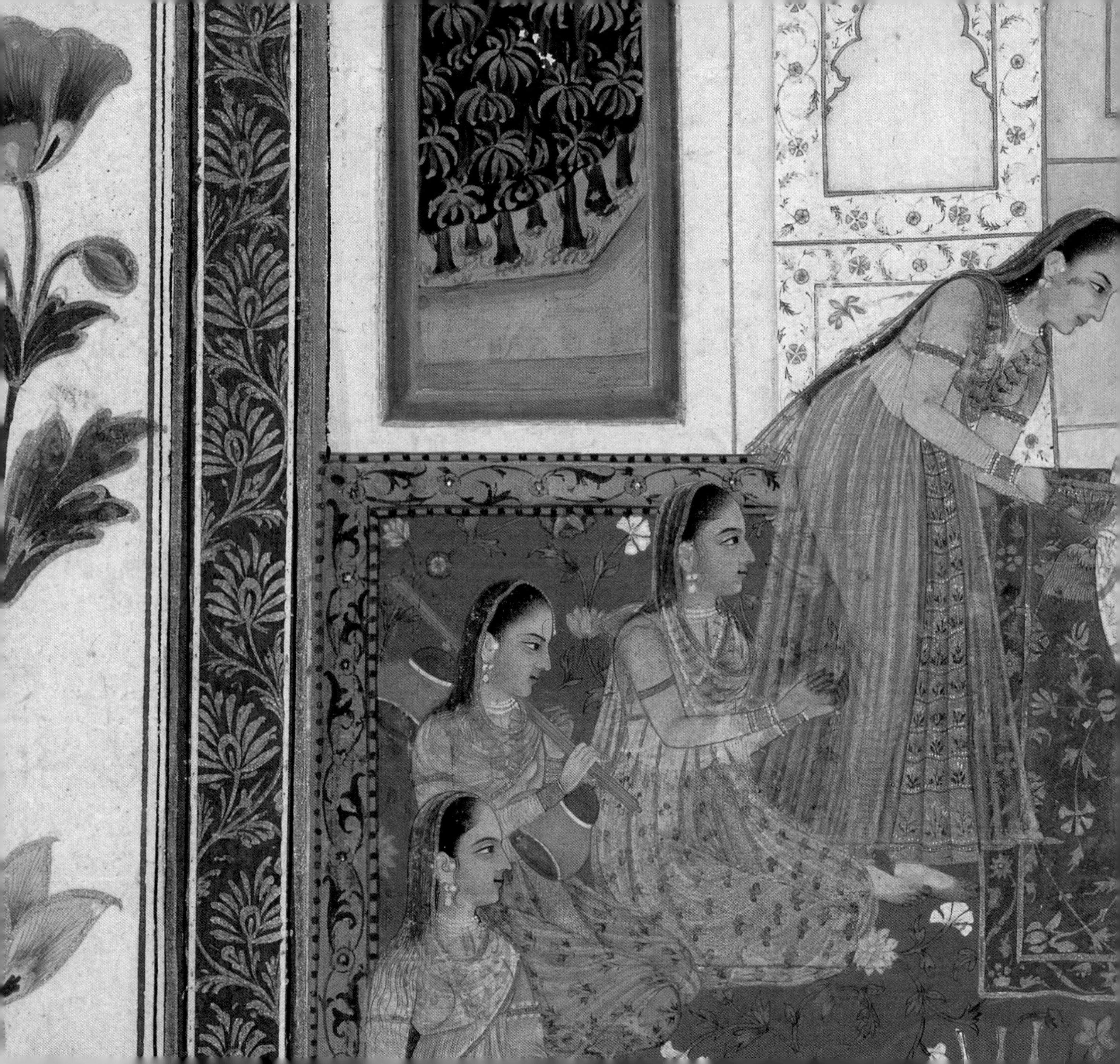

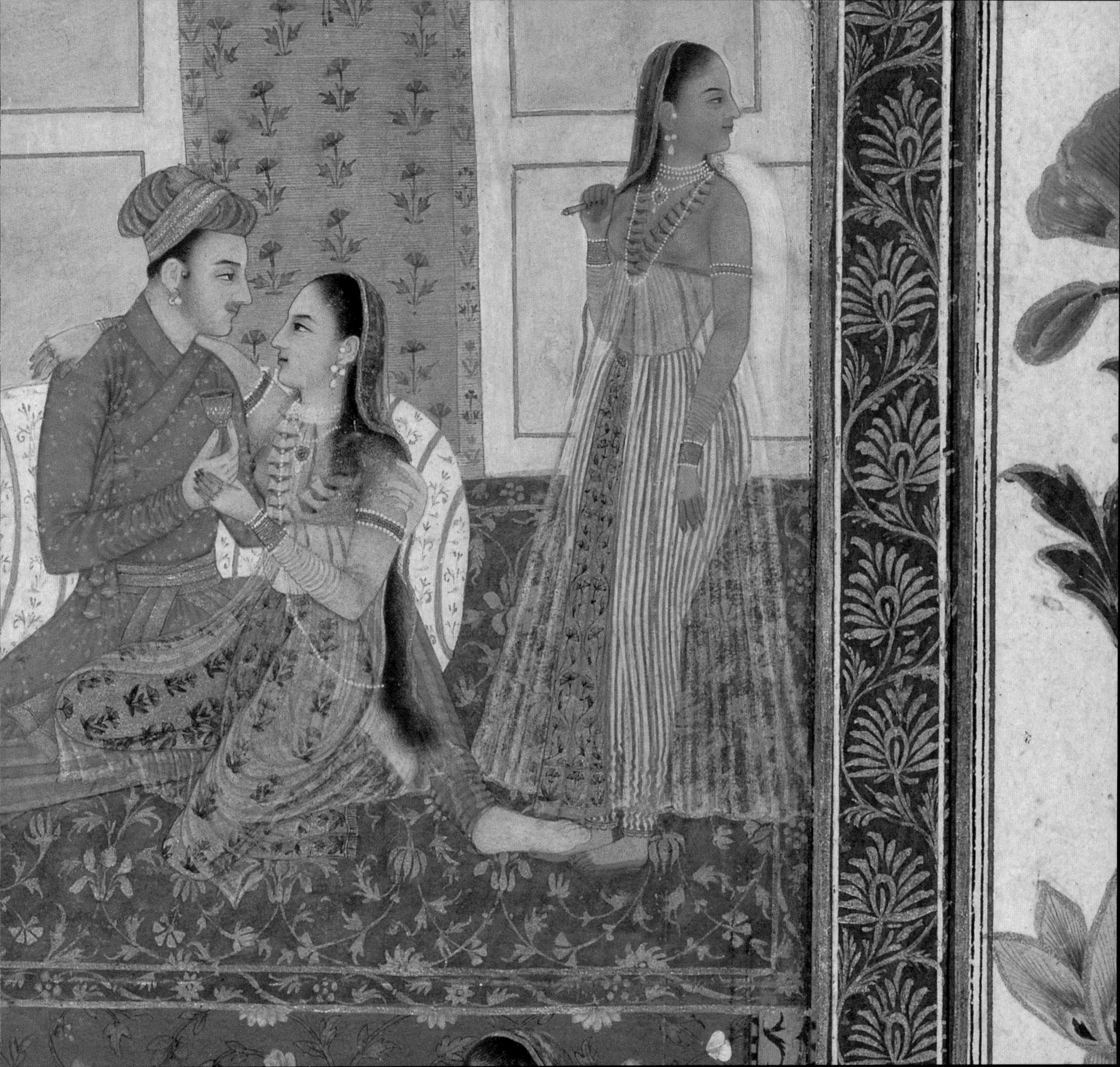

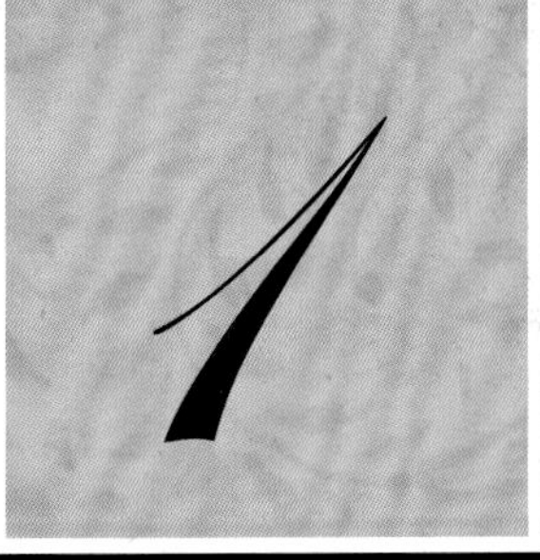

What is the Kama Sutra?

In ancient India sense and sensuality were seen as two sides of the same coin. To embrace and enjoy sex was considered to be an integral part in the journey of life to be enjoyed without guilt. Sexuality was at the very heart of all Hindu culture, including poetry, art, and music. Ancient Hindu sages preached the importance of sexual love; temple walls and religious caves were carved with exquisitely erotic sculptures; and Hindu paintings detailed explicit sexual activities. One Hindu text has famously stood the test of time to become the definitive practical guide to great sex: the Kama Sutra of Vatsyayana.

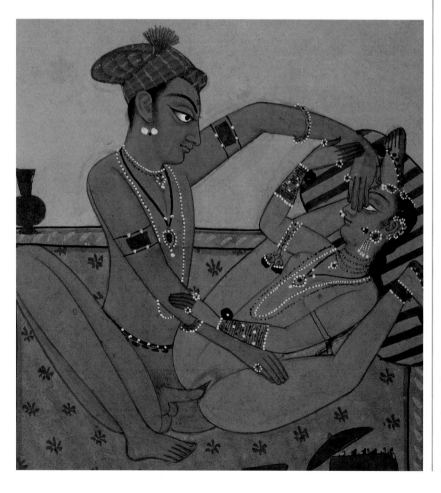

THE DEFINITIVE SEX GUIDE

The Kama Sutra was written by the sage Vatsyayana, probably some time in the 4th century. It is a compilation of the teachings of Hindu sages that were handed down over countless generations, and it had a profound influence on the social mores of Hindu society for centuries to follow. The sexual dictates were just a small part of the work, for the Kama Sutra also laid out the rules for entertaining and housekeeping; the duties of the husband and wife; and the role of the courtesan. However, it is Vatsyayana's vivid descriptions of sexual positions that had a major influence on Hindu artworks and writings over the centuries and, more recently, on Western culture too. Today, the term kama sutra is used to describe any collection of sexual positions, but especially more exotic or extravagant postures.

KAMA SHASTRA SOCIETY

The Kama Sutra was first published in England in 1883, during the notoriously sexually repressed Victorian era. It appeared in limited editions for private circulation to members of the Kama Shastra Society of London and Benares. The translation was the work of the enigmatic Victorian explorer Sir Richard Burton and his friend Forester Arbuthnot, a former civil servant in India. Both men shared a love of erotica and were dedicated to the translation and publication of exotic foreign texts, including the *Arabian Nights*.

< MANY OF THE POSITIONS *and practices described in the Kama Sutra have their origins in ancient tantric and yogic rituals. This artwork shows a woman in the position of the Wife of Indra (*see pg. 126*), combining sex with a yoga breathing exercise.*

SEXUAL REVOLUTION

When the Kama Sutra was published for the general readership at the height of the Western sexual revolution in the 1960s, people were astonished by the variety and descriptions of its lovemaking positions. In the West, sex had been a repressed subject for a long time and was viewed as a preserve for male enjoyment only. Women's sexuality and sexual needs were rarely discussed or even acknowledged. It was widely accepted that women put up with sex to please their husbands and to bear children. Suddenly, the West discovered what the East had known for thousands of years—that women were as orgasmic as men and could derive as much satisfaction and pleasure from sex as their partners. Not only that, the incredulous Western reader also discovered that there were many other lovemaking positions to be thoroughly enjoyed in addition to the male-dominant "Missionary position."

v VATSYAYANA'S VIVID *descriptions of sexual positions have had a major influence on Hindu art. At Khajuraho, in central India, magnificent temples are adorned with erotic friezes depicting every imaginable sexual activity.*

KAMA TODAY

The Kama Sutra is remarkable for its non-judgemental and very pragmatic approach to sexual matters, and a great deal of its teaching remains relevant and interesting to the contemporary man and woman. The Kama Sutra certainly makes it very clear that the woman's satisfaction is as important as the man's (and, fortunately, recent research confirms that most men now share this opinion). A fascinating modern translation by Wendy Doniger and Sudhir Kakar demonstrates that Vatsyayana's text was perhaps more liberal and egalitarian than was previously thought, and that Burton's translation—though a magnificent achievement for its time—is marred by Victorian squeamishness and indirect language that was not evident in the original Sanskrit. The new translators even go so far as to suggest that Burton occasionally adapted the text to incorporate Victorian values. A particularly blatant example is Burton's translation of Vatsyayana's description of what a woman should do when her husband is unfaithful: "She should not blame him excessively, though she be a little displeased. She should not use abusive language toward him, but rebuke him with conciliatory

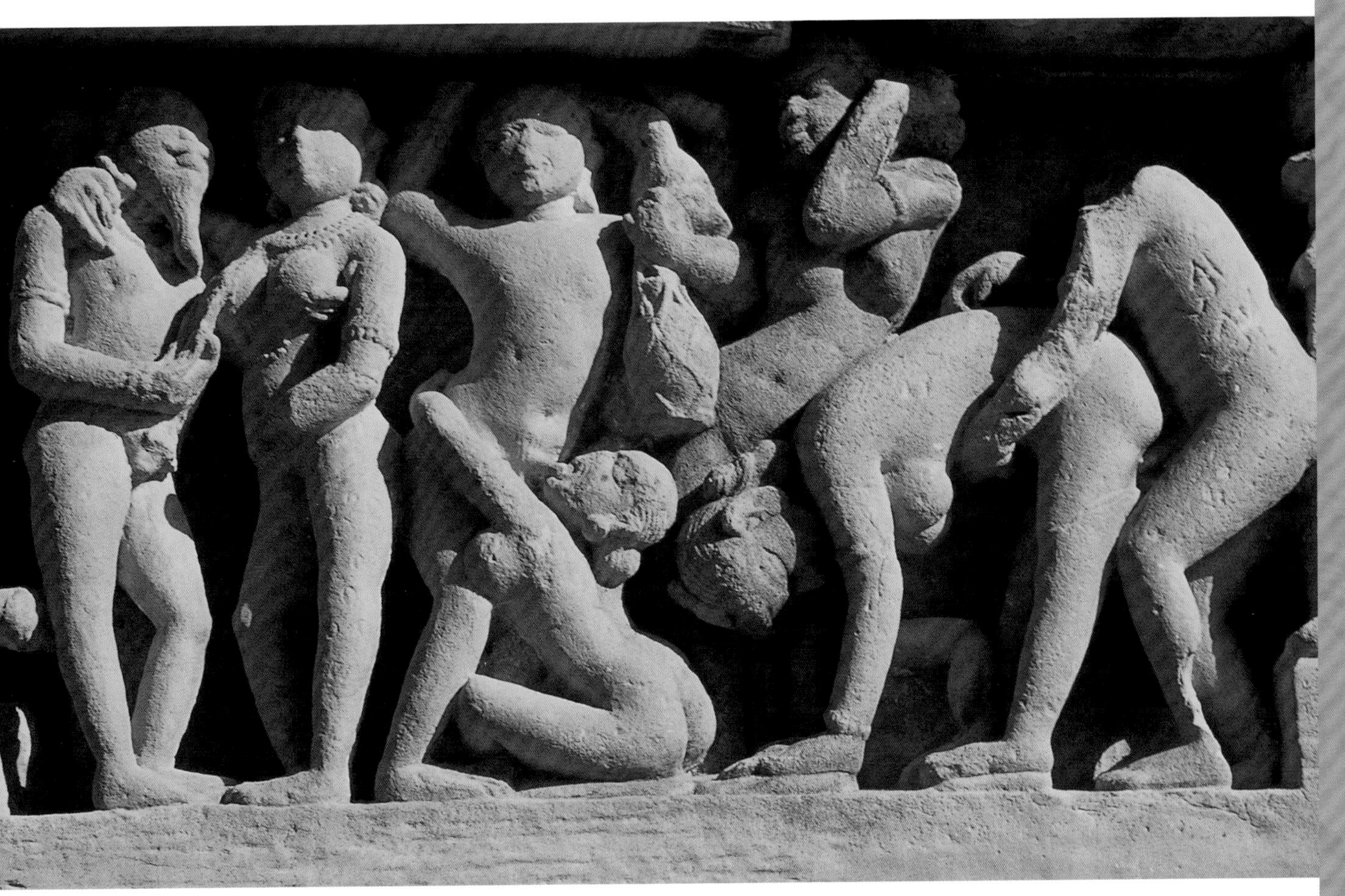

words." The modern translation reveals that Vatsyayana actually advised that the woman should scold her husband with abusive language, whether he is alone or in company. These are two very different interpretations.

ANANGA RANGA

The Kama Sutra is not the only great Hindu work of its kind. The Ananga Ranga, written in the 15th century by the poet Kalyana Malla, specifically targeted married couples in the belief that sexual variety kept a relationship alive and that monotony was the main enemy of marriage. Wise advice even for modern times. This book draws on relevant sexual advice from both these famous Hindu works of eroticism and places it in a modern context.

SEXUAL BATTLEGROUND

Attitudes toward sex are constantly in flux, not only because of generational, religious, and cultural differences, but also because of ever-changing attitudes towards matters of health, economics, gender relationships, and social conditions. Sexual matters that shock one group of people may be regarded as trivial or merely titillating by another. Today, sex is no longer the taboo subject that it once was in the West. The pendulum has truly swung, and sex is all around us in the media, advertising, and the arts. All too often it is portrayed as a selling point without any emotional content. Frequently, it is presented as a battleground between men and women: who dominates, who gets the better orgasm, and who lasts longer. There is little mystery and romance to this modern-day depiction of sexuality. So, in the spirit of the original Kama Sutra, it is the aim of this book to remind ourselves that good sex is developed out of respect for the differences and the similarities of the sexual and emotional needs of men and women.

This book also hopes to put spice and variety back into the readers' lovemaking if it has become a little dull and repetitive. The pressures of modern life can leave little time for good lovemaking; if you are always tired at the end of the day, sex may have become routine or even non-existent. And many partners still take each other for granted and forget to add the sensuality to sex, too frequently forgoing foreplay and concentrating only on the end result.

It is hoped that putting the Kama Sutra in a contemporary context will reignite passion and rapport between you and your partner. If you already enjoy a great sex life, exploring this book with your lover can enhance your lovemaking still further. And if you have not yet met the love of your life, you will find suggestions to help you find a compatible partner.

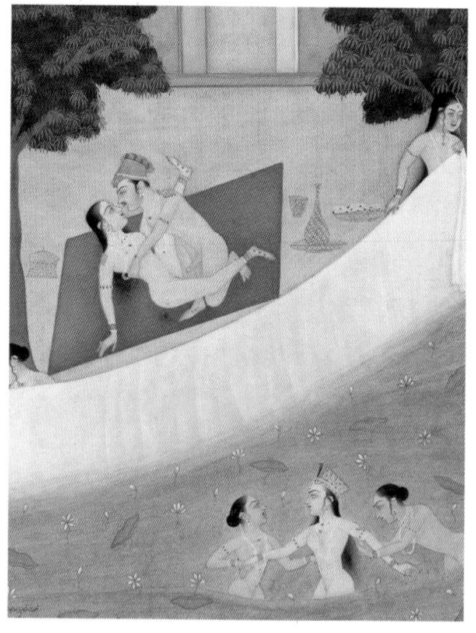

∧ NOT EVERYTHING *in the original Kama Sutra is still relevant to modern couples. In ancient India men often had several wives or even harems.*

NEW APPROACH

The Kama Sutra is not simply a book of sexual positions; it is about pleasure in a much broader sense. It explains the importance of the compatibility of sexual staying power and of matching libidos. It emphasizes how essential it is for the pursuit of love and physical pleasure to stimulate all five senses, and it explains how to prepare yourself physically and mentally to convey the message that you are attractive and ready for sex. It also describes ways of creating an ambient setting in which a loving and romantic relationship can flourish, and it discusses the many pleasures and variations of foreplay that can be enjoyed.

The original Kama Sutra and the Ananga Ranga both make it very clear that certain sexual positions flow naturally into others in what Vatsyayana poetically describes as the "Wheel of Love" (*see* pg.16). The later chapters of this book explicitly demonstrate how lovers can move comfortably between a variety of Kama Sutra sexual positions during a single lovemaking episode without turning sex into a display of gymnastics. Like the Ananga Ranga, this book is specifically targeted toward long-term lovers (or those who are looking for a lasting relationship), because true sexual harmony arises only when two lovers are familiar and comfortable with each other's bodies and enjoy a deep and mutual trust.

> EROTIC *Indian artwork appears throughout this book to place the advice in its original context and to highlight similarities and differences between modern society and that of ancient India. This painting illustrates the equivalent of a "quickie" in the back of a luxury car.*

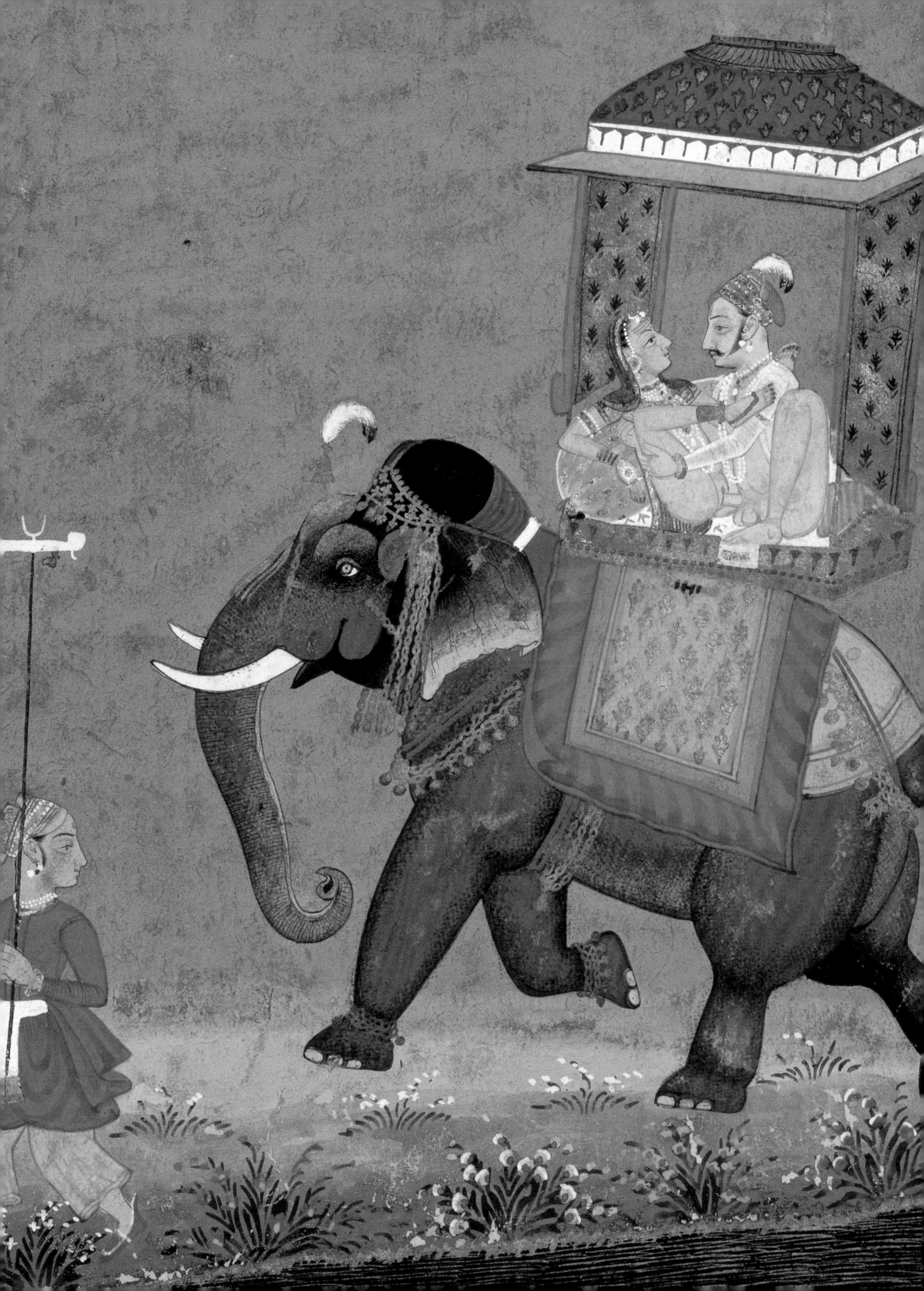

Consciousness of pleasure

Kama sutra translates as "teachings on sensual pleasure." *Kama* is the Sanskrit word for physical sensuality, and *sutra* means a teaching instruction or aphorism. The very fact that the Kama Sutra exists is a testament to how the ancient Hindu civilization embraced sexuality as an integral part of life. The pursuit of pleasure was one of three goals in life, the others being the pursuits of wealth and spiritual growth.

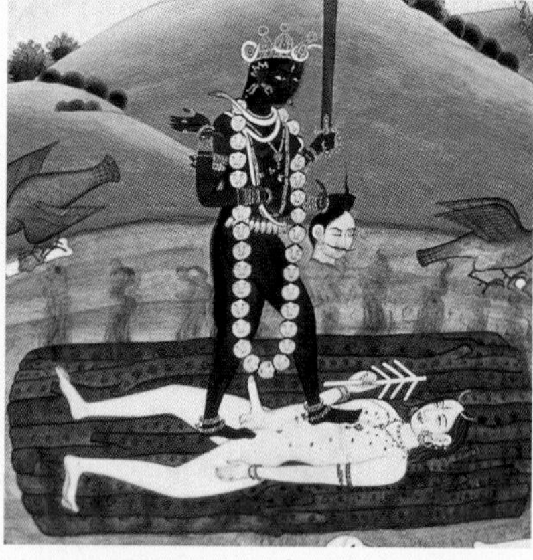

∧ THE TERRIFYING KALI *is the Hindu goddess of destruction. However, as Parvati or Duga, she is also revered as the initiator of creation in the eternal cycle of life, death, and rebirth. Her consort, Shiva, is usually portrayed prostrate beneath her.*

BODY AS TEMPLE

In ancient Hindu culture the body was viewed as the temple of the soul and sexuality as a gateway to spiritual fulfillment through the pathway of the senses. From a spiritual perspective, the five senses were seen as the connecting points between

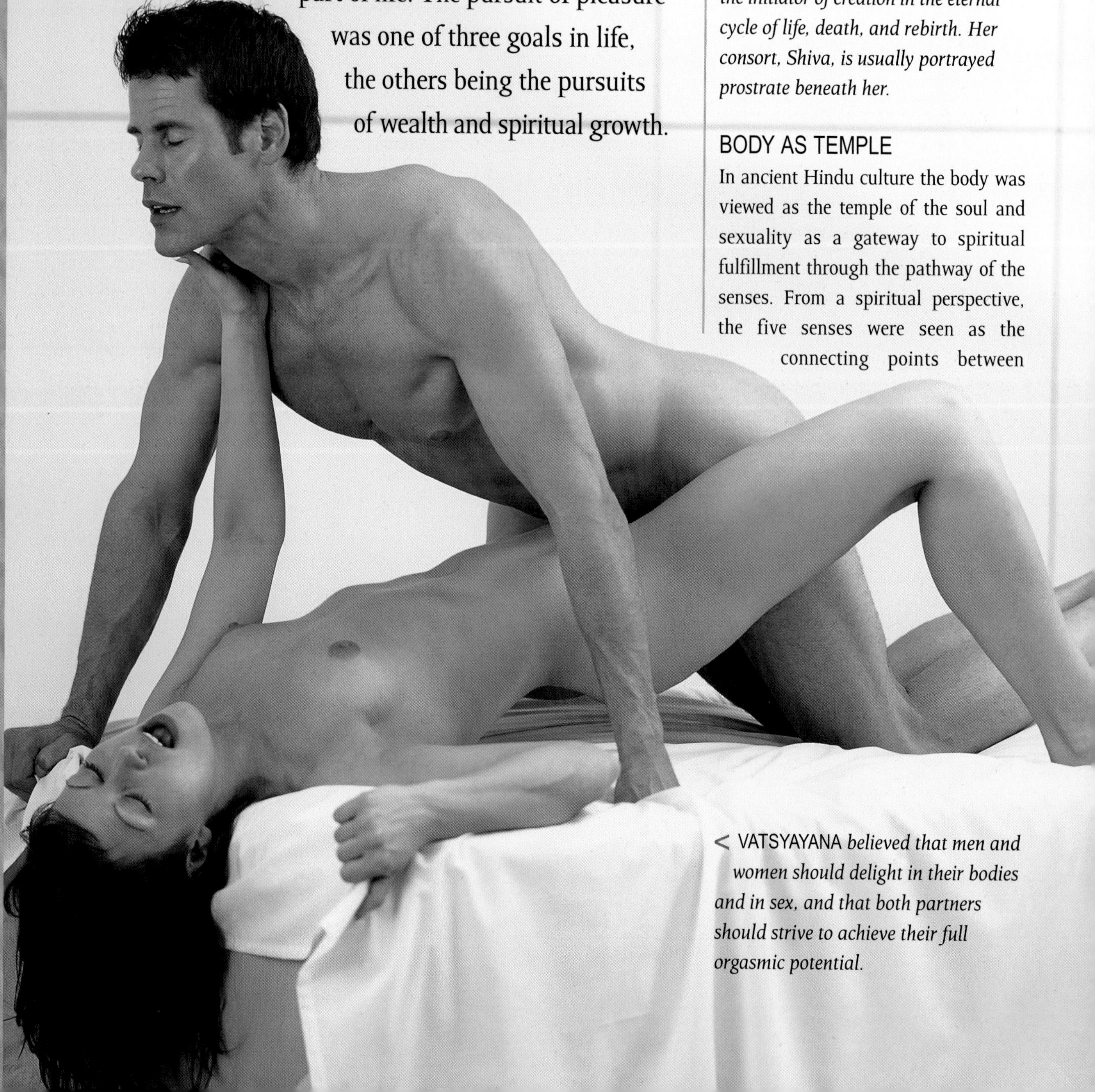

< VATSYAYANA *believed that men and women should delight in their bodies and in sex, and that both partners should strive to achieve their full orgasmic potential.*

Kama

Ultimately, the Kama Sutra derives its name from Kama, the mischievous Hindu god of love, whose flower-tipped arrows pierce the hearts of both mortals and gods alike, forcing his victims to succumb to an irresistible desire for the first person who crosses their path. Like Eros and Cupid of classical mythology, the playful Kama created havoc amongst the mightiest of the gods. So the word *kama* came to represent the pursuit of physical pleasure and sensuality as experienced through the five senses of the body—hearing, touch, sight, taste, and smell. And nothing is quite like the act of sex for engaging all of these five senses and bringing the body to the height of its pleasure.

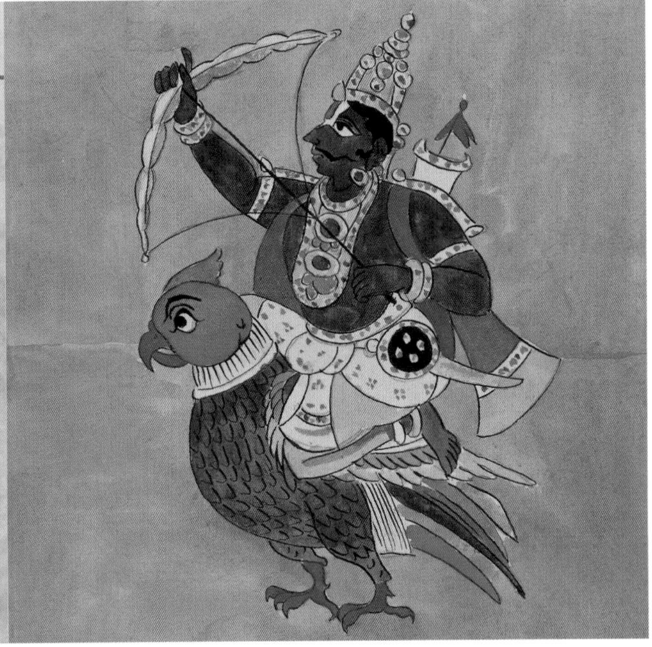

the physical realm of the human body and the cosmic realm of the universe, while the body itself was believed to be a microcosm of all that existed in creation. So, according to the Kama Sutra, the body and all things sensual are to be celebrated and revered as sacred rather than suppressed and reviled as shameful—as has been the case throughout much of our history in the West.

The pursuit of love and sensuality was therefore viewed as a desirable art to be accomplished, and a science to be practiced so that one could gain a mastery over one's physical needs and desires. The ability to experience the happiness of fulfilled sexual union between a man and woman was just as important as the pursuit of wealth, *artha*, and religious merit, *dharma*. While the Kama Sutra derived its text from centuries of teachings of Hindu sages, Vatsyayana delivered his advice in a very straightforward manner. Unlike the ancient Hindu tantric texts on sexuality, he did not couch his advice on sex in spiritual terms, but delivered it in a no-nonsense and straightforward manner. Yet there is no doubt that the Kama Sutra, and much later the Ananga Ranga, emerged from the tantric tradition of ancient India, where sexual acts were performed as ritual practices and where the tantric union of man and woman in lovemaking was seen as an enactment of the cosmic fusion of duality out of which all creation emerges.

HINDU PANTHEON

In Hinduism, every deity has his female counterpart, so every god is depicted with his goddess by his side. There is Shiva and Parvati (or Kali), Krishna and Rhada, Rama and Sita,

< THE LOVE STORY OF KRISHNA *and Rhada is among the most beautiful in Hindu literature. He is often revered as a fertility god, whose flute-playing entrances all who hear it. He is usually represented as a beautiful youth with bluish skin, wearing a crown of peacock feathers.*

Vishnu and Laxmi. Male and female energies, both divine and mortal, are seen to represent the polar energies of the universe from which all duality arises. When these energies merge, universal harmony exists, and when they are separated, creation unfolds. So sexual union, according to Hindu tradition, has great significance, and symbols of the phallus and vagina, known as the lingum and yoni, are represented in places of worship throughout the Indian subcontinent.

> *". . . pleasures, being as necessary for the existence and well being of the body as food, are consequently equally required."* KSI:II

V SCULPTURES *of erect phalluses can be found in temples throughout India. The Shiva lingam and the Shakti yoni (its feminine counterpart) were revered as emblems of regeneration.*

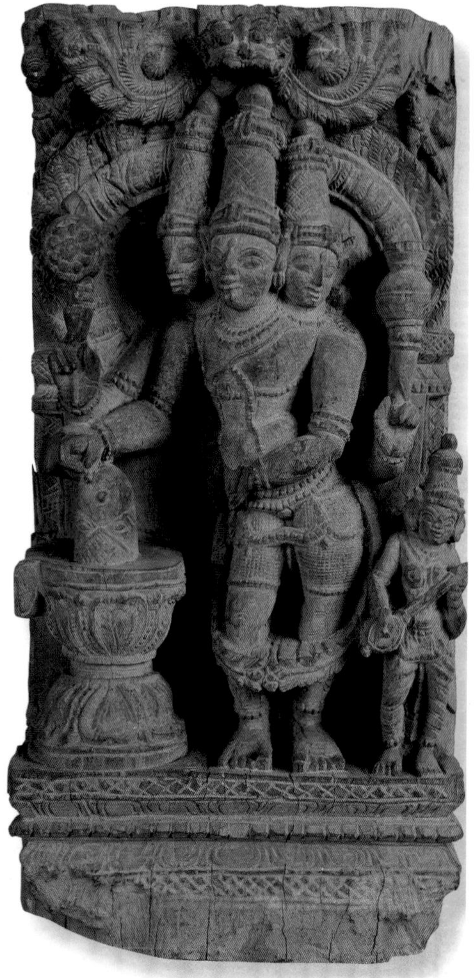

FEMININE ENERGY

Out of this tradition also emerges a respect for woman's sexuality and the necessity for men to respect the female body. In tantric tradition a woman's sexual organs are described in eloquent terms, such as a lotus-bud or a jewel, and her orgasmic potency is worshipped. While Vatsyayana's Kama Sutra is written largely from the male perspective, it readily acknowledges a woman's capacity for sexual joy and even advises men to "place your pleasures second to hers." Like John Gray, the author of *Men are from Mars, Women are from Venus*, in our own era, Vatsyayana believed that by teaching his readers to appreciate the innate psychological differences between men and women he would be promoting greater understanding and respect. He believed that while making love, a man is more inclined to think, "this woman is united with me," while the woman would think, "I am united with this man." This subtle difference in consciousness speaks volumes about the play of emotional and physical dominance and submission in sexuality. Perhaps, however, the modern woman is more confident about playing a dominant sexual role, while the contemporary man may be more at ease being the submissive partner from time to time. Nevertheless, Vatsyayana insists that men and women derive the same pleasure in the sexual act, adding that "men and women being of the same nature feel the same kind of pleasure."

MARS AND VENUS

This version of the Kama Sutra attempts to highlight the varying perspectives of the man and woman in their enjoyment of sex. It hopes that by presenting the male and female perspective on different sex acts in a straightforward and lighthearted way, both partners can learn more about each other's sexual needs and can experiment joyfully with ways to increase the pleasure of their love lives. Sexual positions can stimulate each partner in very different ways. Some of the sexual sequences are male dominated, some female dominated. But sex is not a battleground, it is a playground, and a truly balanced sexual partnership allows a natural and easy transfer between dominant and submissive roles and always leaves room for intimacy, respect, and humor. Lovemaking is about two people who are in love meeting and merging, touching and responding, and losing themselves in the moment and in each other.

> TANTRIC MANDALAS *were used as visual aids to meditation in tantric rituals. The lotus flower in the center is a symbol of enlightenment.*

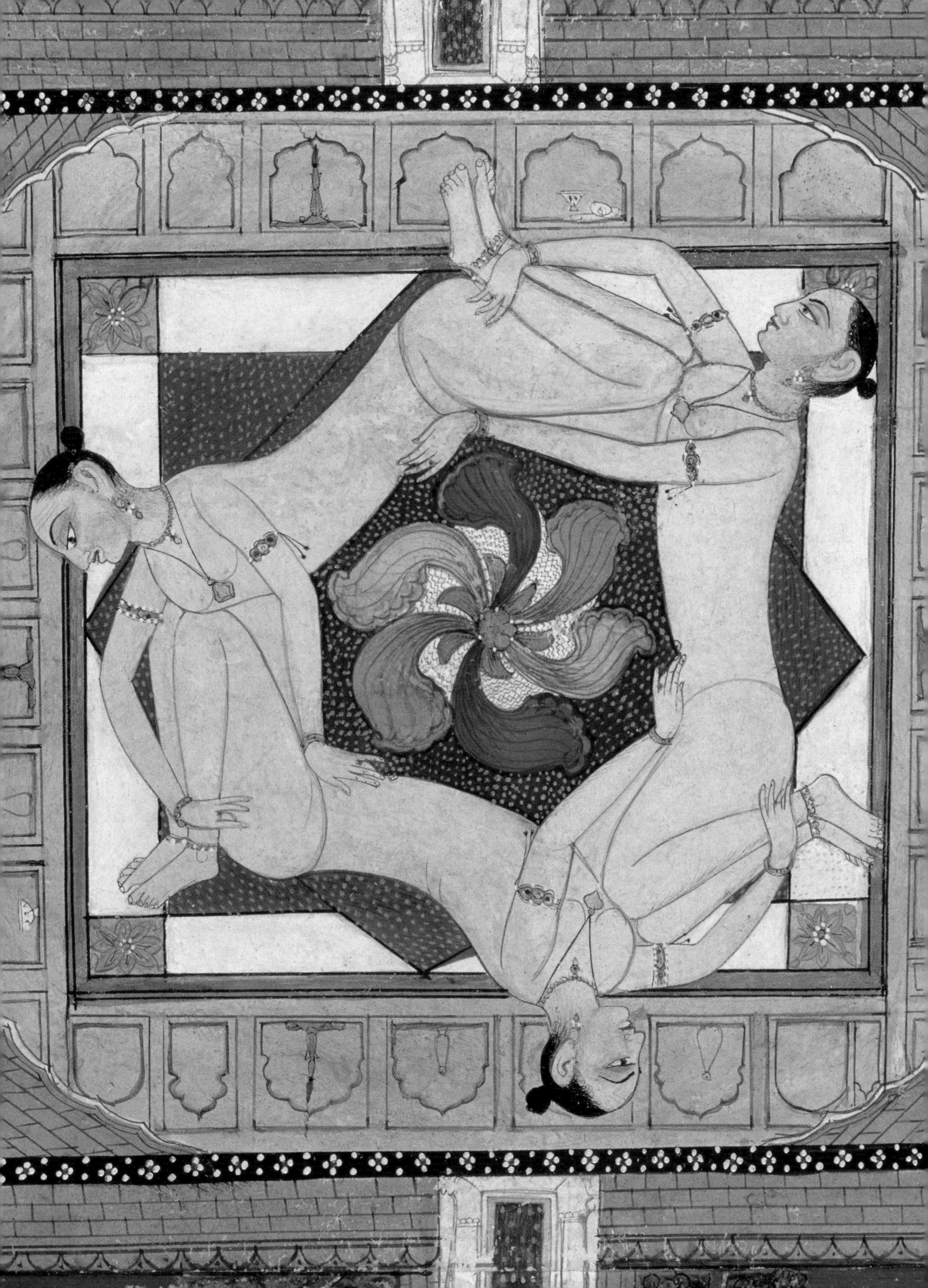

Wheel of love

The Kama Sutra positions are usually presented as a catalog of exotic postures from which lovers can pick and choose when they are feeling a little adventurous. In fact, the Kama Sutra stresses the importance of seeing the positions as steps in a sexual dance, a sensuous *pas de deux* in which the lovers' movements flow naturally and harmoniously from the first tentative steps of arousal to the passionate finale of orgasm.

NATURE OF LOVE

Vatsyayana talks poetically of the wheel of love, the spontaneous, fluid and graceful movement of lovers who have lost themselves in their lovemaking, moving effortlessly from one position to another, in a motion of perfect physical and emotional harmony.

SEVEN ACTS

To reflect Vatsyayana's teaching, this book presents seven sequences in which the positions flow naturally from one to another. All the Kama Sutra positions are included, and there are many others from the Ananga Ranga. Admittedly some are very extravagant and practically impossible to adopt (the Wife of Indra springs instantly to mind). These have been included as curiosities, but it is not recommended that you try them unless you are unusually supple or double-jointed. However, the majority of the positions are relatively simple to adopt and many, such as the Dog position, are almost too familiar for today's sexually wise reader.

DIVERSE MOODS

Each of the sequences has a very different overall feeling and mood. For example, the Clasping position and its variations are intimate, loving, and balanced, whereas the Pressed position and its variations are definitely male dominated and detached. Lovemaking should naturally change from one instance to another because the sexual act ideally reflects the mood and feelings of the moment: raunchy and passionate sex may be enjoyable on one occasion, but might be inappropriate on a day when you are feeling vulnerable and need tenderness from your partner. Passion and intimacy can change each time when two lovers are deeply attuned to one another's moods and needs.

KAMA SHASTRA

Although Vatsyayana clearly intended the Kama Sutra to be a practical manual (or Shastra) for lovers, he also affirmed that during the throes of passion the rule book goes straight out of the window: "When the wheel of love is once set in motion, there is then no Shastra and no order." There is no magical repertoire of movements that is guaranteed to work for everyone. So this book does not suggest that you learn the sequences as you would learn a fashionable dance, but that you explore the movements with your lover as a way of enhancing your sex

> THE TWINING *sequence is based on the Clasping and Twining positions. This is a good way to begin lovemaking because the face-to-face position encourages intimacy, and the full front-of-body contact heightens arousal and facilitates foreplay. The man's erect penis is naturally at the ideal angle for penetration. Moving to the Inverted position makes the sequence sensual and balanced.*

> THE OPEN *sequence is based on the Widely Opened and Yawning positions. Although there isn't full body contact, they are face-to-face positions with good eye contact, so they can still be very intimate and loving. Penetration is deep, which lends a sense of fulfilment emotionally and physically. The Turning position allows the woman space to relax and brings an element of adventure and fun.*

> THE RISING *sequence is centered on the Rising position and its variants. It is the legs-in-the air, raunchy movements that allow both partners to let go of their inhibitions and get a little steamy and vocal. It is a natural progression from the Open sequence if you are feeling passionate. The Splitting position allows you to experiment with new and exciting angles of penetration.*

> THE PRESSED *sequence is based on the very male-dominant Intact and Pressed positions. These positions are not for everyone because the woman is "trussed" in very compact postures that have more than a hint of bondage. However, many women enjoy feeling helpless and dominated at times during sex. The inclusion of the Refined posture allows the woman the chance to rest and literally stretch her legs.*

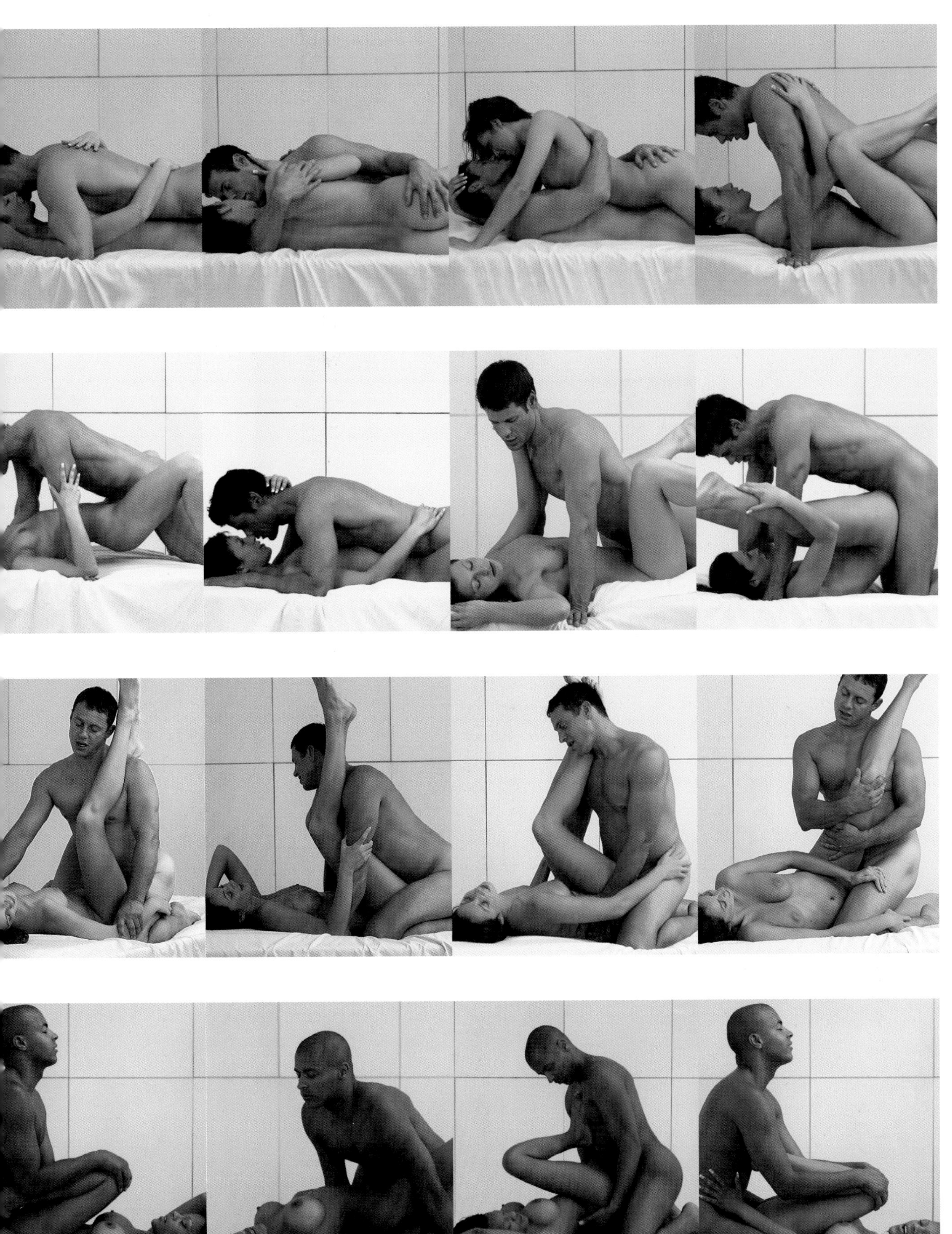

life, and bringing variety into it, perhaps by introducing one or two of the movements into your lovemaking on any one occasion. There are places within each sequence where a number of other, very different possibilities present themselves.

Ultimately, however, it is not the number of impressive techniques or sexual positions that will increase your sexual compatibility. This will come only from intimacy, tenderness, and open communication. Take moments in your lovemaking to be still, to make eye contact with each other, to breathe together harmoniously.

"... when the wheel of love is once set in motion, there is then no Shastra and no order." *KSII:II*

SEXUAL SATISFACTION

In the end there is only one rule to follow when making love, and that is simply that both partners should feel satisfied by the experience, physically and emotionally. Most couples do not expect mind-blowing sex every time. However, when a man is in the dominant role, he needs to exercise a certain amount of conscious control over his thrusting and be aware of his own state of arousal. In man-on-top positions it is all the more important that he always remains aware of his partner's sexual responses so that she receives the right kind of stimulation to achieve sexual satisfaction. Each woman will have her own ideas about what constitutes satisfaction. For many, of course, it will mean being able to achieve their full orgasmic potential. Others say that the most important aspect of lovemaking is emotional and physical intimacy, regardless of whether or not orgasm is reached.

Like good wine, lovemaking usually improves with time as lovers become familiar with one another's preferences and responses. With time, lovers begin to tune in to each other in the same way that dancers do when they continually practise their art together. And good sex is definitely an art.

> THE ANIMAL *sequence is centered on animalistic postures. These are very primal, male-dominated positions, where penetration is deep. Their unique eroticism arises from the detached nature of these positions, as there is little or no eye contact—though the inclusion of the Cat position allows full body contact and a chance to express lusty feline sensuality. Time for a bit of fantasy and role play.*

> THE TOP *sequence is the one place where we deviate from the spirit of the Kama Sutra, because woman-on-top positions were generally frowned upon in Vatsyayana's day. Many women really come alive sexually only when they take full control. She can revel in the full freedom of movement that is available to her in these positions, while the man may welcome the chance to relax and enjoy the very erotic view.*

> THE EQUAL *sequence is centered on the position of Equals and Kama's Wheel. It is the most balanced and loving of all the sequences. The movement of both partners is limited, so the build-up of sexual excitement is slow and sensuous. This is the perfect way to prolong lovemaking post-orgasm if you are not ready to let go of that feeling of oneness that great sex brings.*

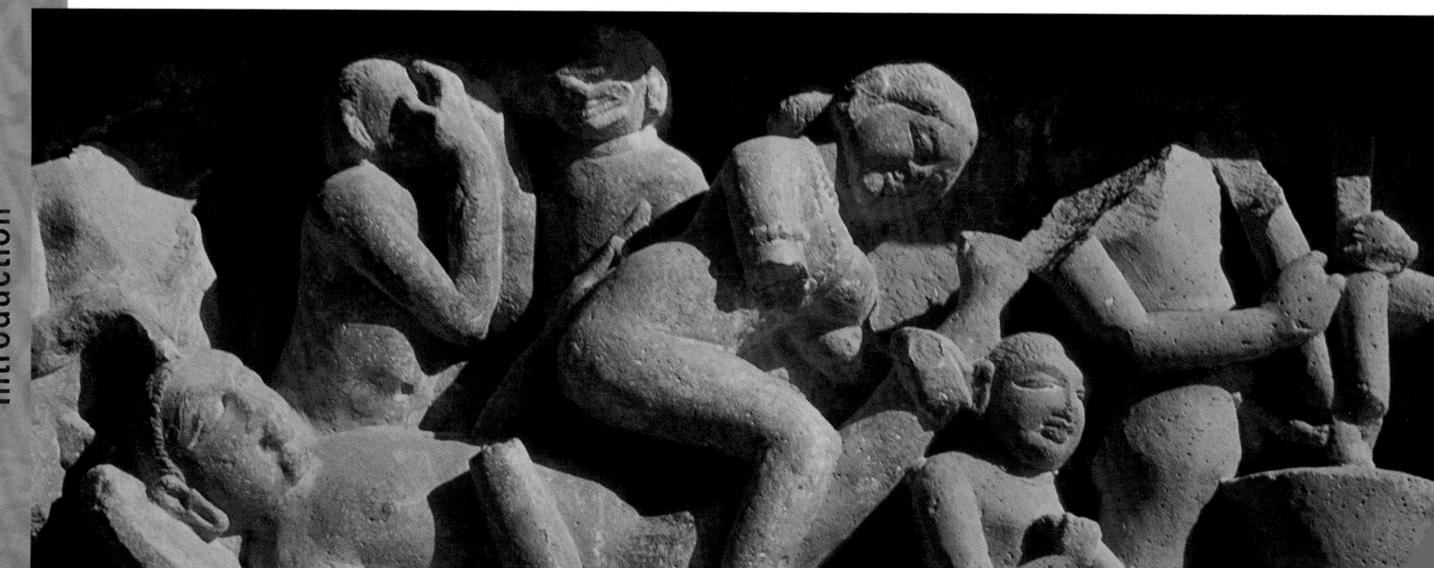

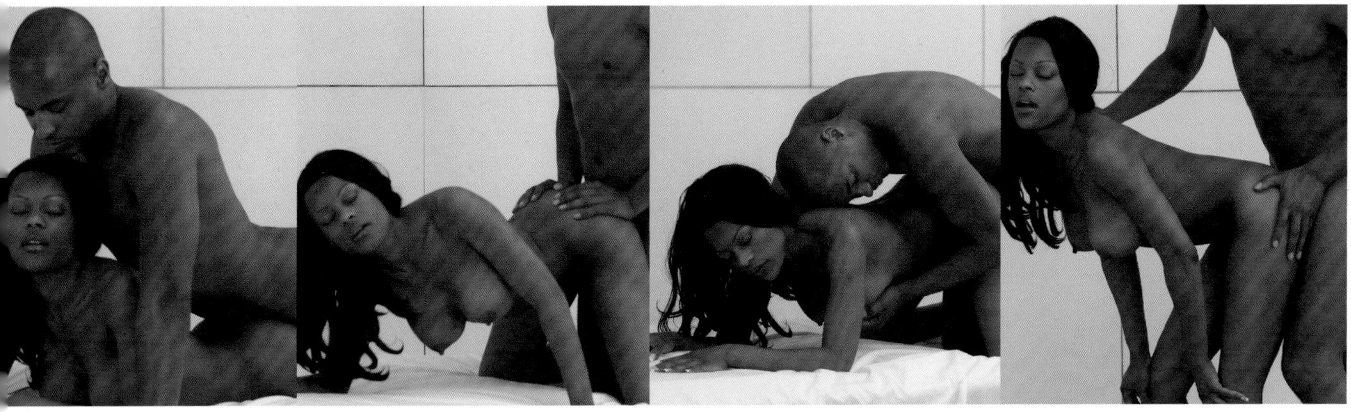

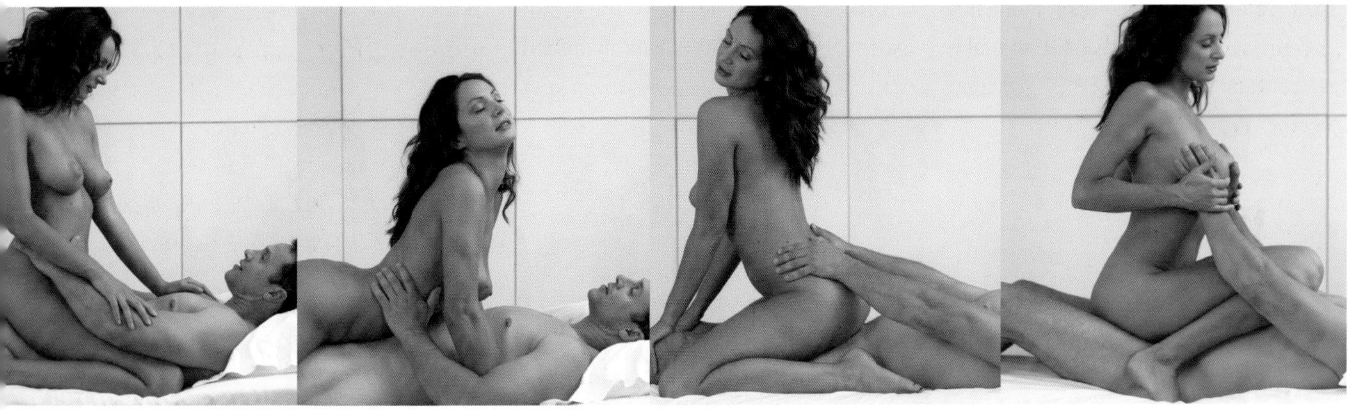

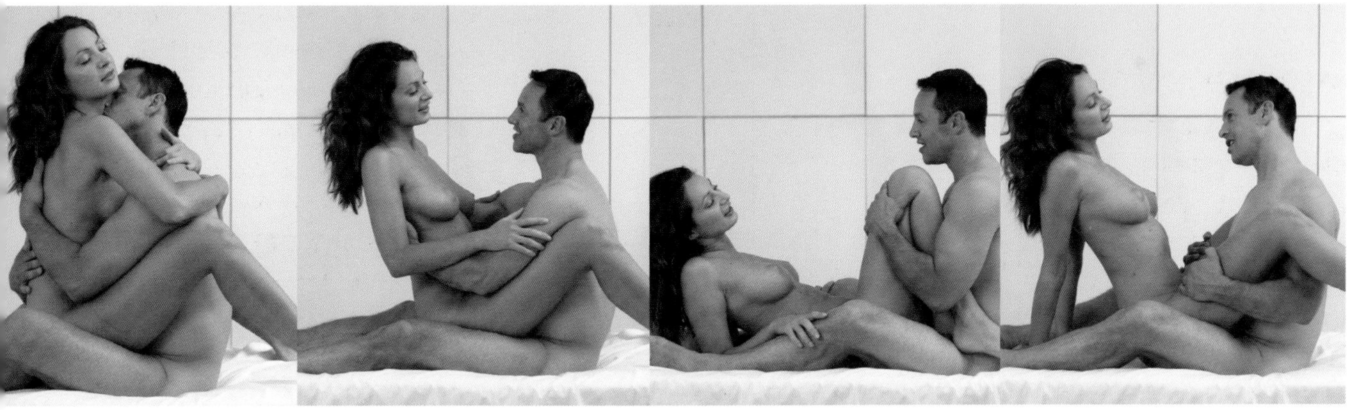

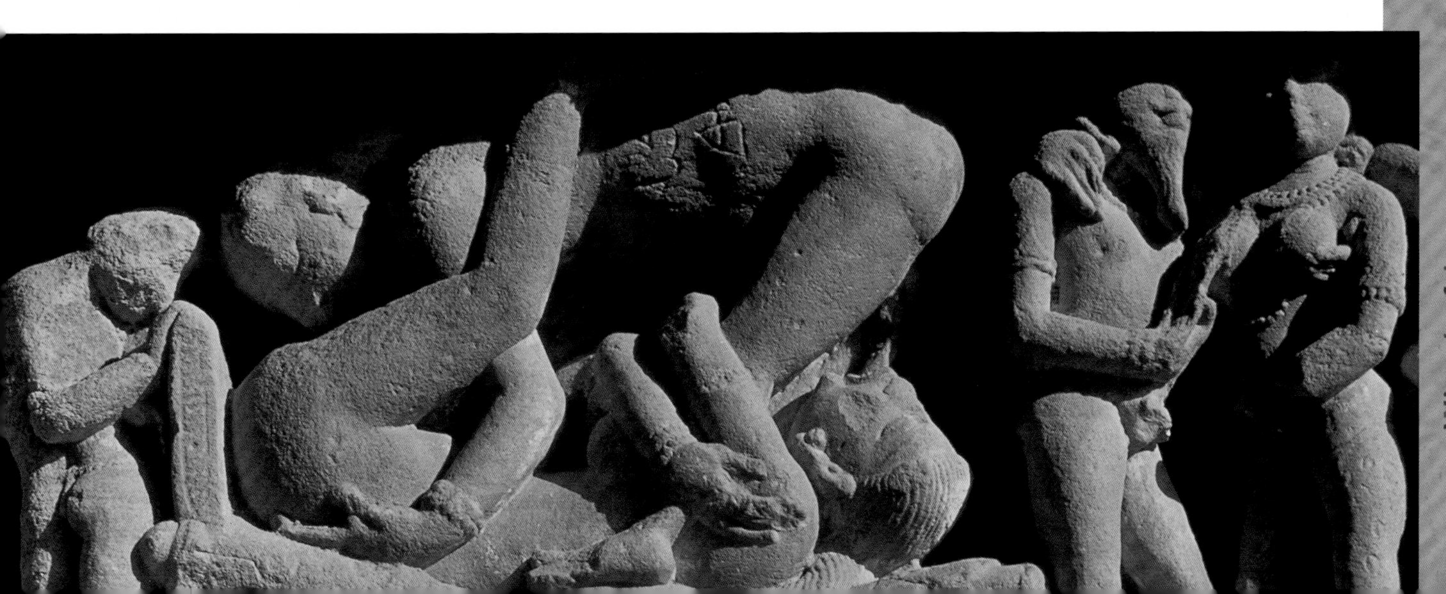

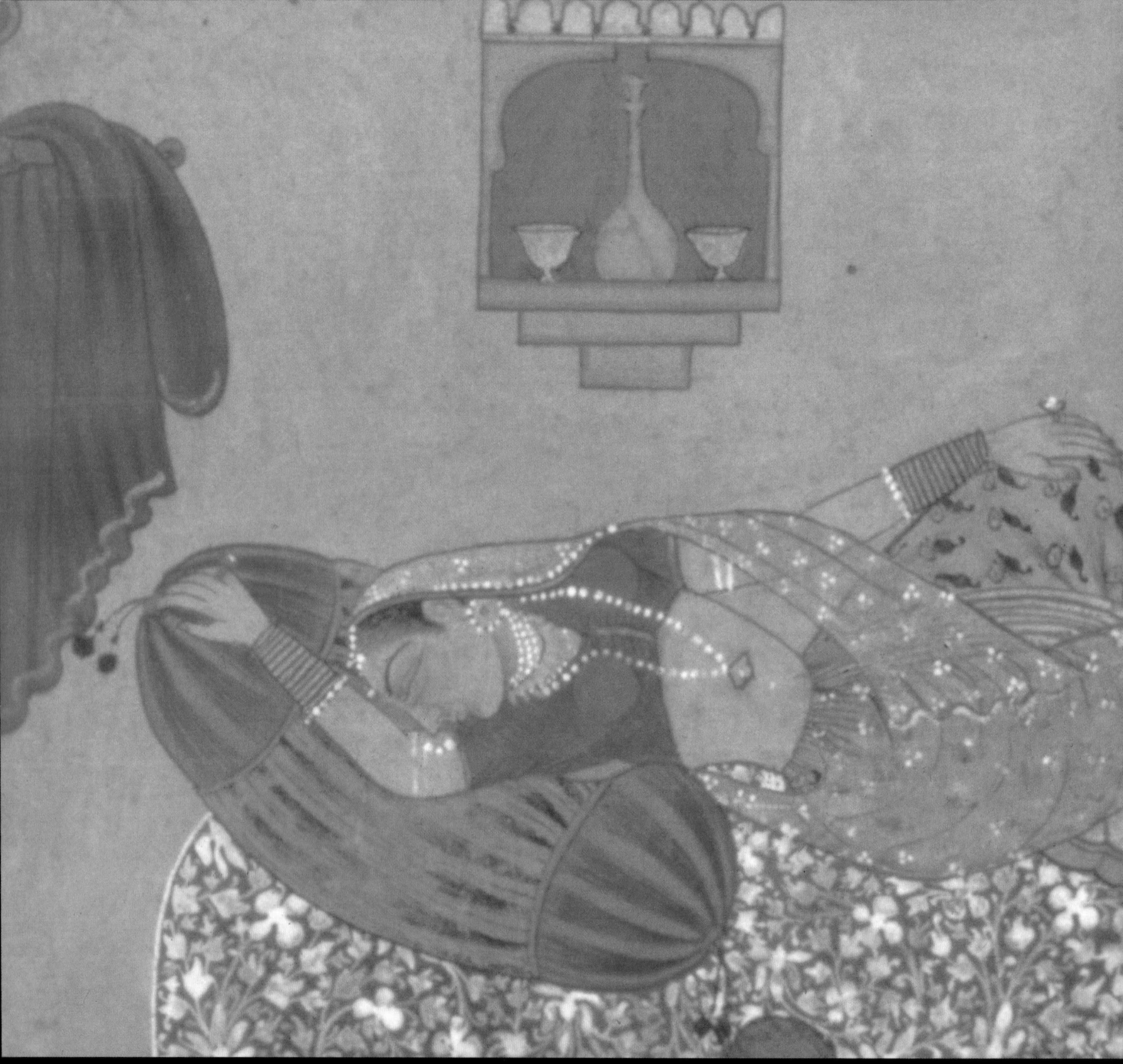

“The love which is mutual on both sides, and proved to be there, when each looks upon the other as his or her very own, such is called love from belief by the learned.”

KSII:I

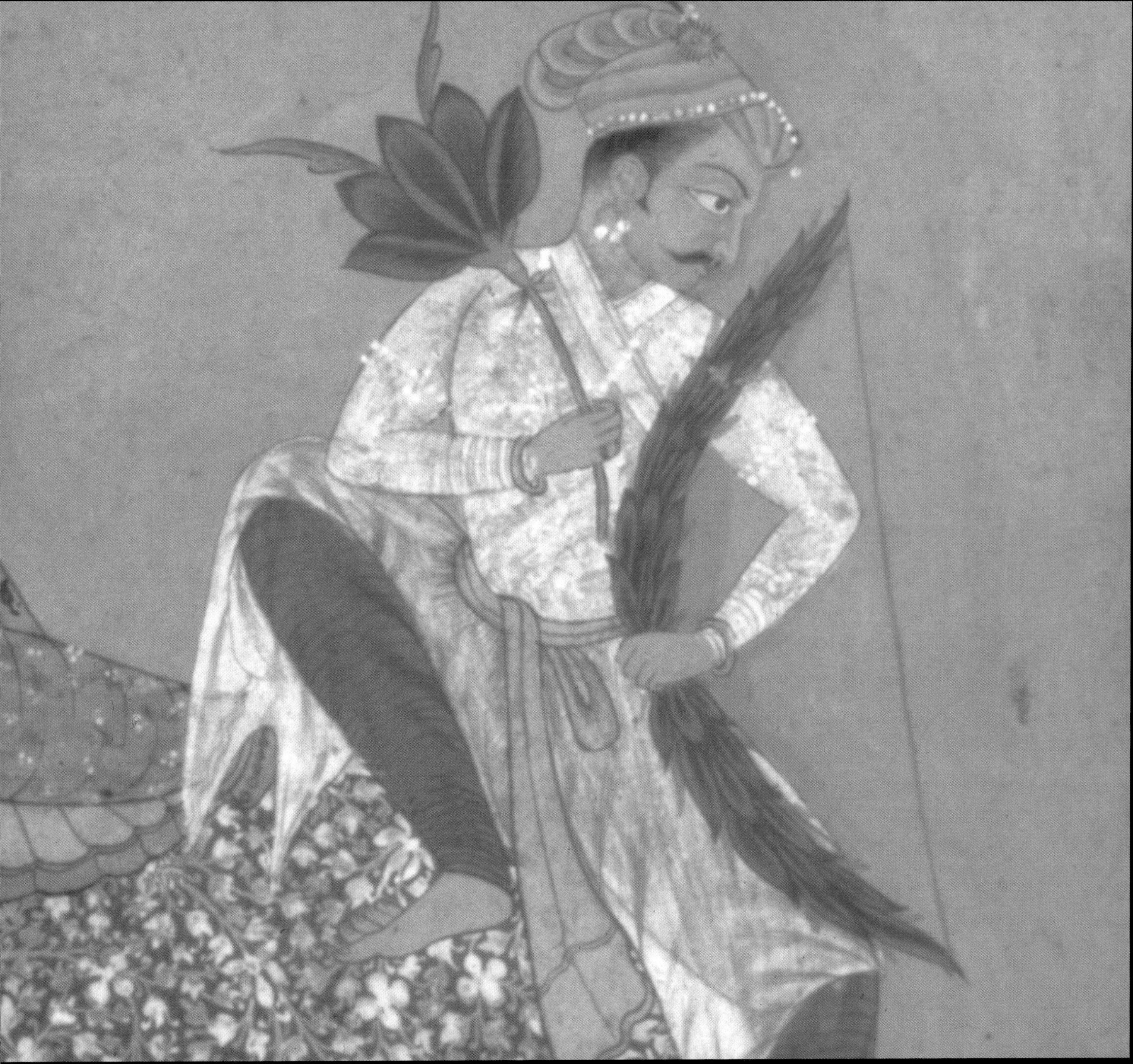

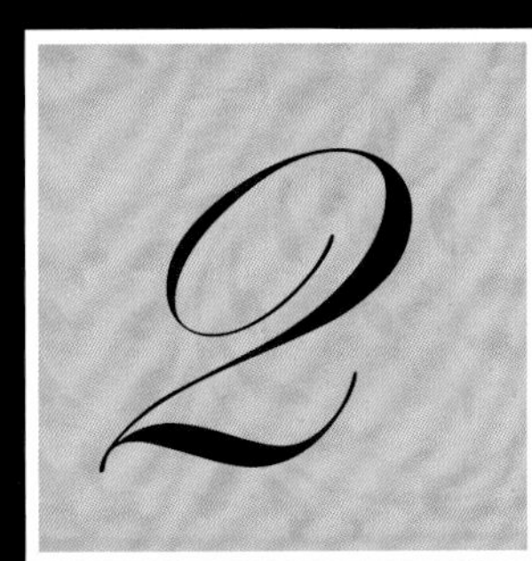

COMPATIBLE LOVERS

Sexual attraction

What really happens when we're attracted to someone? We go through a cycle of stages, from the first spark of desire to the development of a deep attachment. Understanding why we do what we do when we're falling in love can be a blessing, especially when all those feel-good hormones wear off and our rose-colored glasses clear.

FALLING IN LOVE

Why do we fall for some people and not for others? Attraction is a multi-faceted phenomenon. We are drawn to the familiar in others, which is why lovers often describe their attraction as a kind of homecoming. In this case, the love and security we experienced with our parents becomes our emotional reference point. But the opposite may also be true: We may fall for a lover who offers something we feel we didn't receive as children. Our feelings of attraction reflect our store of emotional experiences, which triggers a rush of supercharged hormones.

In the first flush of desire, we can easily make fundamental errors of judgement. Vatsyayana noted that "the forms of bodies" distort a true appraisal of the beloved's character. He advised assessing your lover "by their conduct, by the outward expression of their thoughts and by the movements of their bodies". It's good advice that holds true today. How your lover treats other people is a pretty good indication of how he or she will treat you once those powerful hormones subside.

Social factors also play a part. The Kama Sutra advises lovers to marry within their own caste. Today, there is evidence that matches between people of the same social standing tend to be more successful than those between people from different backgrounds. This is mainly because people with a similar upbringing and education are likely to share the same values.

THREE KINDS OF LOVE

Through the ages, philosophers and writers have identified three distinct types of love: erotic, storgic, and ludic. Erotic love (the term is derived from Eros, Greek god of love) covers much more than physical attraction. Sensuality, mutual understanding, confidence and heart-warming passion are the main elements of erotic love. Storgic is derived from the Greek word *storge*, meaning "natural affection." This kind of love is affectionate and companionable. With its origin in the Latin verb *ludere*, to play, ludic love

V THIS CYCLE OF BODY LANGUAGE *has remained unchanged through time and changes in cultural mores. Trust and awareness of personal boundaries are all-important in burgeoning sexual intimacy. You'll ruin the rapport and trust you've developed if you skip any of the stages in this cycle. The Kama Sutra deems it necessary for you both to work through them all if you are to find confidence and harmony.*

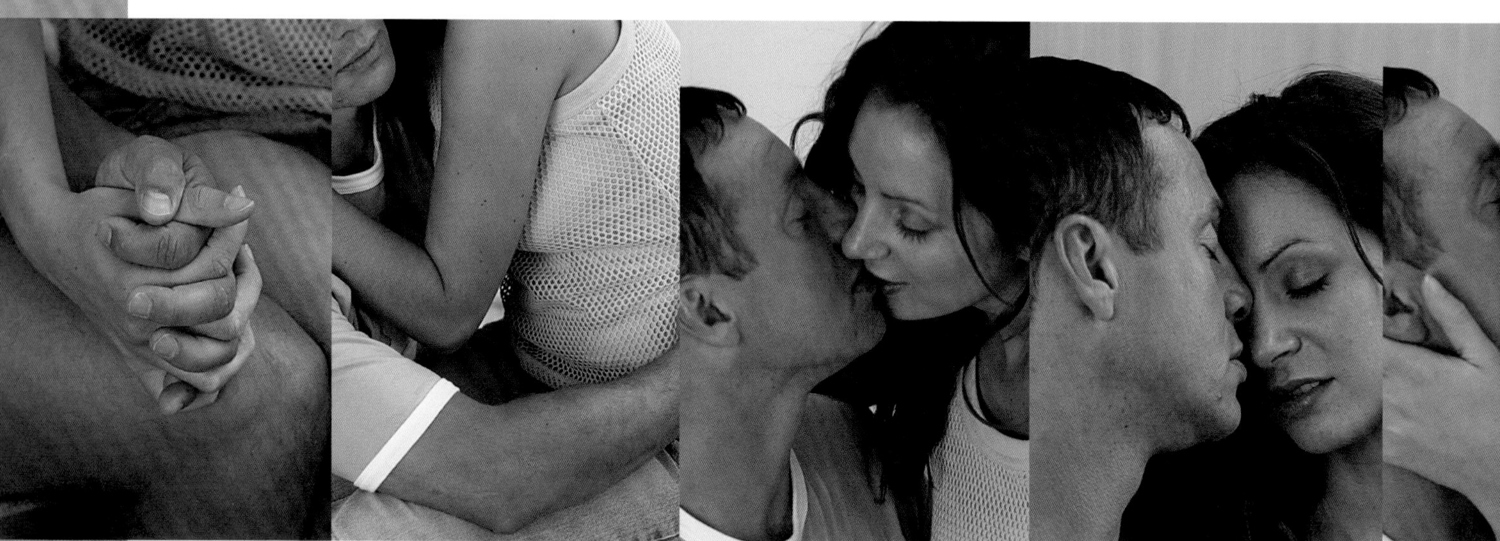

Hand to hand *Arm to arm* *Mouth to mouth* *Mouth to face* *Hand to hea*

Physical types

The Ananga Ranga divides women into four orders, according to their physical appearance and disposition: padmini, shankhini, chitrini, and hastini. These orders are subdivided into three classes, called deer, mare and elephant. Men are divided into three classes—hare, bull and horse (*see* pg.28). The book describes which positions in lovemaking suit the various combinations. It details the hours of the day or night when each type of woman will most enjoy lovemaking, and what kind of touch on which part of the body of each type will bring satisfaction.

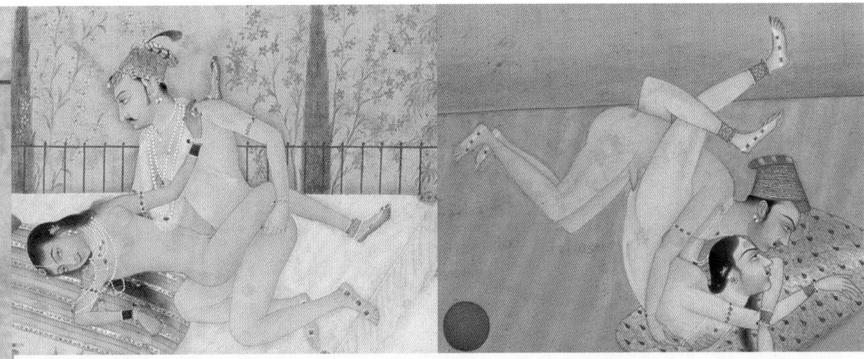

Posture for padmini woman

Posture for hastini woman

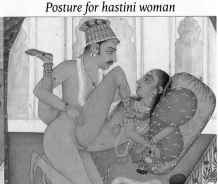

Posture for shankhini woman

Posture for chitrini woman

describes no-strings-attached fun. But it can be bereft of the closeness of erotic love and the security of storgic love.

STAGES OF LOVE

Throughout the passage of time, lovers have gone through a sequence of initial attraction, infatuation, and attachment when they fall in love. Once Cupid's arrow has found a target, desire flares for the first physically passionate stage. Next, we become utterly infatuated, carried along by an addictive cocktail of love chemicals that heighten our physical feelings. For almost two years the body is awash with powerful chemicals. Pheromones are your "come and get me" signature scent. A combination of adrenaline and dopamine intensifies sexual feelings, while phenylethylamine creates a delirious euphoric state. Orgasms produce oxytocin, which promote feelings of attachment. After the two-year mark, these chemicals wane, by which time it is hoped that a bond of attachment will have grown.

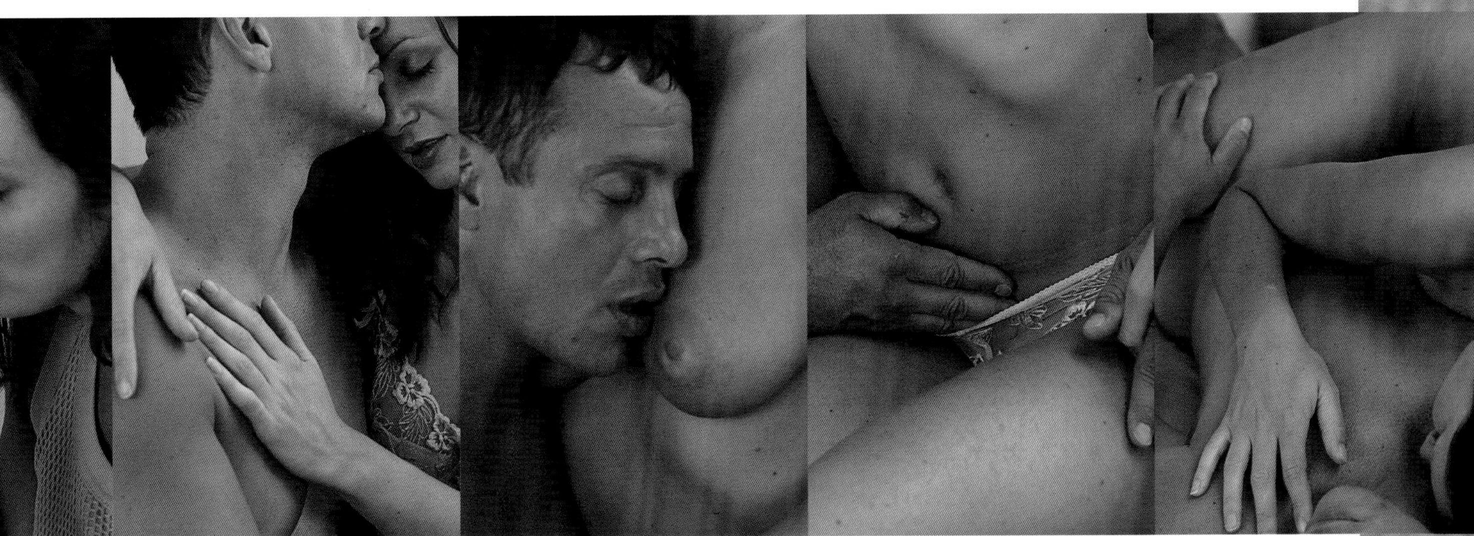

Hand to body *Mouth to breast* *Hand to genitals* *Genitals to genitals*

Wooing and wowing

The Kama Sutra's advice for those pursuing love is still very relevant today. Our 4th-century counterparts were expected to court with great care, to befriend, and to instill confidence, desire, and trust. To this end, they used good conversation, games, gifts, and flowers. These tactics work just as successfully today—and, as equality of the sexes now makes wooers of us all, they don't require men to do all the work.

LOOKING FOR LOVE

If there's no one in your immediate circle whom you feel might make a partner, why not try a reputable dating service? Resist the urge to create an ideal, as the right person may well come in a package quite different from the one you've envisioned.

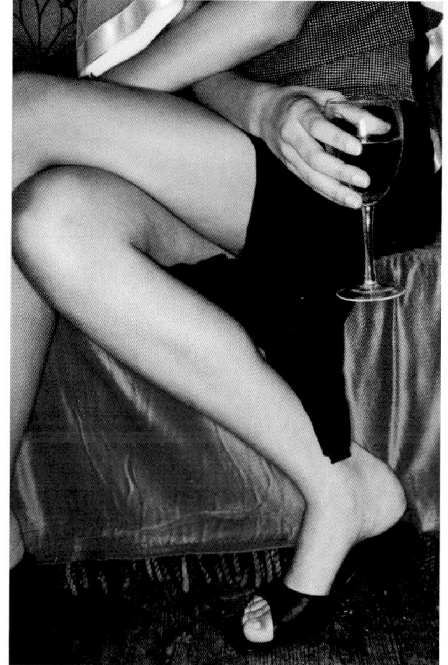

∧ BODY LANGUAGE *speaks volumes before either of you has opened your mouth. Learn to understand its meaning and respond accordingly. For example, when a person crosses their arms or legs, it usually means they are feeling insecure and need reassurance.*

FIRST ENCOUNTERS

Stomach-churning nerves and raging insecurity will probably accompany the first few dates. Break the ice by admitting that you're a bit nervous, to flatter and put the other person at their ease. Your conversational style can make or break a budding relationship. Remember, you're not being interviewed, so relax and ask open questions about safe topics: work,

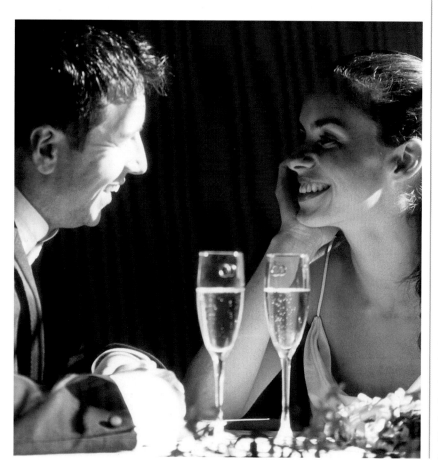

< MIRROR HIS OR HER *body language, hold eye contact a fraction longer than necessary, with obvious intent. And listen. Yes, that's right. Focus on the object of your affection's words as you would a new erogenous zone. There is nothing sexier than someone who knows how to make good conversation. There are only two rules: really listen, and reflect what you've heard in your response.*

Unrequited love

Casualties of unrequited love have been depicted in art, literature, and music since ancient times. Anyone who has the courage to pursue love will have, at some time or another, been spurned by the object of their affections. It's cold comfort to know that you're not the first to experience intense feelings of abandonment and rejection. After an initial grieving period, let go. You may feel you'll never get over your break-up, but the human heart is robust and, given time, it will heal. These painful experiences help us in the long run to appreciate reciprocal love.

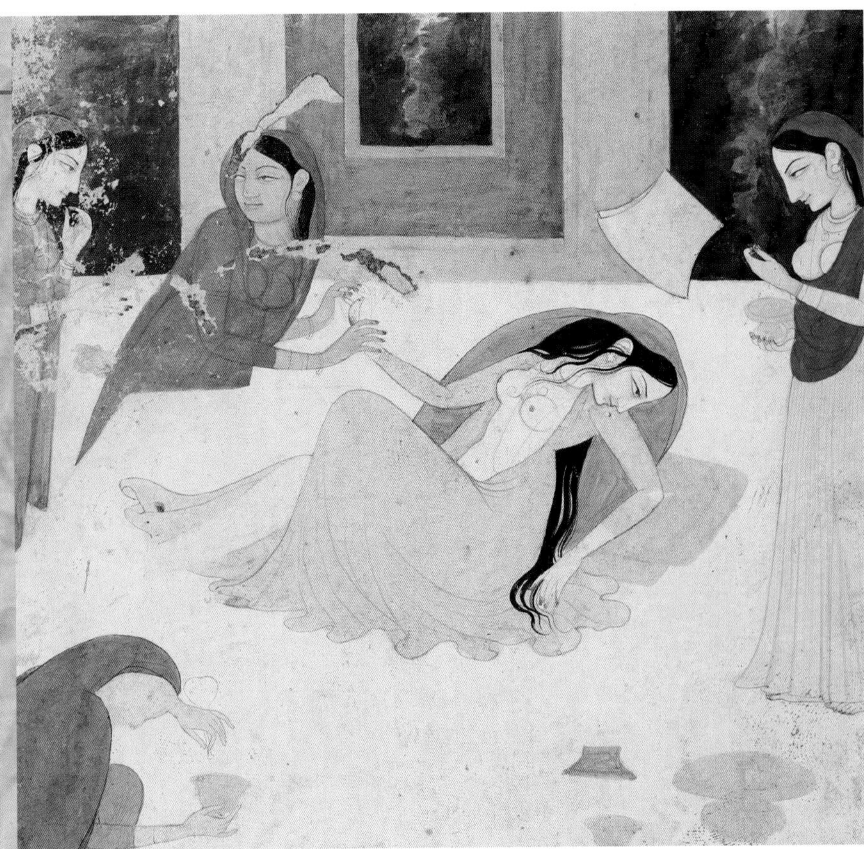

family, interests, or hobbies. The ability to listen is a very attractive quality, especially in men, and she'll find it much more arousing than the non-stop talk of a man who's just looking for an audience. Build on the conversation to create points of mutual interest.

Choose your venue carefully—preferably somewhere quiet, but not overtly romantic. Perhaps you might spend a day at the beach or have a picnic in the park. If you're feeling adventurous, try ice skating, bicycling or some other fun activity that brings out the child in both of you, raising the adrenaline levels and banishing nerves. Follow this with a quiet meal so that you can talk.

KEEPING IN TOUCH

The initial meetings seem to have gone well, but you're anxious to know how the other person feels and whether they want to see you again. You remember all those "rules" about when to call? Forget them: If you've had a good time, then let it be known. This gives the first clear sign that you're a confident person who's both straightforward and honest. Suggest that you meet up again in a few days. This offers your date the opportunity either to confirm interest or to bow out politely. If the answer is a "no," just be philosophical about it; very few of us ever have a 100 percent success rate.

GETTING SERIOUS

If you want your romance to blossom into something more serious, you need to devote time to it. Strike a balance between having your own space and nurturing your new relationship. No one likes to be smothered; neither do they want to feel insecure about when they might hear from you again. And keep being imaginative: Vary your meeting places and times. Show your flexibility by being interested in the pastimes and causes that are important to your new flame. They should return the compliment. If you find each other compelling and the chemistry is there, you'll find a way through those nervous first moments and will be able to enjoy the deliciously euphoric first flush of a passionate romance.

SEXUAL COMPATIBILITY

As individuals we all have specific ideas and boundaries around our sexuality. There can also be differences in belief systems, levels of desire, and expectations. These differences need not end things, but they do require careful negotiation. A sensitive lover not only respects their companion's feelings, but actively reads their moods. As your relationship develops, the level of physical closeness will increase. Remember that—even though you may be champing at the bit—there is no race to consummate the relationship physically. Go at the pace of the slower partner, concentrate on seducing the emotions. Bear in mind that we usually become physically intimate when we feel happy, confident, sexy, and—crucially—stable. If you're the one making the first move, read the signs as carefully as you can. Both partners have the right to say "no" to intercourse, and this should always be respected and not taken as either a rejection or a lack of desire.

KEEPING ROMANCE ALIVE

It is notoriously difficult to tell how people will behave after the initial buzz has worn off. Someone who only last week greeted you at the door wearing a smile and not much else may now be showing signs of wanting to tone it down (which means you need to work hard to persuade them not to!). You may have won their heart, but the campaign to hold onto them shouldn't waiver. It's the little, everyday gestures that keep love alive: notes stuck on the fridge; flowers for no reason other than to say "I love you"; plenty of caresses, cuddles, and verbal assurances of your love and desire. And don't forget to keep kissing each other. Kissing is perhaps the most romantic, personal, and sensual act that lovers share. Keep respect levels high and keep listening, because these are the pillars of a strong relationship. Many couples make the mistake of believing that once courtship is over, romantic gestures and demonstrative behavior can take a back seat; it's all too easy to slip into taking things for granted. However, these small acts are the lifeblood that sustains your attachment to one another through thick and thin.

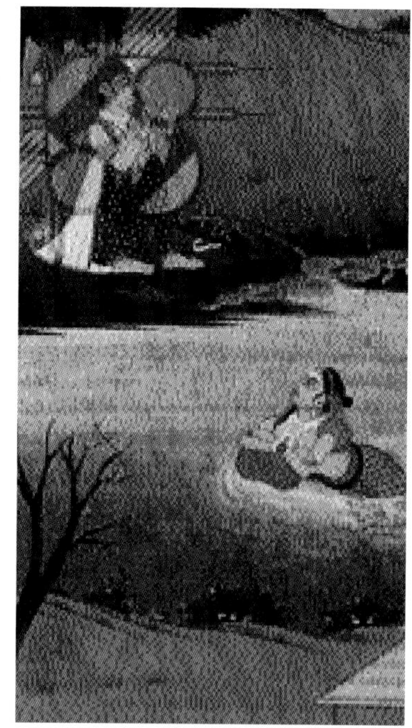

> IF MUSIC BE THE FOOD OF LOVE . . . *Like Krishna, the Hindu god of love, whose flute-playing entranced all who heard it, this man succeeds in seducing the object of his desire across the water with the sound of his music. If only it were that easy . . .*

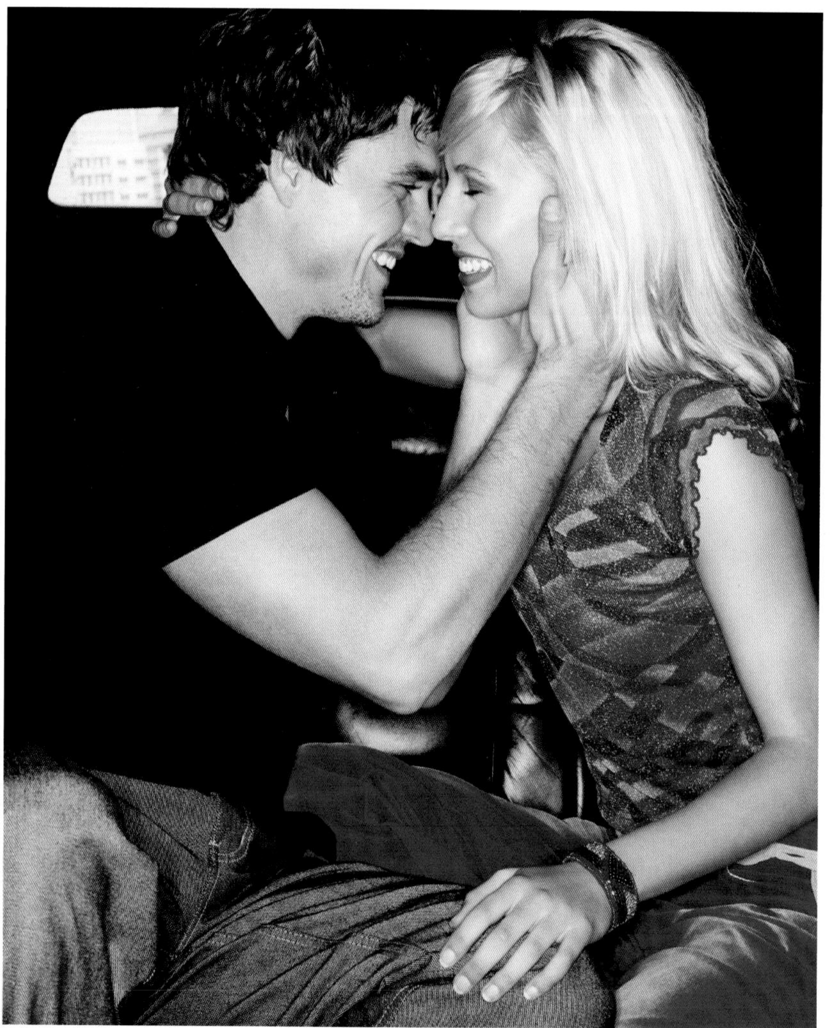

< BEING SIMPLY IRRESISTIBLE *is a matter of bestowing the best of yourself on your lover; make your partner feel adored by being affectionate and flirting shamelessly.*

> IN 4TH-CENTURY INDIA, *riding an elephant while serenading your lover would have been one of many tactics used to enchant and seduce her. Modern lovers may prefer cars.*

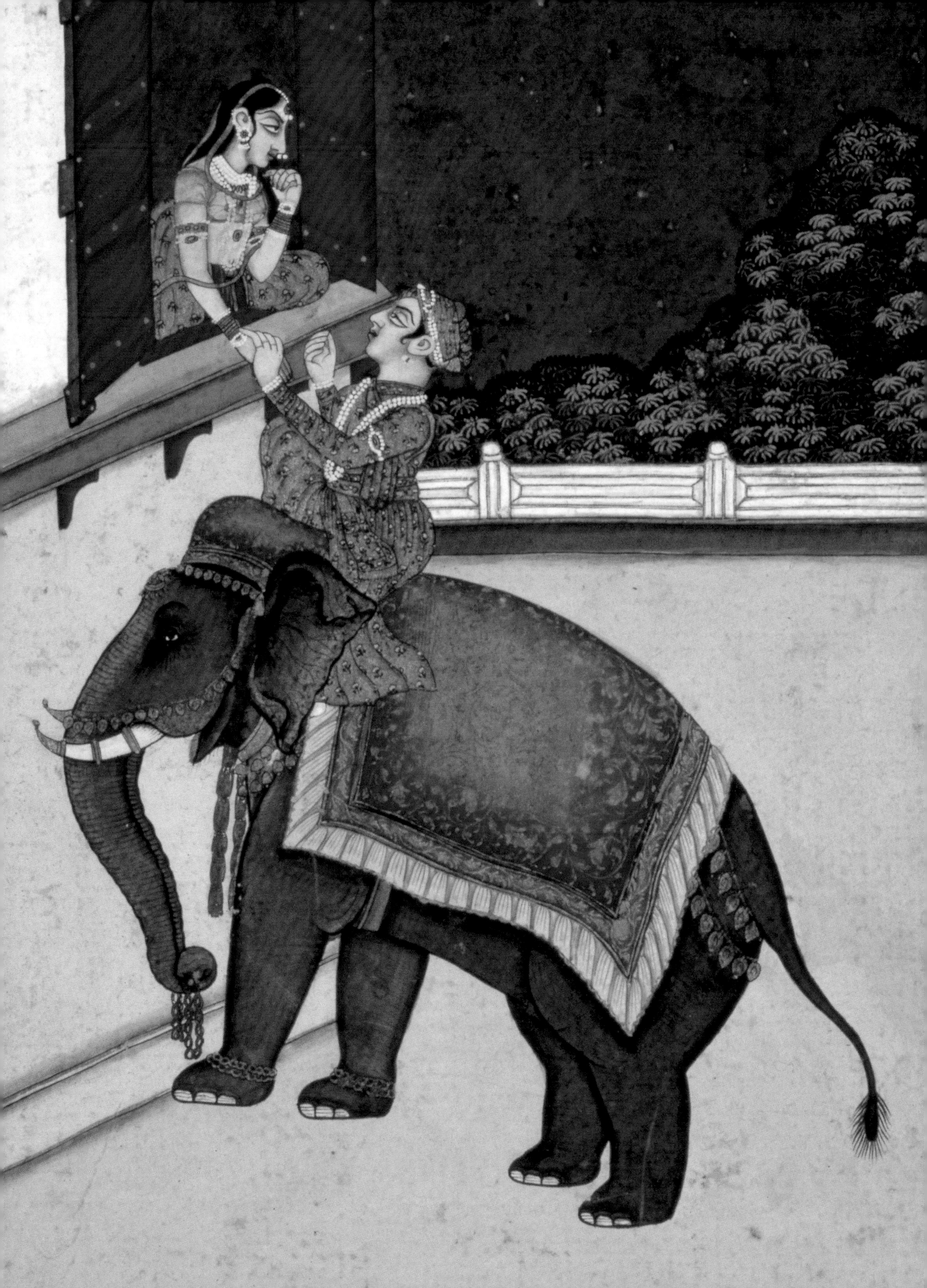

Size matters

The Kama Sutra recognizes three sizes or "classes" of men and women. These refer only to the size of the penis (lingam) and the vagina (yoni), not to body size. The Ananga Ranga describes three orders of men and three of women. These refer to a person's body type as well. In the Kama Sutra, the three types of men are: hare man, bull man, and horse man. They are categorized according to the length of their penis. A woman's size is determined by the depth of her vagina, and the three female types are: deer woman, mare woman, and elephant woman.

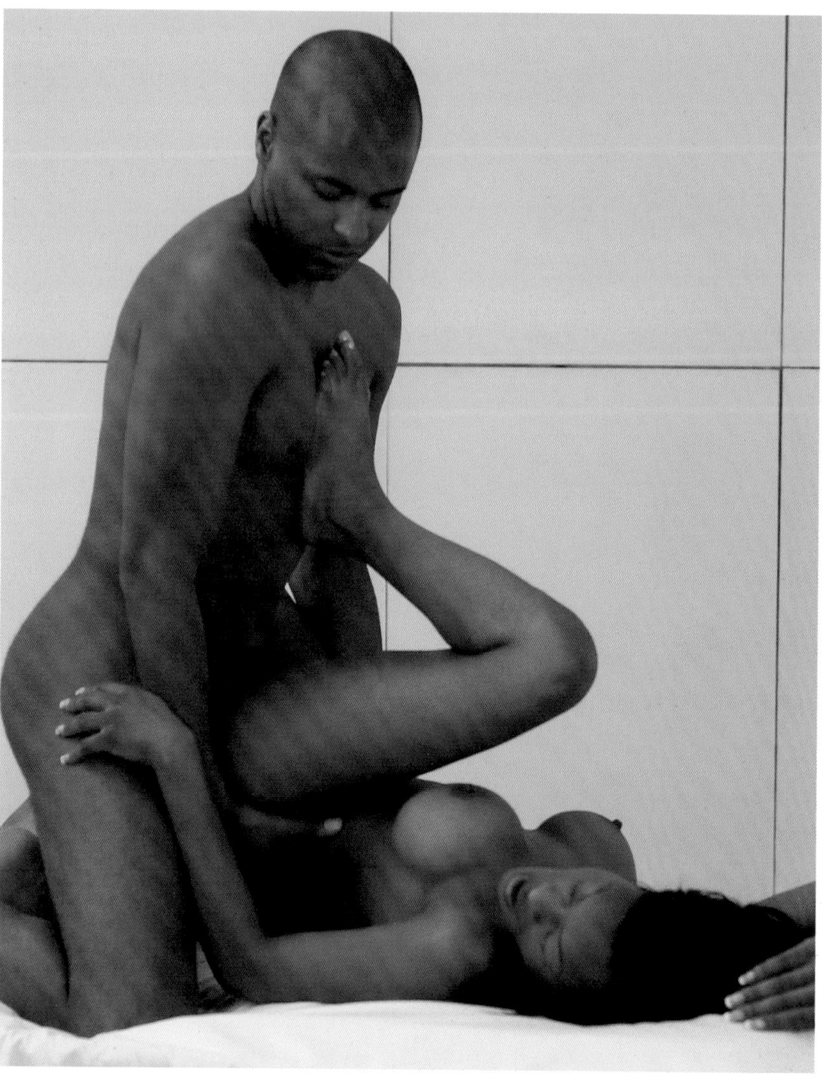

SEXUAL COMPATIBILITY

When a couple are of different genital sizes the Kama Sutra claims they have an "unequal union." It says there are nine kinds of union, of which "equal union"—a horse with an elephant, a bull with a mare, or a hare with a deer—is best. The highest and lowest union, or congress, are considered the worst.

HIGH AND LOW CONGRESS

High congress (or high union) is when a man sleeps with a woman who is one size away from him, for instance a bull man sleeping with a deer woman or an elephant woman. Highest congress is the term used to describe a horse man sleeping with a deer woman. Low congress (also known as low union) is when a woman exceeds the size of the man, for instance, an elephant woman with a bull man, or a mare woman with a hare man. When an elephant woman sleeps with a hare man, it is known as the lowest congress. Vatsyayana believed that high congress was better than low congress as, in the former, a man could "satisfy his pleasure" without injuring the woman; whereas he believed it difficult for a woman to be satisfied with low congress.

MALE AND FEMALE TYPES

When Vatsyayana divides men and women by the length of the lingam (*see* opposite) or yoni (deer woman's yoni is six fingers deep, mare woman's nine, elephant woman's twelve), he also describes in great detail the physical and temperamental characteristics of each

< A MAN WITH *a relatively short penis can add to his and his partner's pleasure by indulging in the Pressed, deep-penetration positions* (see *pg.116*).

type, from size of breasts and feet to propensity to sin. Today, if we categorize people at all we do so more broadly, and in any case we believe that true love will overcome any mismatching.

MODERN MAN

Nevertheless most men worry about the size, shape, or performance of their penis at some point in their life, particularly when they are about to embark on a new relationship. However, almost every size of penis can satisfy a woman. The vagina is about 4in/10cm long, which means that most erect penises are the right length. Very exceptionally a penis may be smaller than this, but the man can still give his partner great pleasure using manual and oral stimulation. Also, it is the circumference, rather than the length, of a penis that is most important to a woman's sexual pleasure.

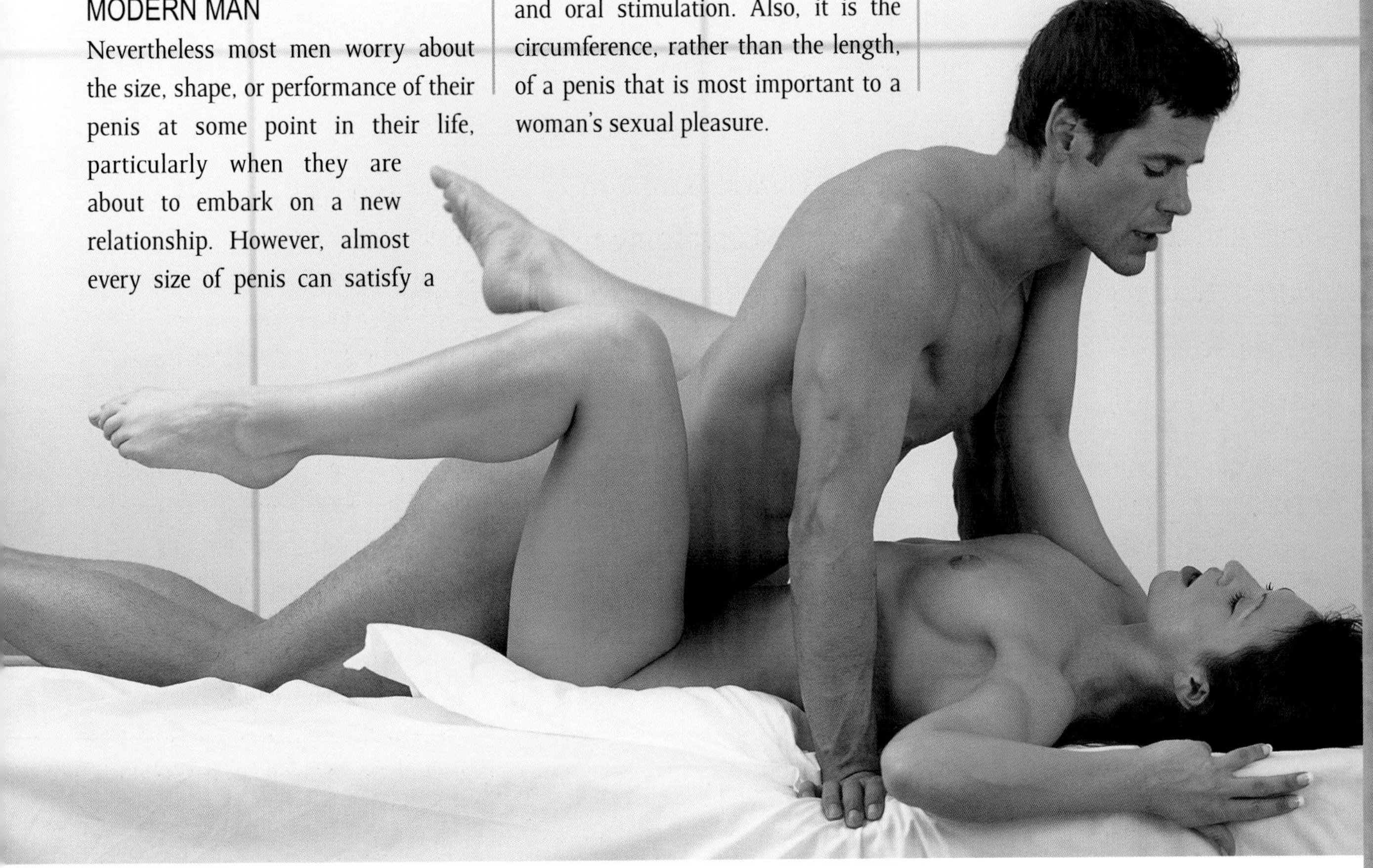

V IF A MAN *has a very long penis, his partner might find certain deep-penetration positions, such as Yawning (see pg.92), uncomfortable. He must take care not to press on the cervix.*

How does your man measure up?

In ancient India the length of the penis was measured in "finger-breadths," where two finger-breadths was about 1 inch/2.5cm. The hare man had a penis "which in erection does not exceed six finger breadths." The bull man has a penis "of nine fingers in length." The horse man "is known by a linga of twelve fingers." The man here has a penis that goes right off the scale. However, any man with a sexual organ closer to the average in size should remember that it is a myth that the man with the largest penis is going to be the best lover. It is only the skill of his lovemaking and his ability to respond to his lover's needs that makes a man a great lover. The size of his penis counts for little or nothing if he hasn't bothered to read the instruction manual!

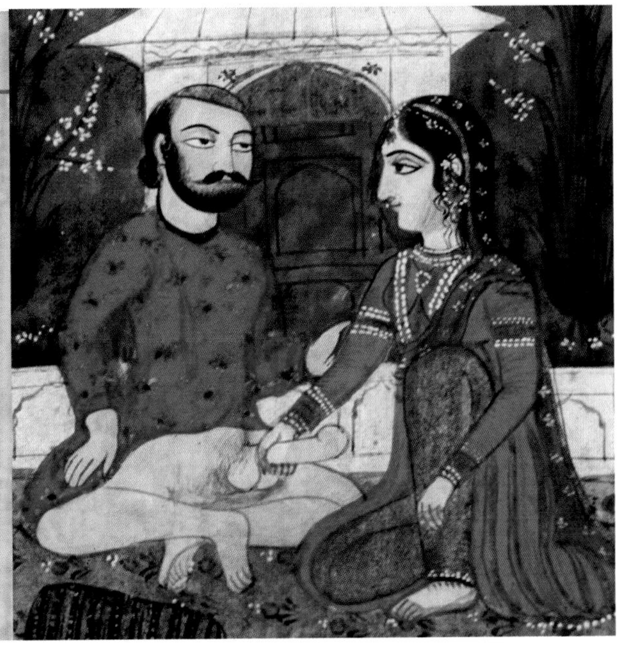

Sexual energy

The Kama Sutra states that "the strength of passion with women varies a great deal, some being easily satisfied, and others eager and willing to go on for a long time." Of course, this relates to both men and women and is dependent on many factors, such as how long you have been together, the stage your relationship has reached, your personal fitness level, and your stamina. Your sexual energy is also closely related to your mental state—at times of stress, illness, or depression, you may find your sex drive is lower than usual.

> VATSYAYANA *suggests that a man with a high libido may desire more than one woman at a time—of course he doesn't consider too closely how much satisfaction this would give to the women in question! The Kama Sutra also states that a man's first lovemaking session of the day is over quickly, but then his passion intensifies and he can go on for longer. With a woman, it says, the opposite is true: Her first lovemaking session is the most intense, after which her passion becomes "weaker." Presumably this is why Vatsyayana suggests bringing in reinforcements.*

MATCHING LIBIDOS

The Kama Sutra acknowledges the importance of couples sharing an equal sex drive, or what he calls the "force of passion" or "carnal desire." Vatsyayana writes about three types of sex drive: "small," "middling," and "intense." He claims that both partners can be truly satisfied only when they are the same type.

It frequently does prove true that couples in disagreement mention unequal sex drives as a problem. It is also the case that most people go through changes in libido levels at different stages in life, and not always at the same time as their partner. There are times, too, in a couple's lives when both partners are too tired for sex, such as while they are bringing up young children. This is unlikely to be a lifelong change, however.

The Kama Sutra and Ananga Ranga emphasize both male and female ejaculation, claiming that those with "intense" sex drives—able to make love more regularly and for more sustained periods of time than others—have different ejaculatory patterns from those with "middling" or "small" libidos.

ENDURANCE

Vatsyayana also describes three types of sexual endurance: "short-timed," "moderate-timed," and "long-timed." These terms refer not only to the time it takes someone to reach orgasm but also to their sexual stamina and the length of time they maintain sexual interest in their partner both before and after orgasm.

> IF THE MAN *wants to delay his ejaculation, he or his partner can use the "Beautrais maneuver." At the brink of orgasm, grasp the testicles and pull down firmly. This action blocks the urethral passage and prevents ejaculation. Repeat as necessary.*

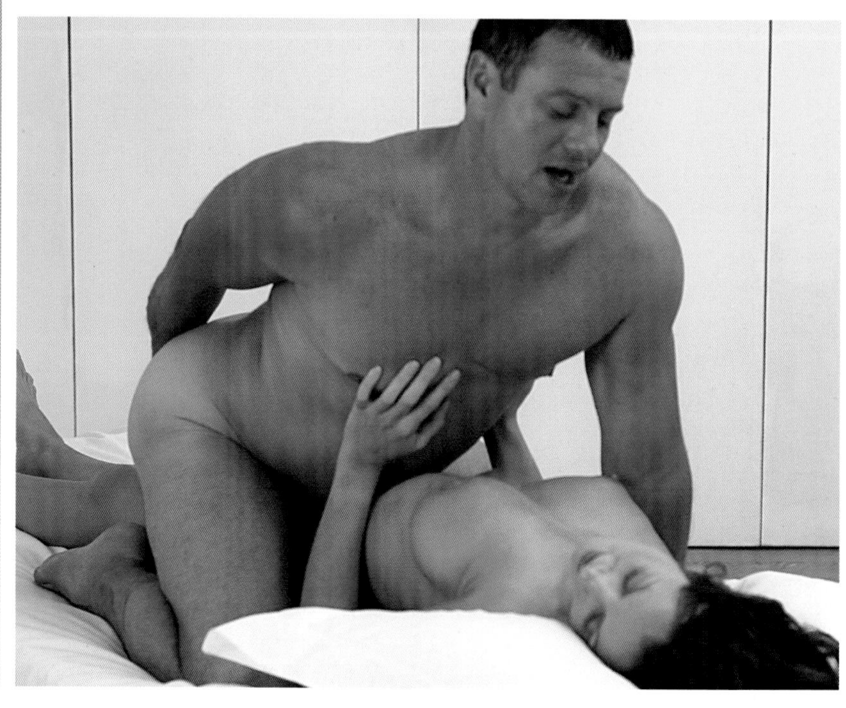

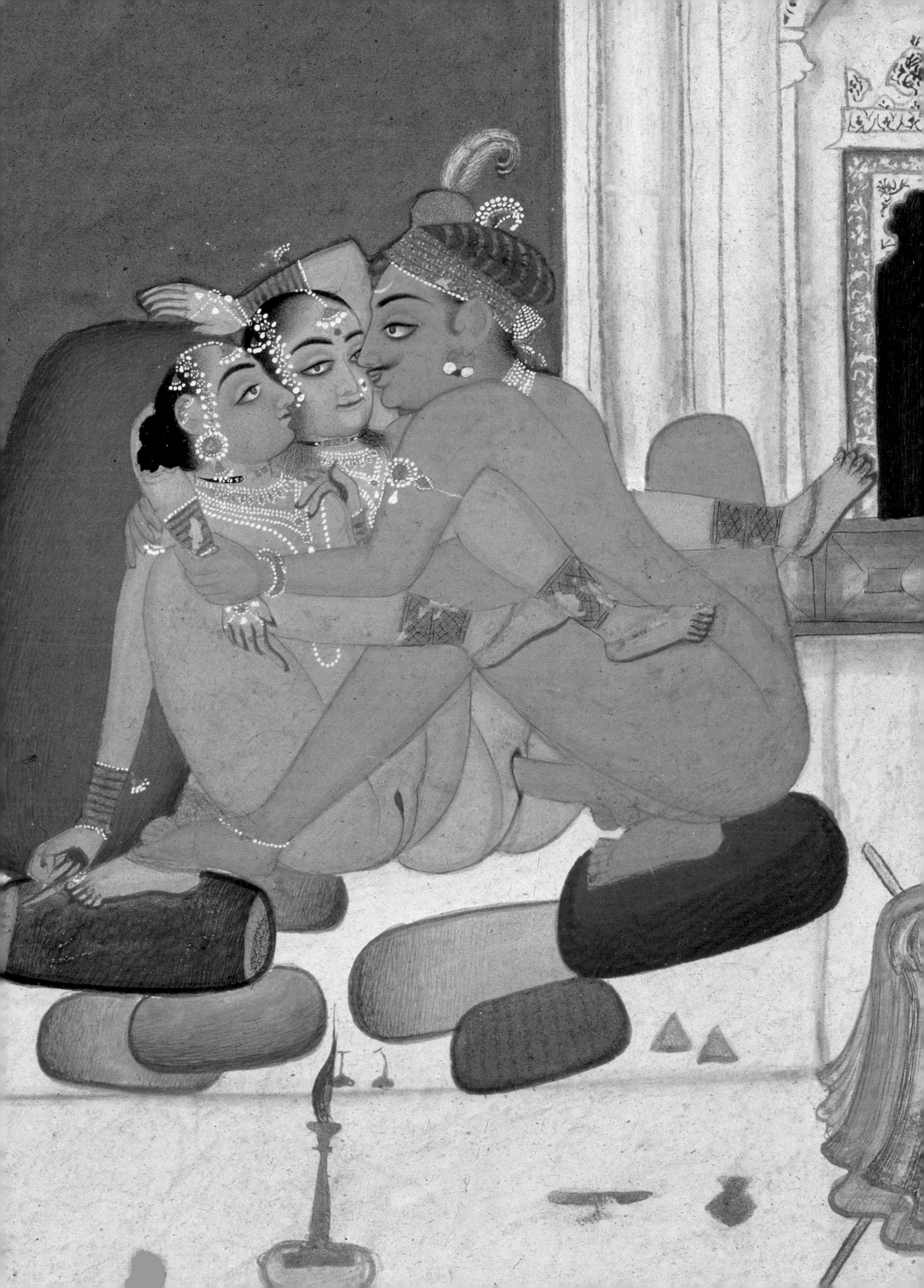

Pleasing your partner

The best sex happens in the best relationships, those that satisfy the emotional and the physical desires of both partners. As well as learning and sharing a wide range of sexual techniques, it is equally important that you share affection, honesty, and trust. If both of you are intent on making sure your lover receives as much pleasure as possible, your sex life will be truly explosive.

UNDERSTANDING EACH OTHER

Even the closest couples can have problems discussing their sexual needs, especially if either or both partners grew up in an atmosphere lacking in intimacy, or where talking about sex was taboo. Hang-ups caused by problems in previous relationships can also create barriers, so it is very important to choose a good time to talk things over and to reassure one another. Talk about what turns you on—and also about what turns you off, but do so objectively without making your partner feel he or she has been doing anything "wrong." Show your lover where and how you want to be touched. Watch your partner masturbate and try to emulate their technique in your lovemaking. If you feel your sex life has become too routine or dull, don't make your partner feel at fault. Discuss it with them, without any blame or hostility, and suggest changes in such a way that they feel like it is an exciting joint decision. Most important of all, make sure you keep the channels of communication open always, especially when you are going through the occasional rough spot. Remember that communication is the key to a successful relationship, even if you feel that talking to each other is the last thing you want to do.

MUTUAL EXPLORATION

A vital part of being a good lover is striving to make—and keep—your relationship enticing. Get to know your partner's fantasies and desires, find out about the dreams that sustain them, in all areas of life, and explore those dreams together. Being a great lover doesn't begin and end between the sheets; it is largely about everyday thoughtfulness and affection. If the intimacy ends as quickly as your orgasms, the relationship will never progress beyond the merely physical. True sexual chemistry should improve and deepen with the length of a relationship. It's a chemistry that intensifies when two people are attracted to one another's personalities,

Communication

A good sexual relationship largely depends on good communication. Your partner will not automatically know what you like and dislike, so it is important that you both talk openly and freely. Let your partner know when something arouses you, as well as when something hurts or makes you feel uncomfortable. Work at creating a relationship where you both feel able to discuss anything.

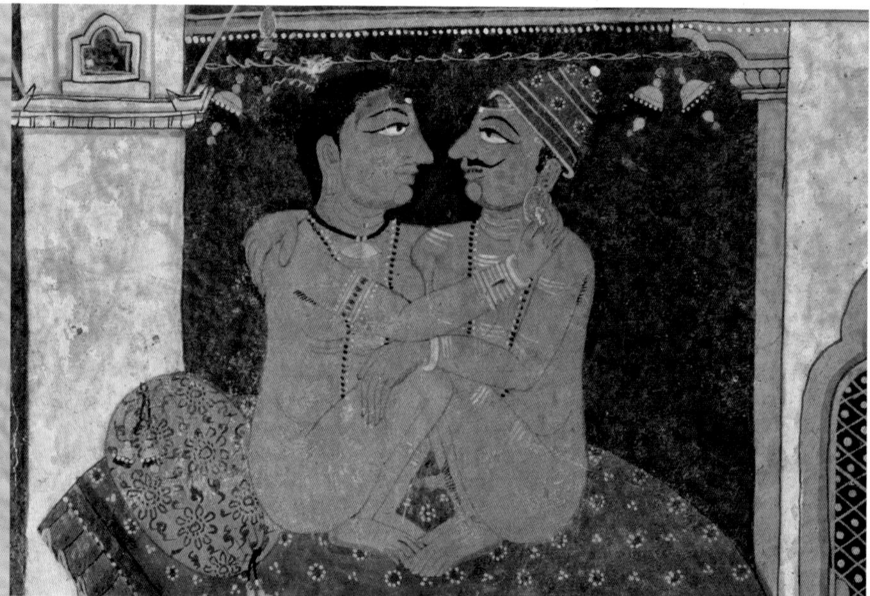

"... if men and women act according to each other's liking, their love for each other will not be lessened even in one hundred years." KSII:V

not purely to physical appearances. In a long-term relationship it is perfectly natural that your libido, and that of your partner, will go through changes at various times of life. These changes may prove deeply frustrating, but they can also be intoxicatingly erotic. Use the opportunity to experiment when you are making love, introducing new positions, tenderly exploring your lover's body with your hands and mouth while keeping constantly attuned to those tell-tale physical signs of enjoyment. Whatever stage you believe your relationship has reached, explore and develop your sexuality together and the journey will be wonderfully exciting.

RECOGNIZING BOUNDARIES

Variety and experimentation can enhance any relationship. Before embarking on anything too wild, however, talk to your partner about what is and isn't acceptable. Lay down ground rules and make sure you are both happy with them. Everyone has boundaries, and these should always be respected. So, if you are not happy with something, say so! Conversely, if something feels fantastic, say so! Never neglect your own enjoyment—you would be doing yourself and, perhaps paradoxically, your lover, a great injustice if you did. Don't say or do anything that you will regret later, or that will emotionally scar your partner. If you are both to really let go during sex, especially if you're indulging in role playing, there must be a genuine and well-established bond of trust. All couples make love differently and (no pun intended!) there are no hard-and-fast rules. Everybody needs to find a sexual pattern that suits them and makes them feel good about themselves. As long as both you and your partner are fully satisfied with the intensity, frequency, and variety of your lovemaking, you are getting it right.

> MANY PEOPLE *are brought up not to talk about their emotions. In a relationship, however, it is vital that you talk to your partner about how you feel. Most women talk to their friends about intimate problems, but men are less likely to do so; this can lead to frustration for both lovers. Always make time to talk and—just as important—to listen to each other.*

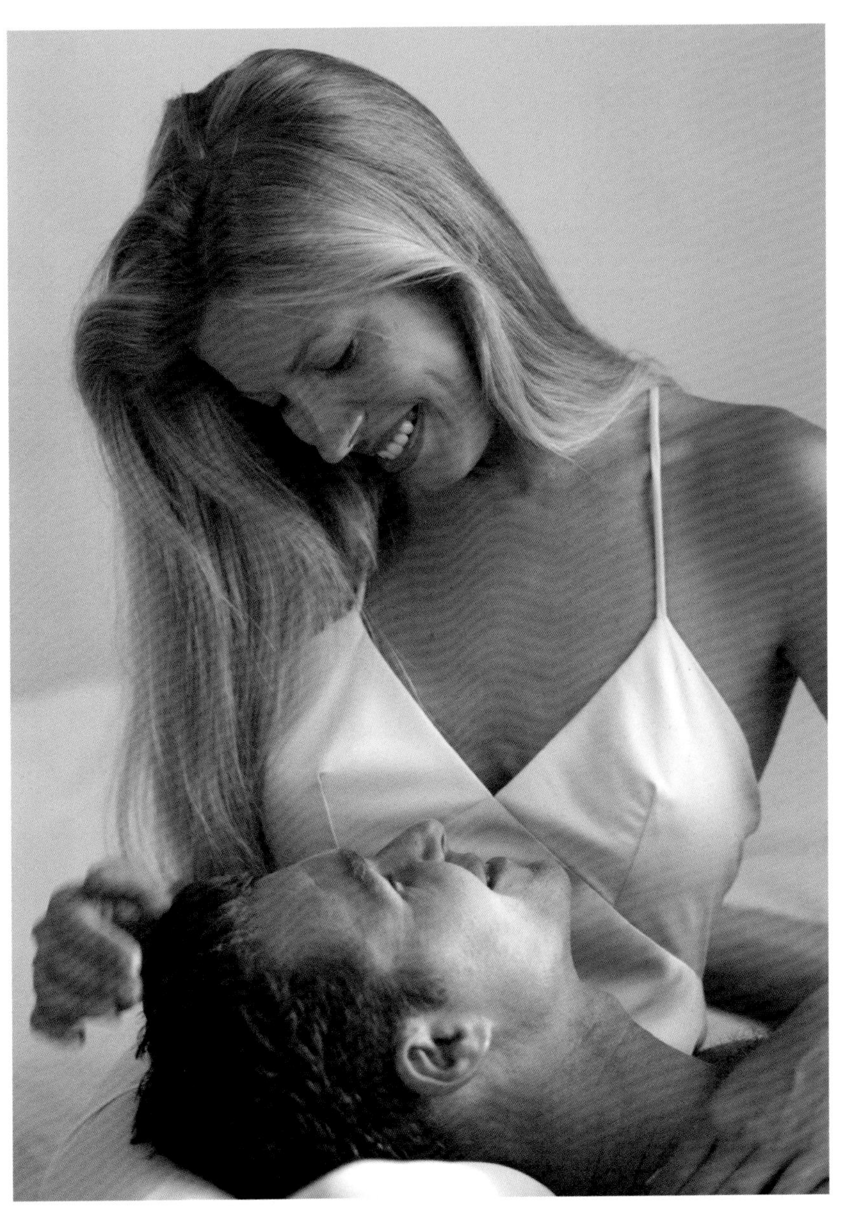

REKINDLING LOVE

When you've been in a relationship for a while, you may begin to feel it's lost some of its spark. However, it is possible to recreate the feelings you had when you first fell in love. Look back to the start of your relationship and remember what it was that was so special about that time. Think of how it felt when you were getting ready to meet one another, or how it was just to sit in companionable silence. Remember how incredible it seemed just to touch one another during a conversation? Concentrate on those early emotions and you will find them again. Why not pretend you are going out on your first date, dress up, go out for a meal, and make conversation as if you didn't know each other?

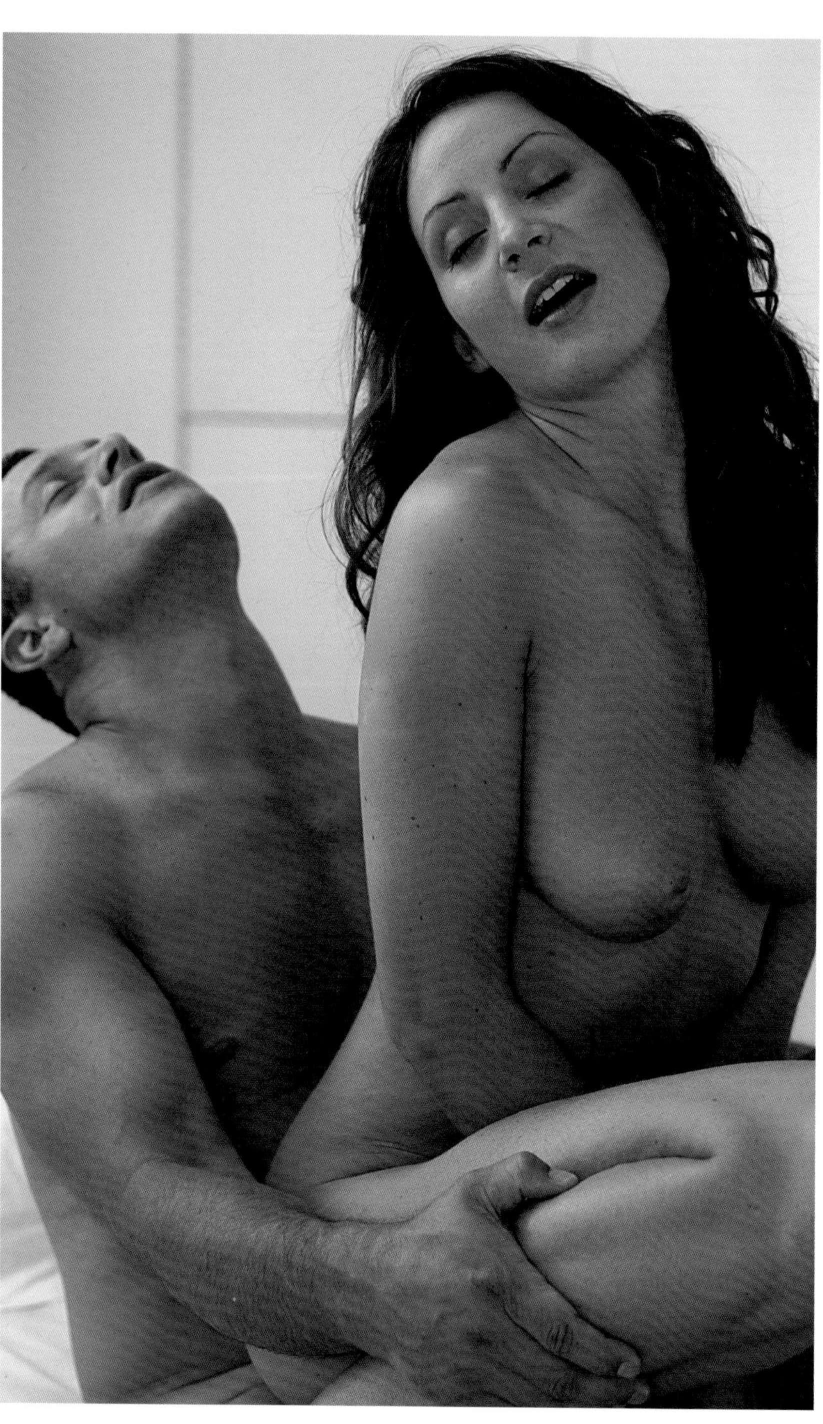

Spice of life

If you have been together a long time and feel your lovemaking is becoming dull, try varying the routine. If you normally wear something in bed, sleep naked, or vice versa. If you've fallen into a habit of making love only at night or only in the morning, make time to have sex in the afternoon or early evening. If you always make love in the bedroom, try other rooms, the garden, or book a hotel. Be more spontaneous: suggest a "quickie" before going out, seduce your partner when he's least expecting it. But before you suggest anything extreme, such as bondage, make sure your partner won't be offended. It is also essential to have complete trust in one another.

<THE KAMA SUTRA *describes the signs of a woman's enjoyment: "Her body relaxes, she closes her eyes, she puts aside all bashfulness, and shows increased willingness to unite the two organs as closely together as possible." Get to know your lover's signals and take delight in learning how to elicit every sigh, moan, and facial expression.*

> THE FINAL PART *of the Kama Sutra is largely dedicated to spells and potions: "If a man takes the outer covering of sesamum seeds and soaks them with the eggs of sparrows and then having them heated them in milk, mixed with sugar and ghee, along with the fruits of the trapa bispinosa and the kasurika plant, and adding to it the flour of wheat and beans and then drinks this composition, he is said to be able to enjoy many women."*

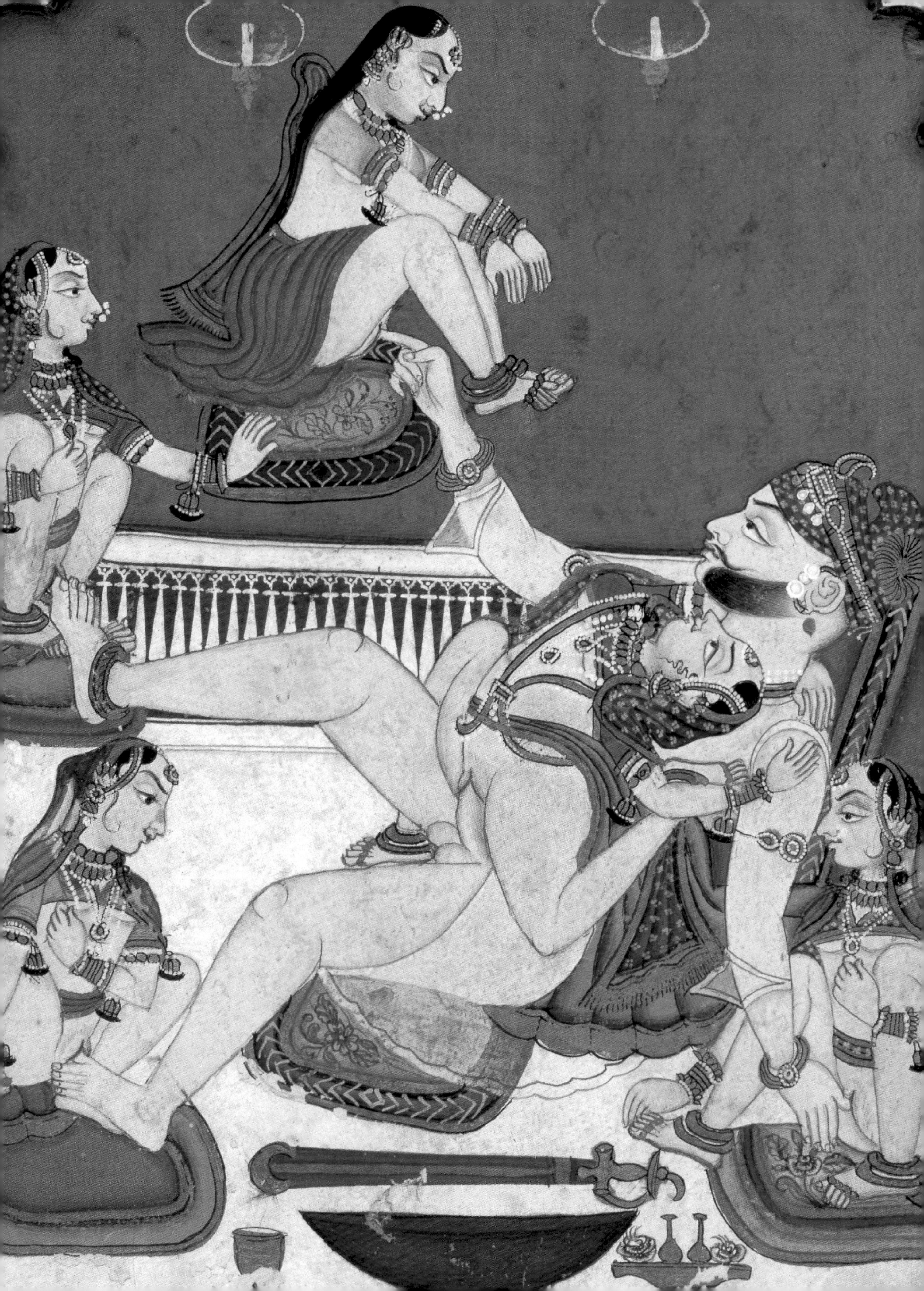

Understanding orgasm

Learning why she takes longer to climax than you (and what you can do about it) or where the G-spot is located; understanding why he always falls asleep at the end whereas she wants to talk—these are crucial steps on the path to becoming better lovers. So read on—here's your chance to discover the facts that will make you hugely successful between the sheets.

> THERE ARE MANY WAYS *you can improve your ability to reach orgasm. Start by focusing your mind on sex, because the brain creates desire. Stay together—you're more likely to learn how to match your sexual responses. Develop your pelvic floor muscles. Use plenty of lubrication. Still having trouble? Stress and relationship problems affect your ability to climax. Check any medication you're taking—like alcohol, tobacco, and drugs, some medicines dull sexual sensation.*

WHAT HAPPENS?

Orgasms are the fireworks that go off at the height of arousal. But if the Earth doesn't move every time you make love, don't worry. Orgasms come in different forms, depending on many factors, from our health to the state of our relationship. Orgasm is the final stage of an important process of arousal. Desire is the first stage: The brain is the first part of your body to become aroused. From then on differences emerge between the sexes in the length of responses. As the Kama Sutra says: "The ways of working as well as the consciousness of pleasure in men and women are different." The man can quickly combine desire with the next stage, physical arousal, and can be turned on by the visual stimulus of his lover's body—or part of it—while she tends to desire the whole person.

GETTING PHYSICAL

What happens next? Blood rushes to the genitals, you start sweating, nipples harden, muscles tense, your heart beats faster, your breath quickens, and your blood pressure increases. All this makes the body overtly sensitive to touch. The next stage, a plateau stage, generally occurs when you are both engaged in coitus, but this stage is significantly shorter for him than it is for her. This is why he may ejaculate before she has had a chance to reach orgasm. The good news is that he can learn to prolong the plateau phase by intermittent thrusting. Knowing her sexual responses really well helps him to control the ejaculatory reflex. (This is the unsung pleasure of a long-term relationship.) Orgasm itself is a release. Men will reach a point of no return, when they physically can't stop their ejaculation. However, as Vatsyayana notes, women differ in the orgasm stage: "The fall of the semen of the man takes place only at the end of coition, while the semen of the woman falls continually." This is recognition of the fact that, once a woman is fully aroused, one or more orgasms are entirely possible and desirable.

After orgasm, he will want to be quiet and perhaps fall asleep, while she will want to snuggle up and talk. This is because men shut down quickly, while women's bodies take longer to return to their pre-sexually aroused state. For this reason, the considerate lover will try to ensure that his partner reaches climax before, or at the same time, as he does.

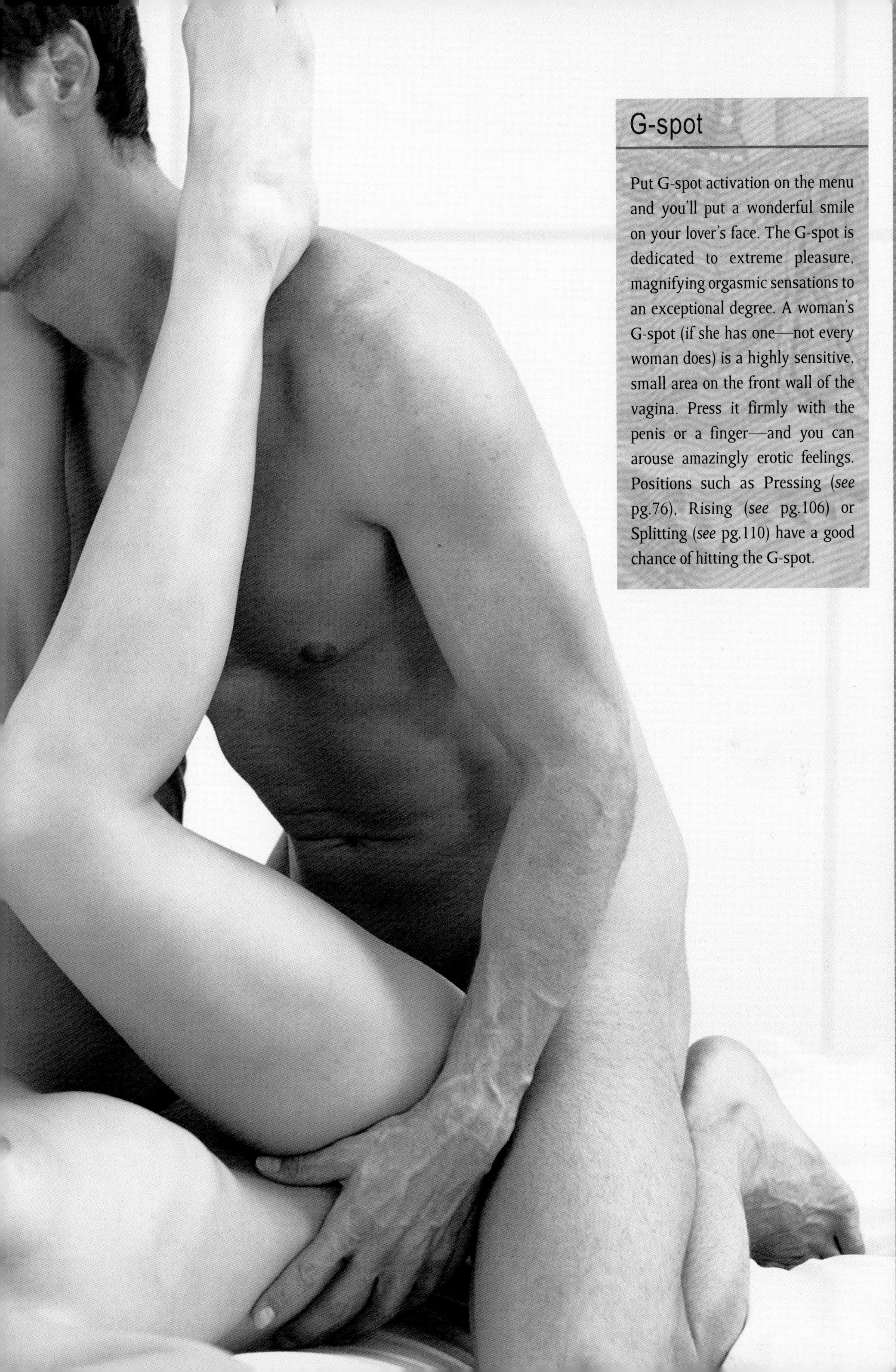

G-spot

Put G-spot activation on the menu and you'll put a wonderful smile on your lover's face. The G-spot is dedicated to extreme pleasure, magnifying orgasmic sensations to an exceptional degree. A woman's G-spot (if she has one—not every woman does) is a highly sensitive, small area on the front wall of the vagina. Press it firmly with the penis or a finger—and you can arouse amazingly erotic feelings. Positions such as Pressing (*see* pg.76), Rising (*see* pg.106) or Splitting (*see* pg.110) have a good chance of hitting the G-spot.

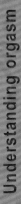

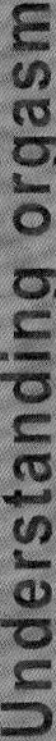

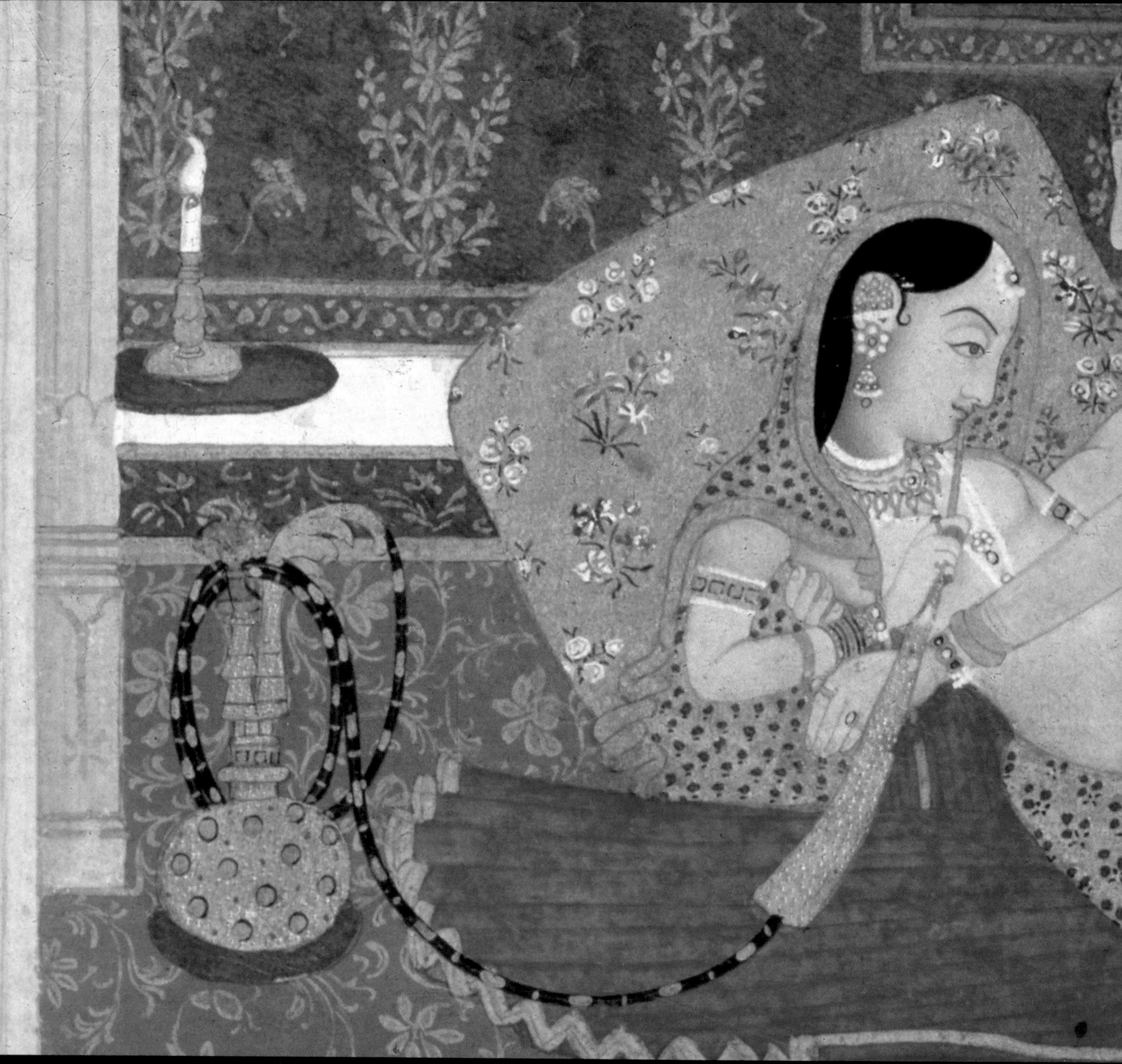

"Kama is the enjoyment of appropriate objects by the five senses of hearing, feeling, seeing, tasting, and smelling, assisted by the mind together with the soul."

KSI:II

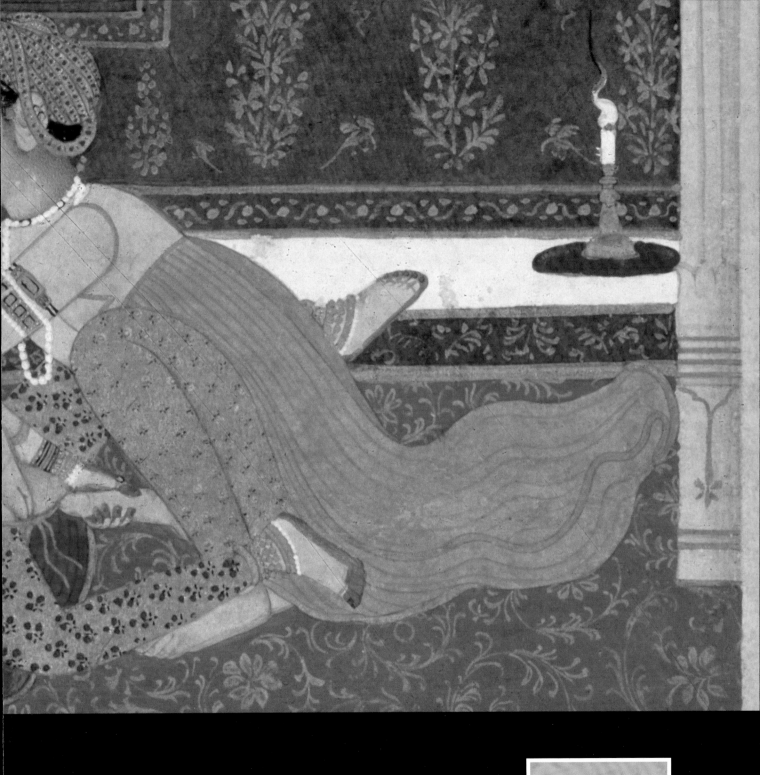

3

Enhancing sensuality

The Kama Sutra considers a good lover to be an accomplished person who takes time to appreciate the really good things in life. Educated, interested in current affairs, engaging, sensuous, and vital, the ideal lover is adept at squeezing every drop of pleasure out of life. However, Vatsyayana makes it clear that the student of *kama* must always retain mastery of the senses, and not be enslaved by them.

SELF-IMPROVEMENT

Although the Kama Sutra is, as its translators concluded, "a treatise on men and women, their mutual relation, and connection with each other," it is not simply about relationships. It also stresses the importance of heightening the appreciation of pleasure through self-improvement. Vatsyayana provides a long list of arts and sciences to be practiced, many of which we highly value today—for example, singing, playing musical instruments, and dancing. The list also includes some more obscure skills, such as the art "of teaching parrots and starlings to speak."

MASTERY OF PASSION

In dealing specifically with his "rules" for sexual relationships, Vatsyayana warns on more than one occasion that they are not necessarily suitable for all people under all circumstances: "An act is never looked upon with indulgence for the simple reason that it is authorized by the science, because it ought to be remembered that it is the intention of the science that the rules it contains should only be acted upon in particular cases."

To leave no doubt as to his intentions in writing the Kama Sutra, he concludes by stating: "This work is not intended to be used merely as an instrument for satisfying our desires. A person, acquainted with the true principles of this science [*kama*], and who preserves his dharma [spiritual wellbeing], *artha* [worldly welfare], and *kama*, and has regard for the practices of the people, is sure to obtain the mastery over his senses.

In short, an intelligent and prudent person, attending to *dharma* and *artha*, and attending to *kama* also, without becoming the slave of his passions, obtains success in everything that he [or she] may undertake."

Hedonistic pleasure

The Kama Sutra was written mainly for the aristocratic and wealthy members of Hindu society, who had plenty of time to indulge in their hobbies and hedonistic pleasures. This macho man seems to have lovemaking and hunting at the top of his list of activities—not necessarily in that order and maybe occasionally both at once. The modern woman would be deeply unimpressed if her partner interrupted their lovemaking to take a potshot at next-door's cat.

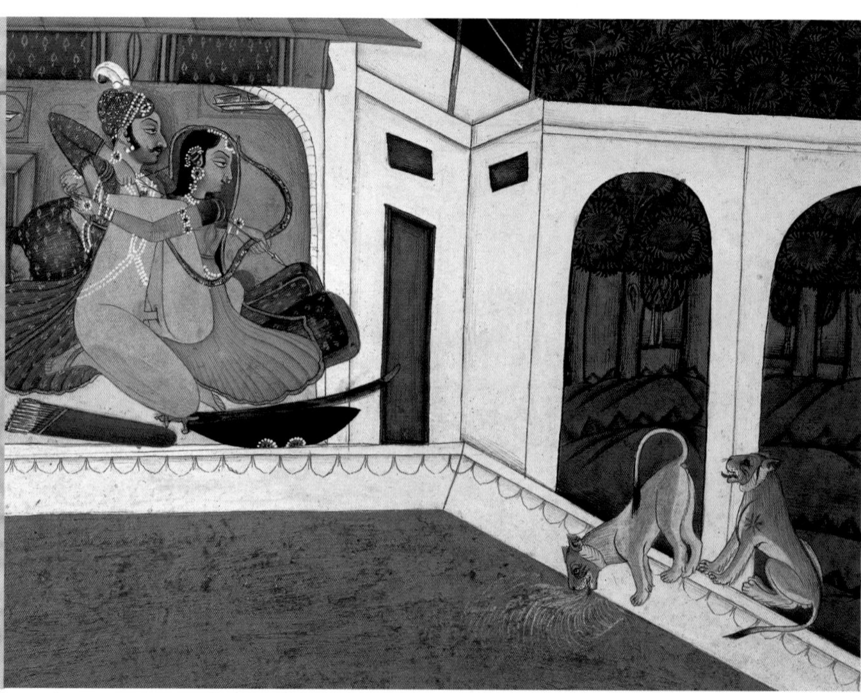

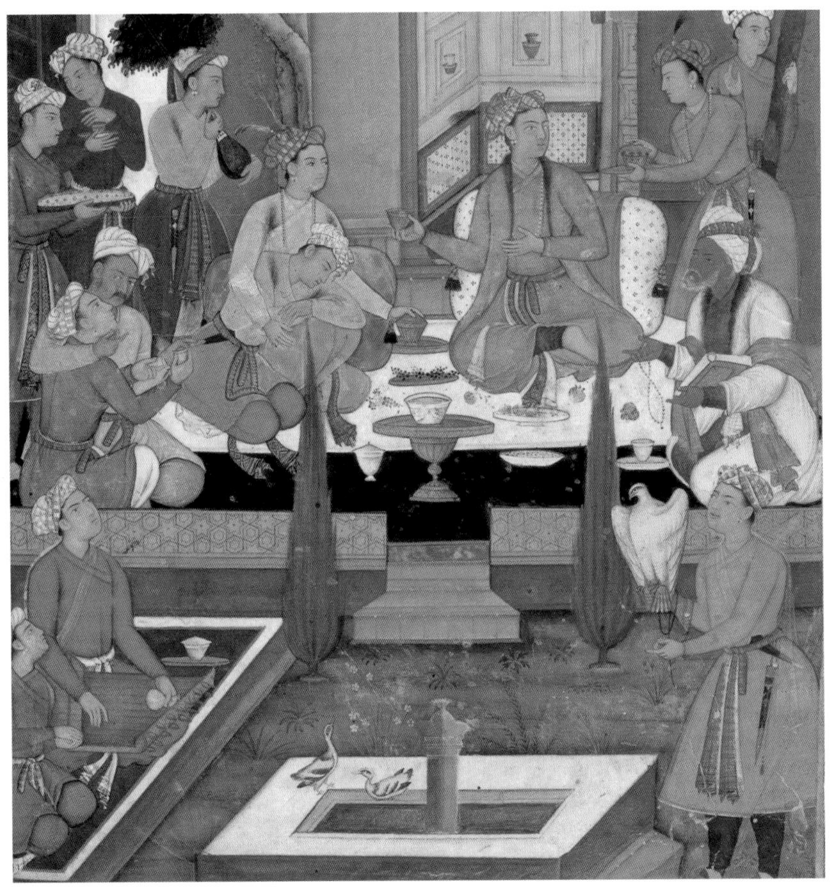

< THE KAMA SUTRA *painstakingly lists the intellectual, physical, and sensual spheres in which a 4th-century Indian gentleman would have to excel if he was to be considered a real catch. He would gather around him friends and attendants to enjoy fine food and drink, while listening to music or discussing arts and sciences. Often they would play intellectual games: breaking codes, solving riddles, and improvizing poetry.*

V THE PLEASURES OF FOOD *and the flesh are closely related. Nothing is more sensuous than combining them. Feeding your lover delicious treats gives out two messages: 1) you want to nurture and protect her; and 2) food tastes really good when taken from your fingers. Using a blindfold removes the dominant sense of sight so you can focus entirely on the sense of taste.*

ENHANCING THE SENSES

Although we know of people who can be described as "the slave of his passion," in the West—where so many exciting consumables are available—we are perhaps far more in danger of becoming the slave of fashion. In today's world, it is the relentless and unthinking pursuit of *artha* that is most likely to prevent us from leading balanced lives. In this respect, *kama* provides an antidote.

According to Vatsyayana, "*Kama* is the enjoyment of appropriate objects by the five senses of hearing, feeling, seeing, tasting, and smelling, assisted by the mind together with the soul." By appreciating how to control and develop our senses, we can learn to escape this constant barrage to our senses that is endemic in 21st-century everyday life. In your love life, the five senses can all be brought into play to stir and to heighten the emotions.

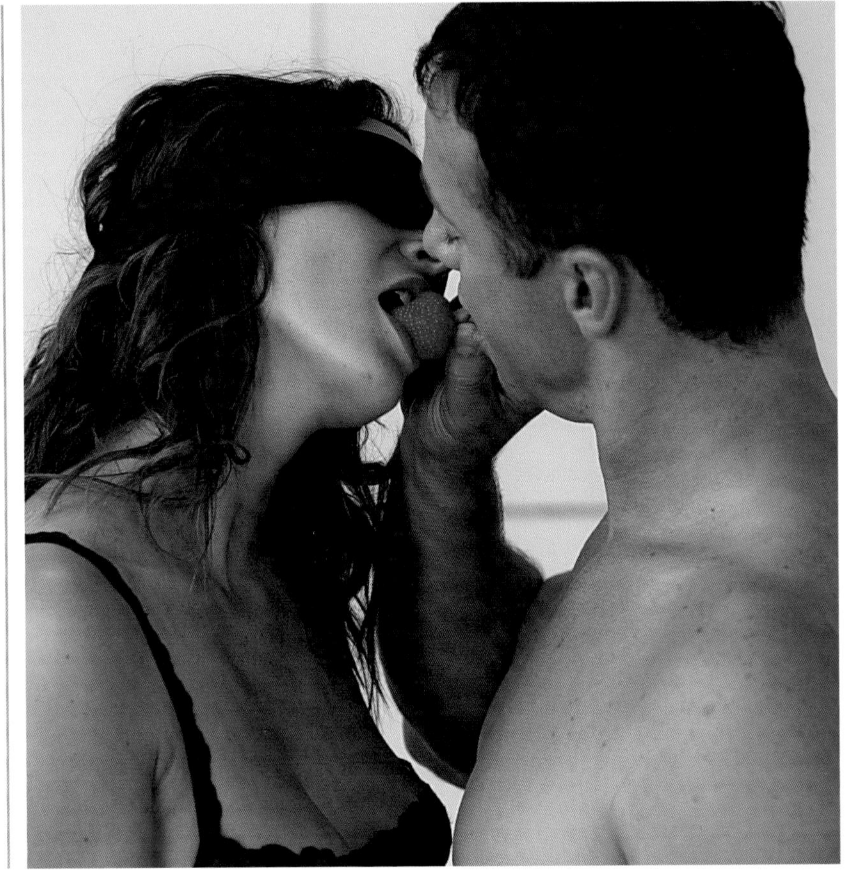

THE FIVE SENSES

How often have we heard the expression "Love at first sight"? We take it for granted that first impressions are nearly always visual. Truth is, we must keep ourselves looking good for our partners always, way beyond the first flush of passion. Wear that shirt she likes so much, arouse his interest by letting him have glimpses of his favorite underwear (on you). And remember those little things you can do to make the look of a room unashamedly romantic—soft lighting, mirrors, comfy cushions, a flickering fire.

Use the power of sound to your advantage: Create a barrier between yourself and the outside world. Cocoon your lover with sounds that soothe and arouse. Make time for silence. Get out into an open, natural space.

Your skin is your largest body organ. Put it to good use. Love it. Sensitize it to pleasurable sensations with massage. Get into contact with your own skin, and chances are you'll then know exactly what feels lip-bitingly good for someone else. Feel textures around you, educate your sense of touch: the smooth coldness of a pebble, the rough, ticklish lick of a cat's tongue. Notice how much emotion can be passed through the touch of your hand on your lover's body.

Our sense of smell gives us direct access to the primitive, emotional part of the brain, which is why, throughout history, perfumes have been used to seduce. Use sandalwood, for example, to elevate awareness of the physical senses, while relaxing the body and mind. Learn about the power and influence of aromatic oils, and use them to enhance the romantic atmosphere.

Food and sex have always been top of the list of things that make living an enjoyable experience. Certain foods are said to have aphrodisiac properties: bananas, carrots, asparagus, oysters. Then there's chocolate and good wine. Enjoy the sense of taste as part of your sexual experience: licking jam off your lover's fingers after a midnight snack will always rate higher than a meal at a fancy restaurant with someone you'd rather not be with.

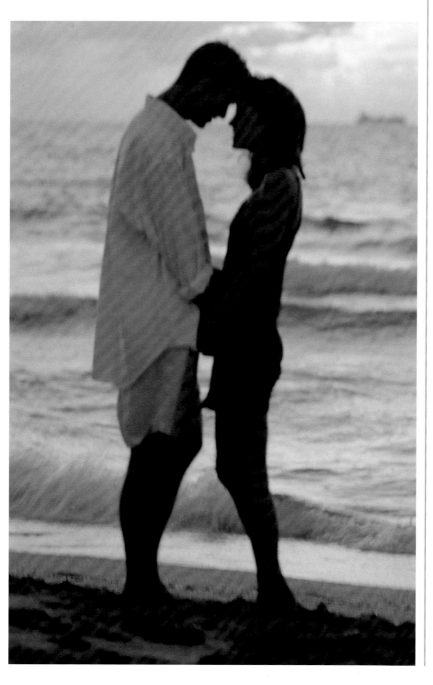

< BRING YOUR SENSES ALIVE: *Get outside with your lover. Go someplace you can walk in bare feet, feel the sun and the wind on your body, and generally revel in the heightened physical awareness that being outside brings to your senses.*

> VATSYAYANA *encouraged men to go on picnics "accompanied by public women and followed by servants." They should later return home, "bringing with them bunches of flowers."*

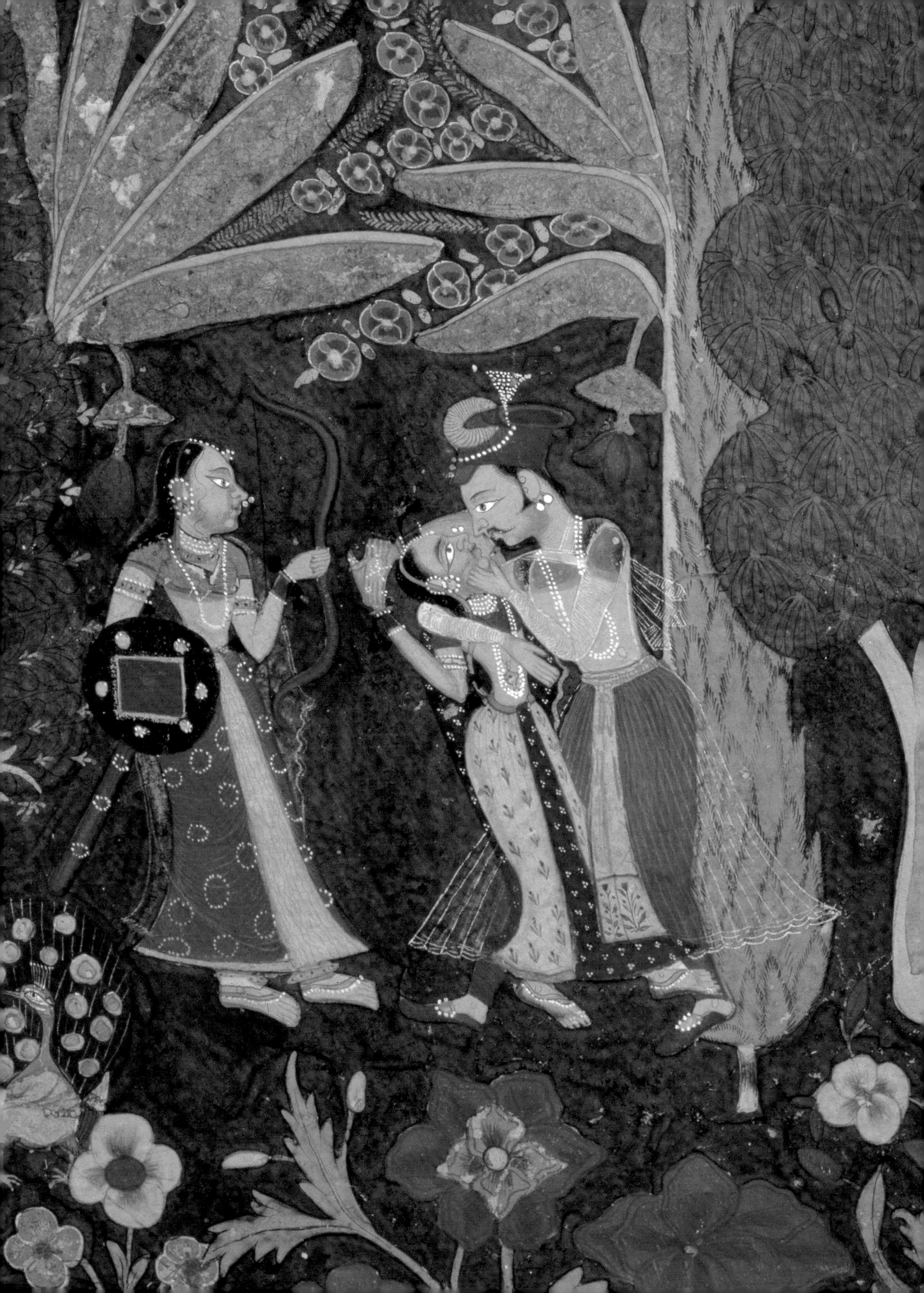

Setting the scene

Vatsyayana's detailed description of the ideal bedroom (*see* below) would need little adaptation today. It exudes elegance and sensuality. The description of the bed itself hints at the lively nature of the Kama Sutra lovemaking techniques. There's no mention of headboards, footboards, or his-and-hers reading lights: the bed is a place for love, with pillows at either end and accessible from all sides.

SENSUAL MATERIALS

Plenty of big, soft pillows or cushions are essential for good lovemaking: Placed strategically under the body, they can make certain positions far more comfortable and allow for deeper penetration. Follow the Kama Sutra's suggestions and place pillows at the bottom as well as the top end of the bed for free-ranging lovemaking. It goes without saying that bedding should be fresh and clean. Luxurious, deep-piled

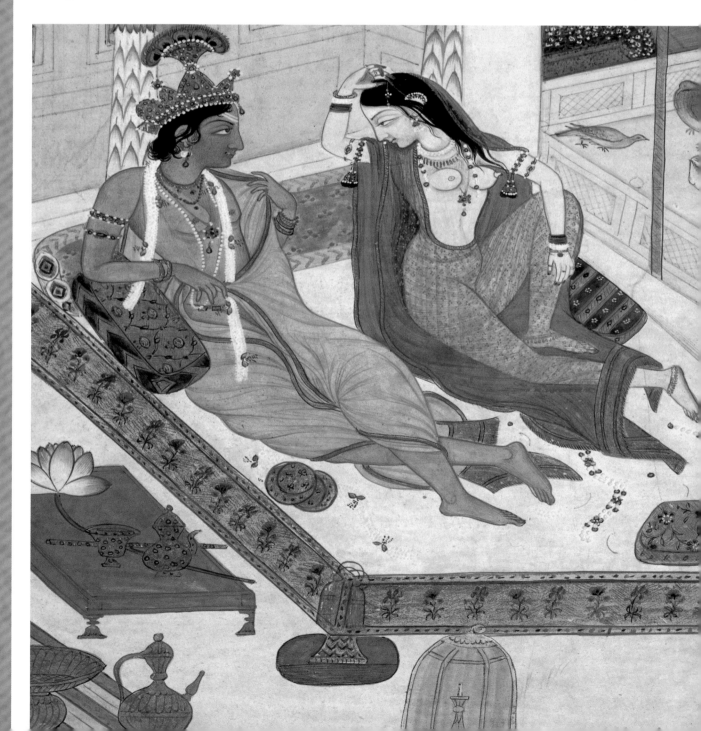

rugs on the floor are useful if the action spills off the bed. Velvet, silks, satins, and other exotic materials can feel wonderfully sexy against naked flesh, so be sure to incorporate them into your overall scheme for the bedroom.

Petals strewn on the bed may perhaps seem a little over the top nowadays, but certainly a vase of flowers will add elegance, beauty and fragrance to any room. In the absence of scented flowers, you can use perfumed candles or incense sticks. Alternatively, burn essential oils such as frankincense or cedarwood in elegant aromatic burners to stimulate the arousal of sexual energy.

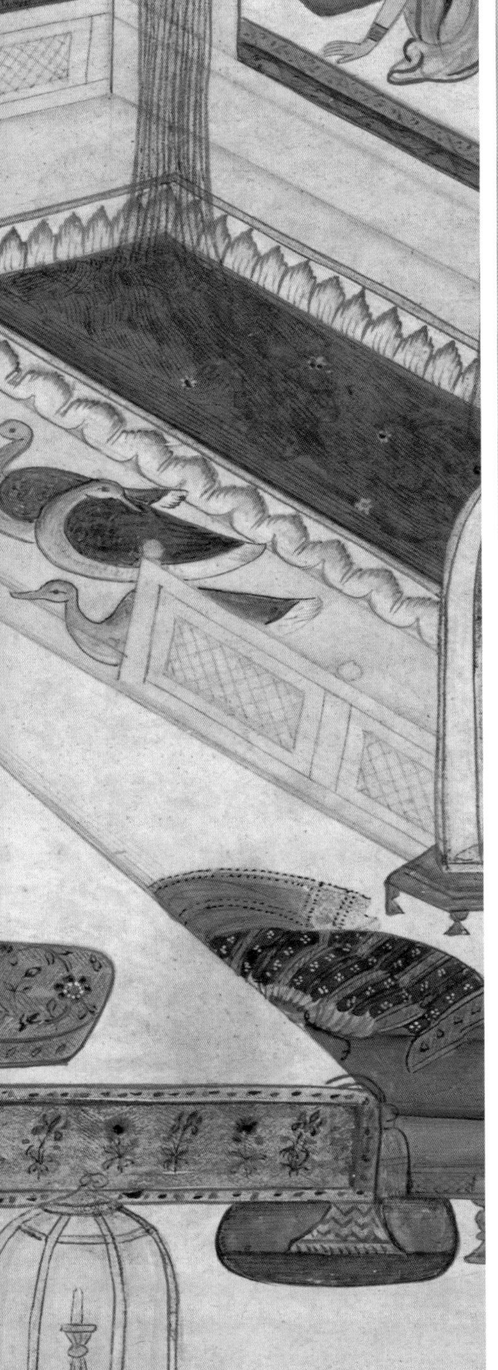

LOW LIGHTING

Candlelight is ideal for creating a sexy ambience, and the flames of an open fire will cast a warm, orange light over your lover's body. As well as a romantic, flickering glow, a fire will provide the warmth you need. Alternatively, use low table lamps rather than a central ceiling light. On a shoestring budget, you can simply replace the bright central bulb with a colored red or orange light.

THE NECESSITIES

Ointments and lubricants, sex toys, condoms and the like should all be placed within easy reach so that you're not forced to rummage around in the heat of passion. Drinking water is a must if you're planning a long, raunchy session. And wine and tidbits of food are good for maintaining energy levels and can be incorporated into sex play.

< VATSYAYANA'S DESCRIPTION *of the ideal bedroom is still magical: ". . . the outer room, balmy with rich perfumes, should contain a bed, soft, agreeable to the sight, covered with a clean white cloth, low in the middle part, having garlands and bunches of flowers upon it, and a canopy above it, and two pillows, one at the top, another at the bottom. There should also be a sort of couch besides, and at the head of this a sort of stool, on which should be placed the fragrant ointments for the night, as well as flowers, pots containing collyrium and other fragrant substances used for perfuming the mouth, and the bark of the common citron tree."*

However, the 21st-century lover may well choose to ignore Vatsyayana's recommendation: "Near the couch, on the ground, there should be a pot for spitting . . ." Music is the food of love, but make sure the choice of music suits the mood; if in doubt, go for soothing, ambient music.

PLAYING GAMES

The suggestions Vatsyayana makes for accoutrements for the bedroom include games and diversions such as dice and caged birds. Certainly there are some games today that can help make foreplay more interesting: strip poker or strip chess, for instance, can be fun. Each time a player loses a hand or a chess piece, he or she has to remove an article of clothing. To add an extra element of excitement and anticipation, agree on a particularly risqué forfeit for the overall loser. Or try a sexy version of Scrabble, where only sex-related words are allowed. You might be surprised by the extent of your lover's vocabulary, and ideas for subsequent activities may present themselves.

BEYOND THE BEDROOM

Of course, the bedroom is not the only place suitable for sex. Spontaneity is always exciting, and to this end the kitchen, living room, and bathroom can all be used from time to time. Away from home, the anonymity of hotel bedrooms can sometimes give you both the freedom to break out from your normal routine.

And then there's the great outdoors. Lovemaking takes on a whole new sensuality when you commune this closely with nature. If you have a secluded garden—or you find yourselves alone when walking in the woods or fields—all you need for comfort is a rug or a jacket to lie on.

Bathing and beautifying

Getting ready to go out and attract or meet a mate involves the time-honored tradition of cleaning, preening, and pampering. The early days of a relationship are always characterized by a focus on presenting one's body in the best light possible.

BODY BEAUTIFUL

It seems that throughout time civilized lovers who are contemplating sexual intimacy have preened, plucked, smoothed, shaved, waxed, painted, moisturized, buffed up, and polished. While modern man tends not to do quite so much of the above as modern woman does, he should, like his 4th-century male counterpart, know that looking and smelling good are an absolute must.

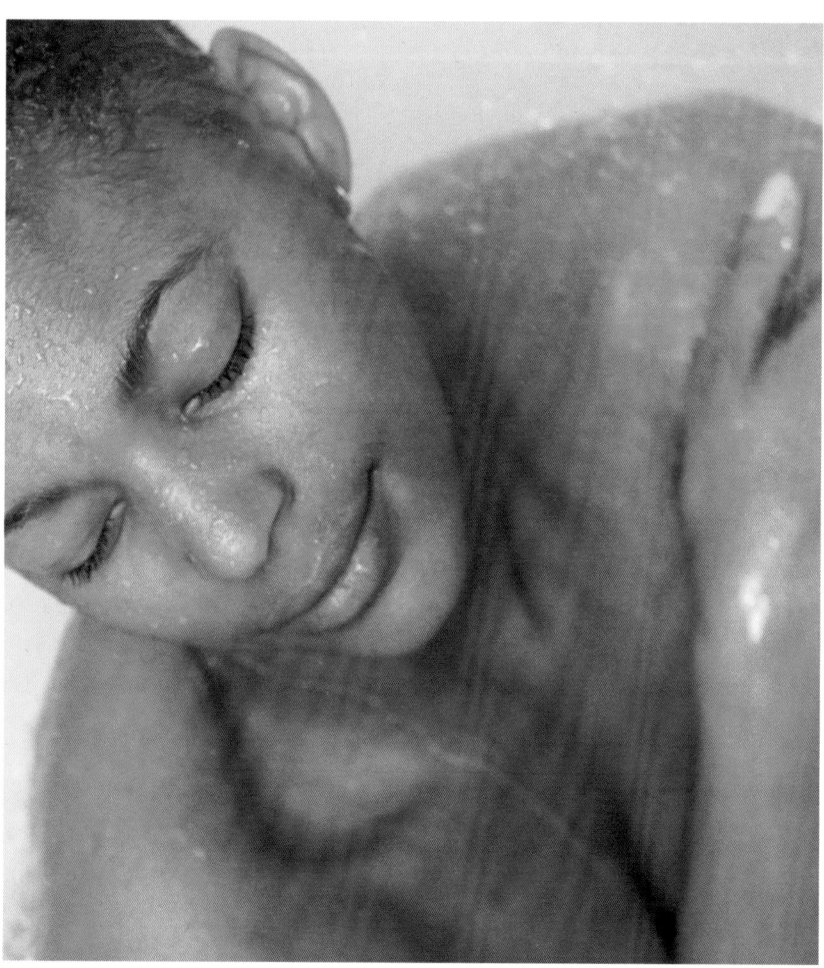

The Kama Sutra is unequivocal regarding male hygiene: "He should bathe daily, anoint his body with oil every other day, apply a lathering substance to his body every three days, get his head (including his face) shaved every four days, and the other parts of his body every five or ten days. All these things should be done without fail, and the sweat of the armpits should also be removed."

And it didn't stop there. Cosmetics and jewelry also featured: "The householder . . . should wash his teeth, apply a limited quantity of ointments and perfumes to his body, put some ornaments on his person and collyrium on his eyelids and below his eyes, color his lips with alacktaka." Yes, in those days you certainly put your best foot forward to seduce. Somehow, these rituals have been lost on modern man, which is a pity, as women love well-groomed (but not vain) men. Men take note: It is a myth that a sweaty body is an overpowering aphrodisiac to women. In truth, sweat post-sex is manly and ultra sexy; beforehand it's just plain smelly and offensive.

Not all bodily smells and secretions are unpleasant or dirty. In fact, fresh genital secretions perform a starring role as a natural aphrodisiac. So give nature a chance. Being freshly washed, with fresh breath, clipped nails and a winning smile is all that is necessary. Indeed, most of us find the person who

< OUR LOVE OF WATER *is primordial, whether we're talking about skinny-dipping in a lake or swimming pool, a luxurious soak in the bathtub, or an invigorating shower. Sharing a bath or shower with your lover can evoke a real sense of intimacy, as you both engage in a caring, as well as a sexual, role.*

Bathing together

The cool, all-over kiss of water's liquid touch is fundamentally relaxing and somehow enables us to feel and to get closer to each other. Bodies become light and graceful. If privacy allows it, making love in water is an intensely sensual experience, especially if you are in the open air. In 4th-century India, lakes, ponds, and rivers were used by the whole community, both for daily ablutions and as places for strict religious practice. For this reason, any sexual shenanigans in water were frowned upon. Nevertheless, the suggestion is made in the Kama Sutra by one sage, Suvarnanabha, that lovers use the buoyancy of water to help them perfect difficult sexual positions.

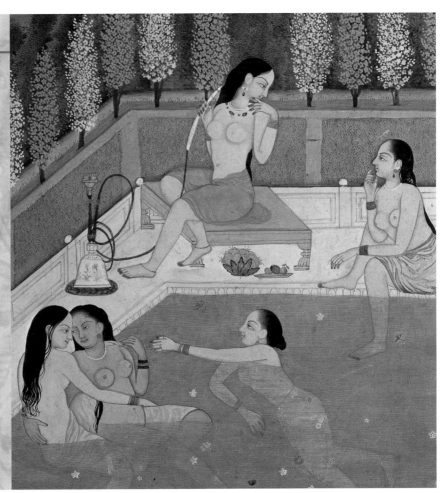

goes no further than this infinitely more desirable than someone who spends their life in the salon. Also, if you've doused yourself in an array of products, those poor pheromones will be difficult to detect.

There are one or two things that women can do to make their man as comfortable as possible. Take care not to scratch him with your jewelry, keep your nails trim and smooth, don't overpower his senses with strong perfume (just a dab will do), and condition your pubic hair to make it less abrasive. And there's one thing he may never tell you—that your loving stroking of his chest, thigh, arm or calf is in fact far from pleasant or sensual for him. It may well be extremely irritating—it feels like all the hairs are being pulled. And lotions, massage oils, and creams only make this worse.

Bear in mind, too, that there are some grooming rituals that beautify and prepare the body for intimacy that you will probably want to perform in private and others that can be shared. Keep to yourself all references to that rash you had or how much your bikini wax hurt. Share a bath or shower only when you're fully prepared to be enjoyed by your lover, having performed all necessary hygiene and beautifying rituals in privacy beforehand.

BATHTIME BLISS

You know when you're really starting to accept and care for each other when you bathe together. It's intimate, caring, erotic, sensual, and incredibly good fun (not to mention astonishingly good foreplay). A candlelit bath is probably one of the most romantic ways to luxuriate and delight in the sensuality of being together. Wet, soapy bodies look stunning in the flickering, soft light of the candles. In fact, the scene is almost primal: fire, water, and sex.

Bathing is also an excellent time to find out more about how your lover likes to be touched. Explore areas of your bodies that may not normally get enough attention, or are too ticklish when dry, such as feet. Washing each other's backs and shampooing hair are actions that echo the physical care we were given as children. While, on an emotional level, bathing reinforces the caring, loving side of intimacy, it also acts as erotic play.

Massage

Massage—or, in Burton's translation of the Kama Sutra, "shampooing"—serves many beneficial purposes: It can calm the nerves, reduce stress, alleviate pain, and boost the cardiovascular system. Massage can also be highly erotic. Its soothing, rhythmic strokes relax the mind while stimulating the skin and awakening the body's responses. In skilled and loving hands, it can be the ultimate prelude to lovemaking.

TENDER, LOVING CARE

In the Kama Sutra, Vatsyayana describes massage as a "sign of a woman manifesting her love." There is a strong sense of playfulness about the description: "She occupies herself with shampooing his body and pressing his head . . . she works with one hand only, and with the other she touches and embraces parts of his body . . . She places one of her hands quite motionless on his body, and even though the man should press it between two members of his body, she does not remove it for a long time."

In another chapter of the book, Vatsyayana gives a surprisingly tender account of massage as part of the process of a groom "winning the confidence" of his bride: "On the second and third nights, after her confidence has increased still more, he should feel the whole of her body with his hands, and kiss her all over; he should also place his hands upon her thighs and shampoo them, and if he succeed in this he should then shampoo the joints of her thighs. If she tries to prevent him doing this he should say to her, 'What harm is there in doing it?' and should persuade her to let him do it. After gaining this

V THE PERFECT TIME *for a sensual massage is following a luxurious bath when you are already warm, relaxed, and naked. All you need is a basic carrier oil, such as sunflower or almond, but you may like to blend in a few drops of one or two recommended essential oils. Rosewood, sandalwood, jasmine, rose, and ylang ylang are popular.*

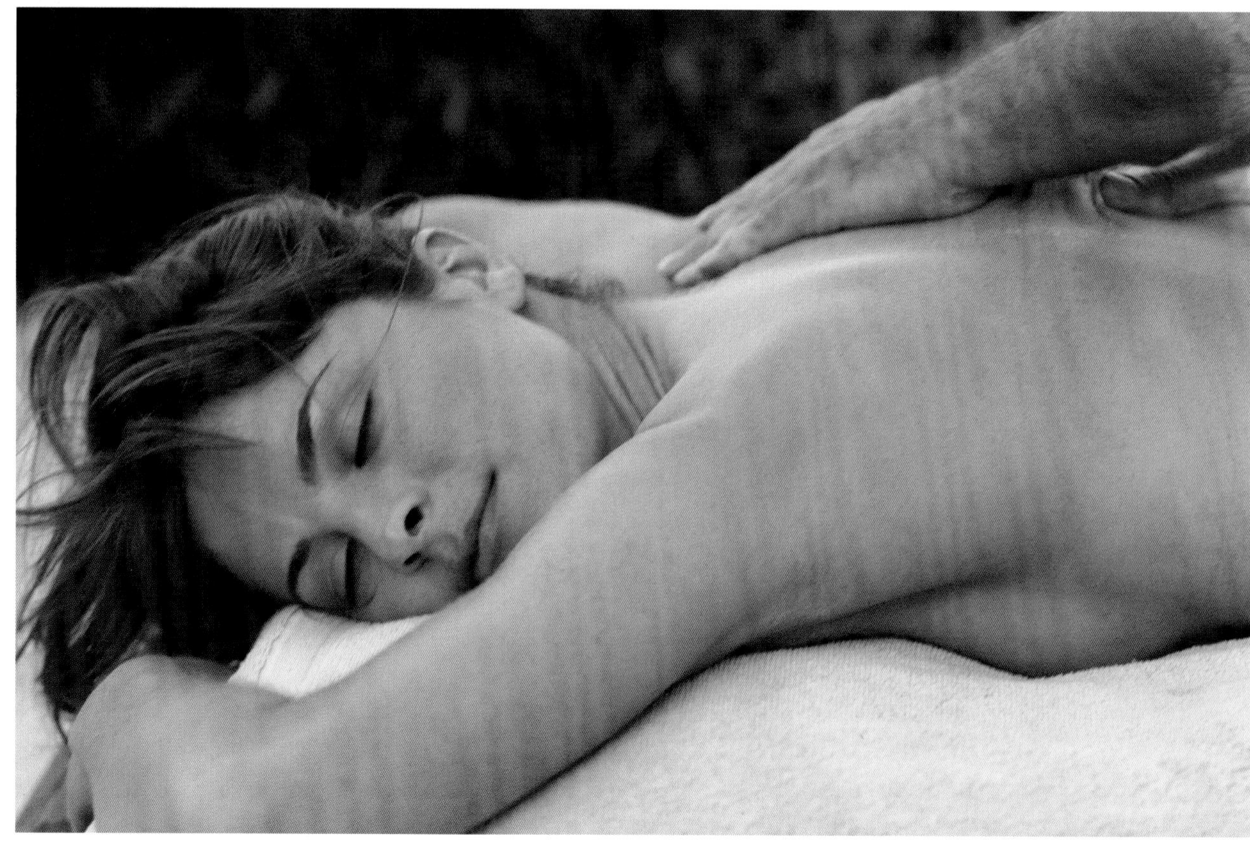

Foot massage

Female attendants pamper a wealthy woman by playing music and fanning. One of the attendants massages her mistress's foot using the ancient art that is known today as reflexology. A foot massage eases away stress and soothes the body, giving you the chance to chat and relax together. Soft strokes over the feet have a calming effect, while stronger pressures boost low energy levels. Pay attention to the toes because touch here is surprisingly sensual. The toes tend to retain tension, which adds stress to the posture. Stretching them brings relief to the whole body. After pressing gently over the toe, pull gently along its length from the base to the tip.

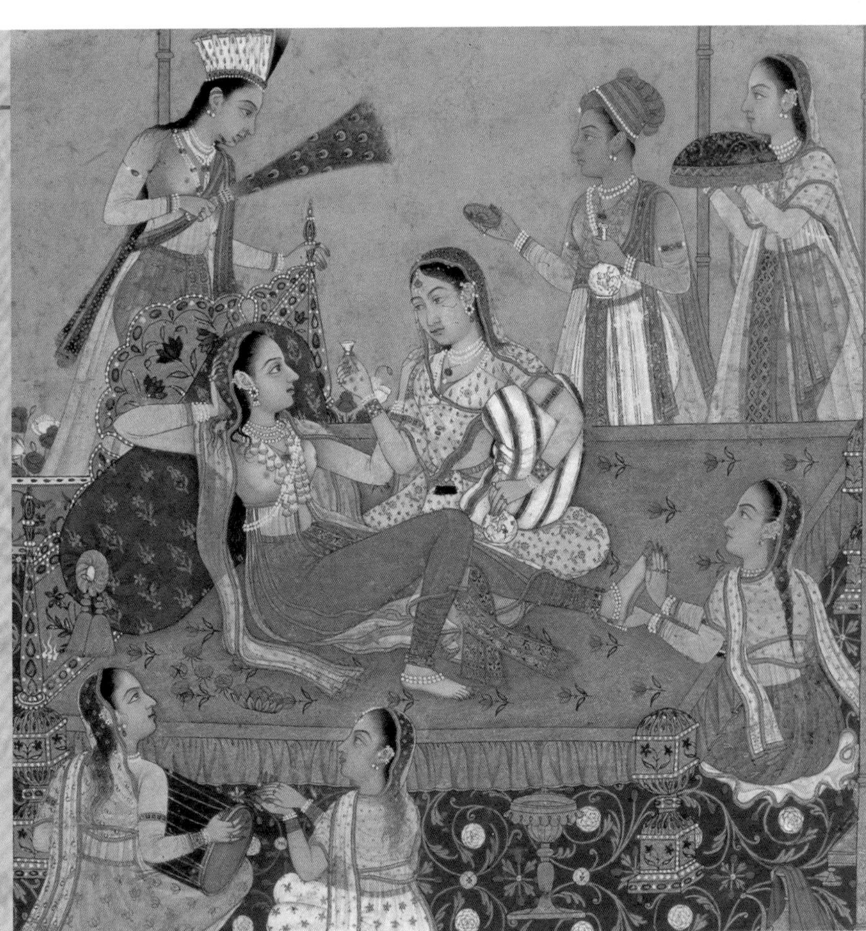

point he should touch her private parts, should loosen her girdle and the knot of her dress, and turning up her lower garment should shampoo the joints of her naked thighs."

Knowledge of massage is definitely one of the arts of love that you should add to your repertoire, whether you teach yourselves from a book or take a massage class or workshop. Between modern lovers, massage can still be the ideal medium for building confidence and trust. The perfect time for a massage is following a long, luxurious bath when you are already warm, relaxed, and naked.

THE TECHNIQUE

A basic, flowing, full-body massage is not difficult to master, but there are a number of golden rules. First, create a sensual environment, as you would for all lovemaking (*see* pg.44) but remember that a warm temperature is even more important because one of you will remain inert (in case your lover feels cold, have some soft, thick towels on hand to cover the body areas you are not working on). Be sure to warm your hands and the massage oil before placing them on your partner's skin. Make sure that one hand remains in contact with your partner's skin at all times, and use continuous, soft, rhythmic motions.

Use a relatively firm pressure at first in flowing, circular strokes. Use kneading motions over muscular areas such as the buttocks, thighs, and shoulders. Use a more moderate pressure once your partner has relaxed to enliven the skin and arouse feelings of passion. Finally, lighter brushing motions can feel very exciting and sexy. You don't have to use the palms of your hands: the man can use his fingernails and his breath; the woman can use her hair. Finally, never use circular motions on bony areas, and always massage away from the spine—never toward it and never directly on it.

Once you have mastered the basic techniques and have grown a little in confidence, you can let your intuition take over. Practically anything you do will feel wonderful if you stick to the golden rules above and take things slowly, using gentle, circular motions to relax the body and gentle kneading of the muscles to relieve tension.

Finally, remain attentive to your partner's reactions to particular strokes so that you learn what pleases or arouses most. Remember that what feels fantastic to you may do absolutely nothing for your lover.

Dressing to thrill

Dress to attract and to seduce. Here's how: Flaunt your body by emphasizing every curve in tight, sexy clothes, especially those that showcase the chest, genitals, and bottom. Choose clothing that is either easy to slip off or difficult to remove—so you can use it to taunt and tease the object of your desire.

DRESSING UP

"When the wife wants to approach her husband in private, her dress should consist of many ornaments, various kinds of flowers, and a cloth decorated with different colors, and some sweet-smelling ointments or unguents. But her everyday dress should be composed of a thin, close-textured cloth, a few ornaments and flowers, and a little scent, not too much." So said Vatsyayana. Today, however, things have changed: There are no hard and fast rules to the art of seductive dressing—we are all of us turned on by different images, sensations, and associations.

ROLE PLAY

Ask your lover what they find irresistible. Bondage may not excite her, but pretending to be a high-class courtesan may. Educate fingers to appreciate and differentiate between textures and sensations. Blindfold your lover and ask him to guess what materials you're wearing. Then get out the costume box and let your imagination run riot—feather boas, leather, cashmere, cotton, fake fur, rubber, latex, silk. Once you have a good idea of what pushes their buttons, you can use clothes that will really enhance arousal. Dressing up allows us permission to play with our sexual identities, freeing us up from our workaday selves. She may be a businesswoman by day, but a '50s sex-siren in the bedroom. He's an ordinary working guy, but at bedtime he's a superhero in latex. You get the idea.

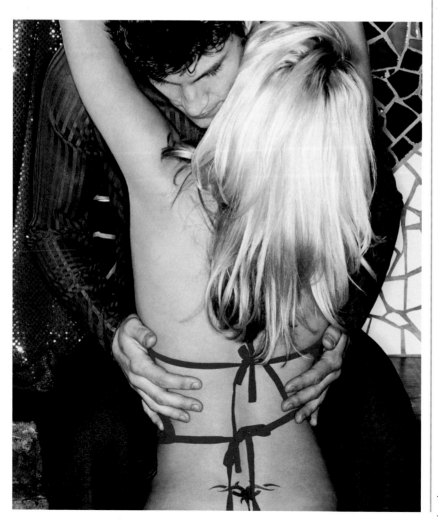

< TODAY WE WEAR *less and less to attract a mate. Women realize that acres of flesh on show does attract men. Men are also becoming body conscious, wearing their clothes to show off their bodies in a more provocative way.*

> AT THE TIME THE KAMA SUTRA *was written, women dressed in an incredibly sexy fashion, wearing floaty, diaphanous clothing and often exposing their breasts completely. A married woman judged her success in life by how much pleasure she afforded her husband—which explains the fashion for provocative and seductive dress for women of all ages.*

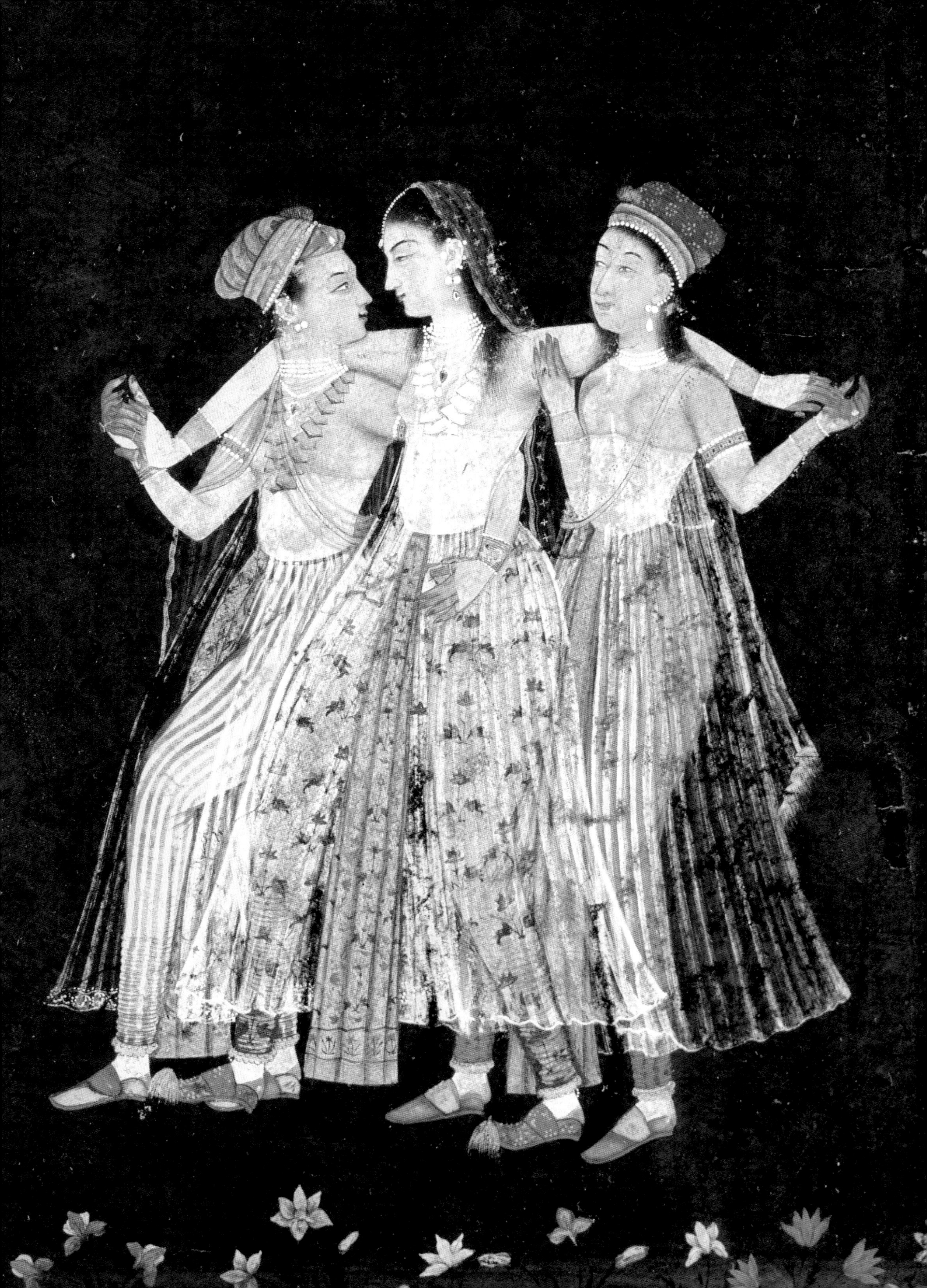

Fantasy and fetishes

Indulging in acts we perceive to be taboo gives us all a certain thrill. Because desire is created in the brain, acting out our innermost, almost forbidden thoughts is deeply erotic. Meanwhile, as more and more of us experiment with bondage, leather and latex, the fetish scene is becoming almost mainstream.

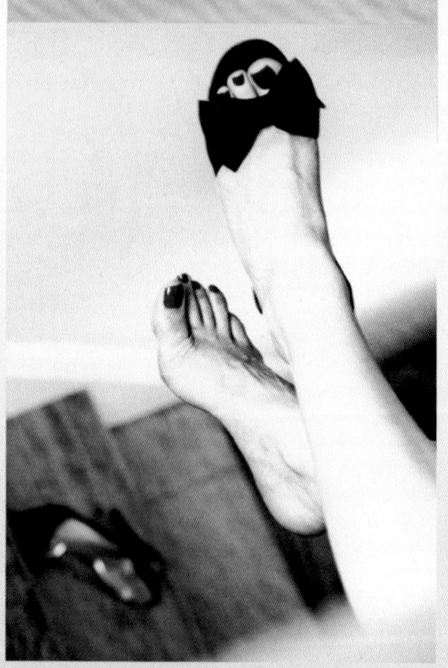

Ever wondered why playing doctors and nurses, firemen and teachers make us horny? Many find authority sexy, and uniforms project a strong, powerful image, which is why they're such a turn on. Share fantasies that involve dressing up in costume or playing your favorite characters from the silver screen. Above all, enjoy the sexual intimacy that enables you to play and explore yet another facet of lovemaking.

UNDRESSING TO THRILL

Underwear for sex needs to do more than cover your modesty and hold your bits in place. It needs to arouse your lover to distraction by emphasizing and sexualizing your body. Women are lucky in the underwear stakes—they have a huge selection to choose from; for men, the choice is not so good. This means he has to think a little bit harder about how he uses his clothes (perhaps a tight-fitting shirt or undershirt that has to be peeled slowly over manly shoulders) or he can order more risqué items from specialist shops.

If you feel shy about undressing in front of your lover, make it something you both do, as part of foreplay. This way you won't feel your body is being scrutinized. Or don't bother about getting undressed—remove only those items of clothing that really get in the way (this is something that gets top erotic marks). Play that game where you have to remove each other's underwear with your teeth (excluding the bra clip)—a guaranteed way for you to end up in a steamy, semi-dressed, giggling heap.

But if you really want to turn your lover into your sexual slave, strip for them. That's right, stripping is on the Top 10 fantasy list for both men and women. The main secrets of how to strip with aplomb are: practice, prepare, set the ground rules, tantalize, tease.

To practice, parade around in front of a full-length mirror and remove your clothes slowly. Look at your body, see what angles suit it best, touch yourself. Learn how the professionals walk: Hold your head high and push that chest out, then put one leg in front of the other, mentally following a figure of eight. Remember to keep outer garments, such as a jacket, on for some

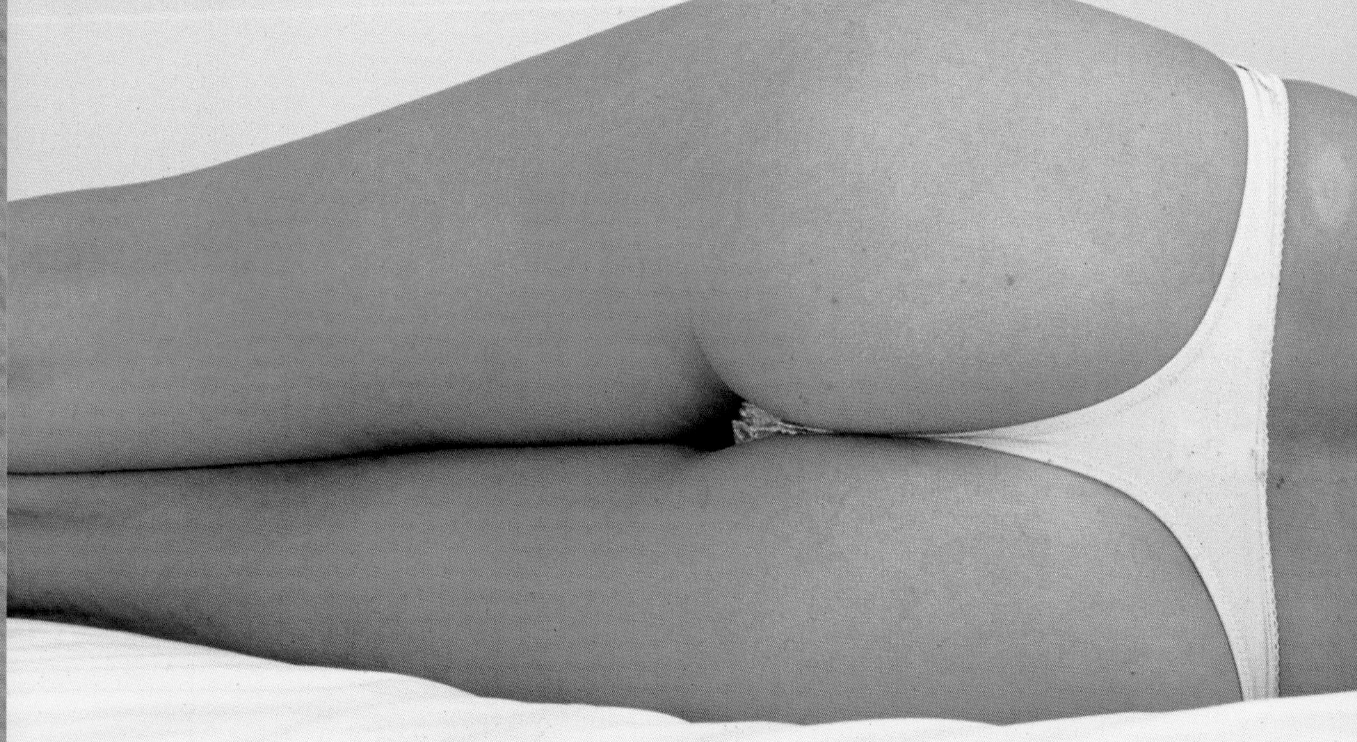

time and, when you do remove it, use it to keep the good bits covered a bit longer. You want to tease your lover, not win points for speed of disrobing. Think of yourself as a prize that you are presenting, little by little, to your lover. The first rule is that your lover can't touch you; the second is that you have to maintain eye contact. A tip: The seductive way to remove panties is to slide your thumbs under the material, pull them away from the body and bring them down, slip them off, and brandish them. Ready? Now it's showtime!

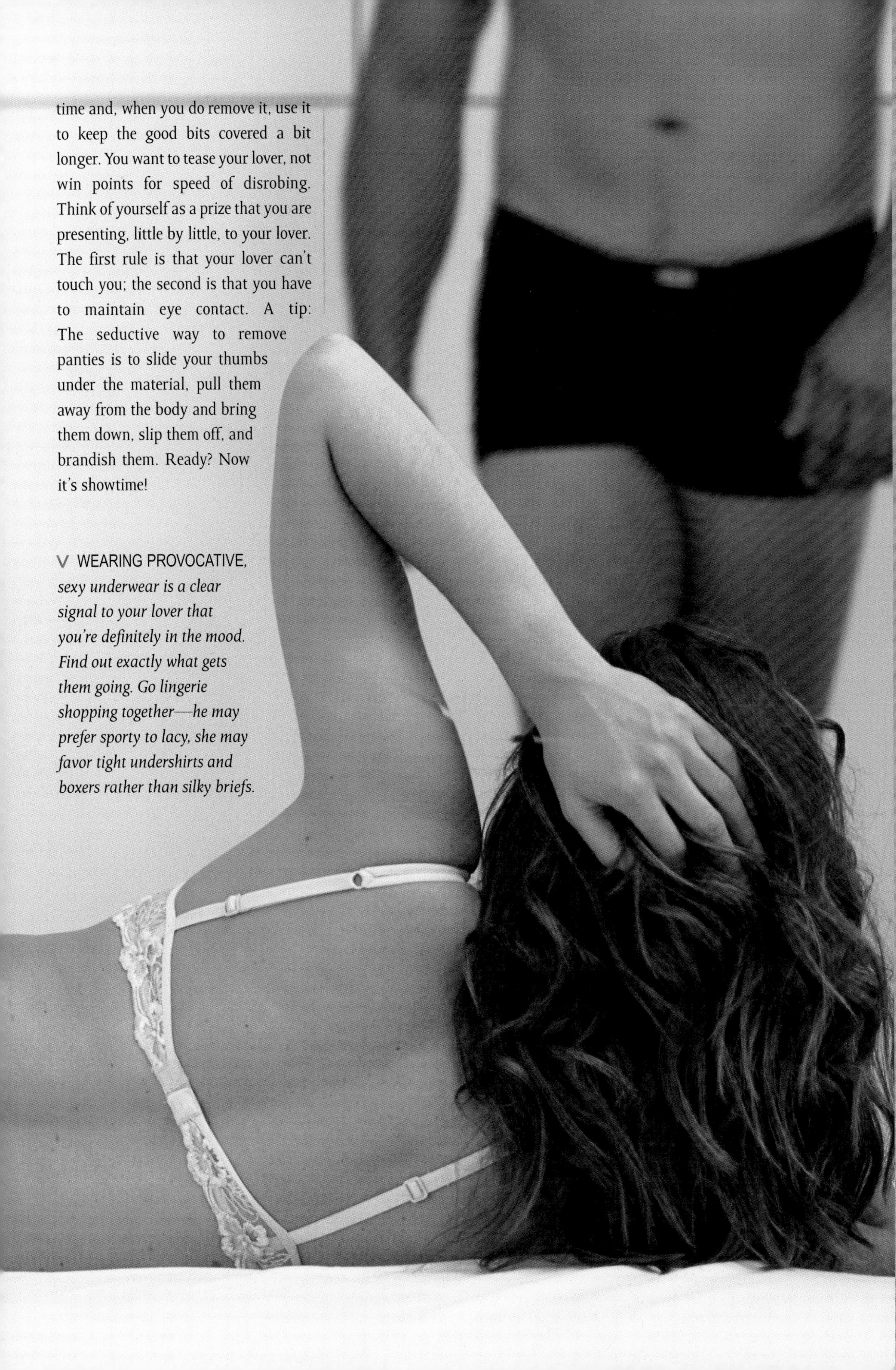

V WEARING PROVOCATIVE, *sexy underwear is a clear signal to your lover that you're definitely in the mood. Find out exactly what gets them going. Go lingerie shopping together—he may prefer sporty to lacy, she may favor tight undershirts and boxers rather than silky briefs.*

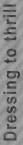

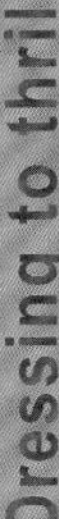

The embrace

The embrace is a powerful tool with which to entice a new partner. In a loving relationship it is the surest way to express deep affection and desire. Vatsyayana describes four types of embraces to use in the sex act: two standing positions—the "twining of a creeper" and "climbing of a tree"; and two supine positions—the embrace of "sesamum seed and rice" and the "mixture of milk and water."

SEDUCTIVE EMBRACE

"When a man under some pretext or other goes in front of or alongside a woman and touches her body with his own, it is called the 'touching embrace'." Some people are naturally more tactile than others, so it is sometimes difficult to know whether this kind of embrace is an advance or not. That is why it can be effective. If someone is interested in a suitor's advances, she will reciprocate; if she is not, she will shrink away and may even flash an unequivocal look of distaste—unspoken rejection.

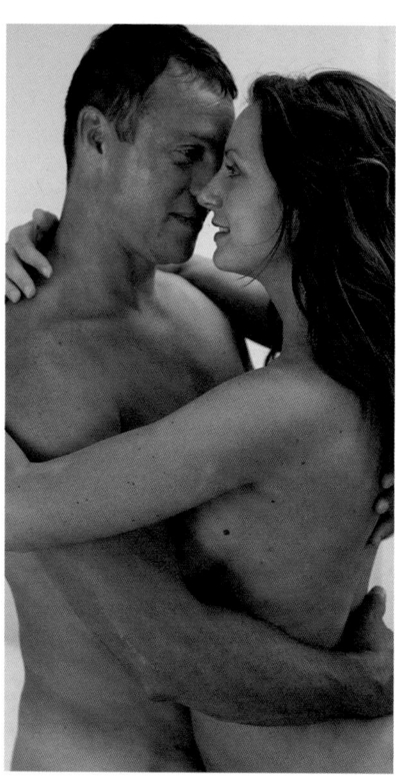

∧ VATSYAYANA *also describes "four ways of embracing members of the body," one of which is "the embrace of the breasts."*

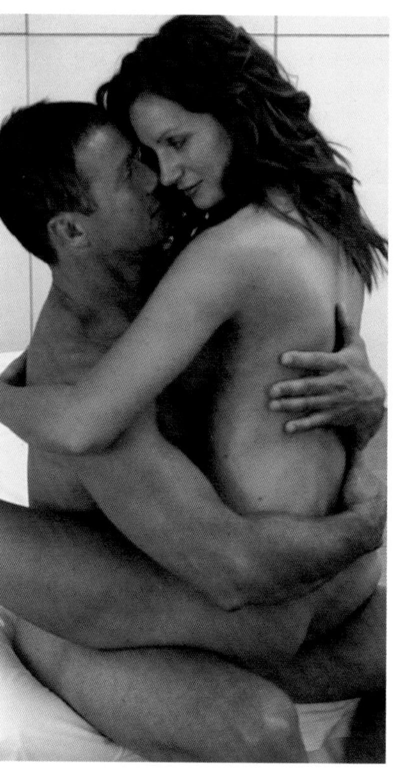

∧ THIS VERY LOVING *"milk and water" embrace, "as if they were entering into each other's bodies," can initiate potent woman-on-top sex.*

"When a woman in a lonely place bends down, as if to pick up something, and pierces, as it were, a man sitting or standing, with her breasts, and the man in return takes hold of them, it is called a 'piercing embrace.'" The "lonely place" is key here; if a man were to "take hold of them" each time a woman's breasts brushed against him on a crowded train, he would be in serious trouble. But, in the appropriate place, wearing a sexy and revealing top on an initial date is a very effective way to display your interest in a potential lover.

SEXUAL EMBRACES

Vatsyayana describes two types of embrace for lovers who "know the intentions of each other," that is when a relationship of some sort has been given the green light but real intimacy is still some way off. These "rubbing" and "pressing" embraces describe those moments when tentative lovers take every opportunity to rub their bodies together as they walk along side by side, and even occasionally trap their lover, perhaps in mock protest about a teasing comment, and "press" them against a wall or a tree.

During lovemaking, embracing and kissing are ways of reassuring your partner that you are interested in them for more than just their body, and it is an element of sex that most women, in particular, regard as indispensable. While the inability to embrace lends a detached and cold element to certain sex positions, notably the animal positions, it is the ability to embrace that gives other positions, such as the Lotus position, their special intimacy.

> "MILK AND WATER" *is the ultimate romantic and loving embrace, where the lovers seem inseparable, dissolving into one another.*

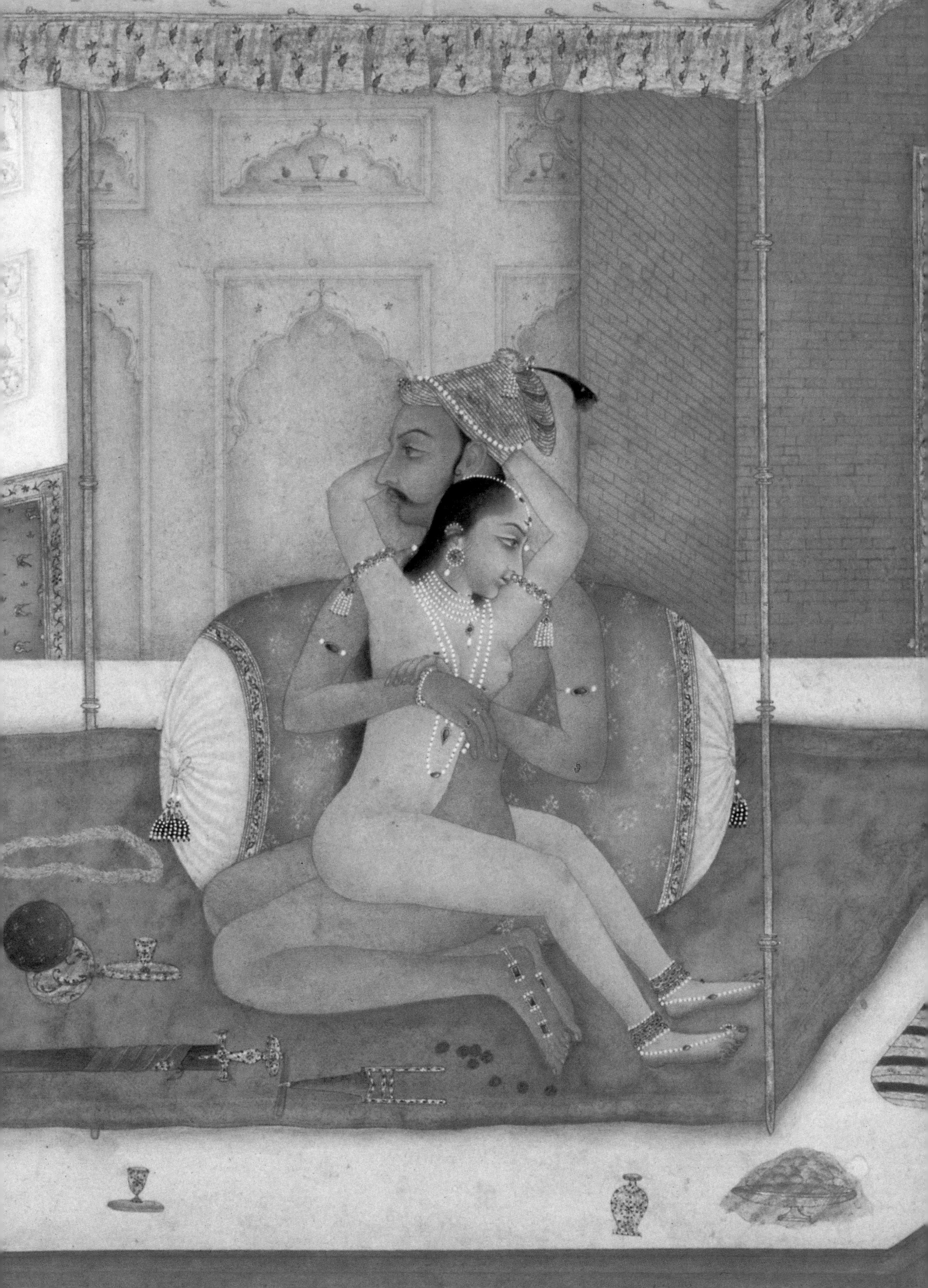

Kissing

Kissing is probably the most romantic, personal, and sensual act shared by lovers. It is an essential ingredient of any loving relationship—in foreplay, during intercourse, and at any time as a way of reaffirming love. The Kama Sutra treats kissing as an art form in itself, and Vatsyayana identifies almost as many different variations on the kiss as varieties of sexual postures.

THE ART OF KISSING

The kiss is a versatile weapon in your sensual armory. It can be friendly and affectionate or totally, knee-tremblingly passionate. It can be a greeting or a farewell, it can soothe or excite, distract or awaken. At one end of the scale is the quick peck (where a hand may be placed on the shoulder, if only to stop you from bumping heads), at the other end, the full-on embracing kiss during intercourse, where you couldn't get any closer unless you climbed into each other's skin.

Of course, kissing isn't confined to the lips. Vatsyayana is quite specific regarding the regions of the body that should be kissed, and identifies many of the body's most erogenous zones: "The following are the places for kissing: the forehead, the eyes, the cheeks, the throat, the bosom, the breasts, the lips, and the interior of the mouth." He goes on to mention that "the people of the Lat country kiss also on the following places: the joints of the thighs, the arms and the navel" but warns that such customs are "not fit to be practiced by all." Nowadays, every square inch of the skin is fair game.

TONGUE BATHING

Kissing the most sensitive parts of the body heightens arousal and anticipation. "Tongue bathing" (exploring your lover's body with your tongue and kisses) is a great way to pleasure your partner, although you must be aware that certain parts of the body are more sensitive than others and so require a different touch. Vatsyayana, of course, was very aware of this fact, which is why he categorized kisses according to pressure and duration: "Kissing is of four kinds:

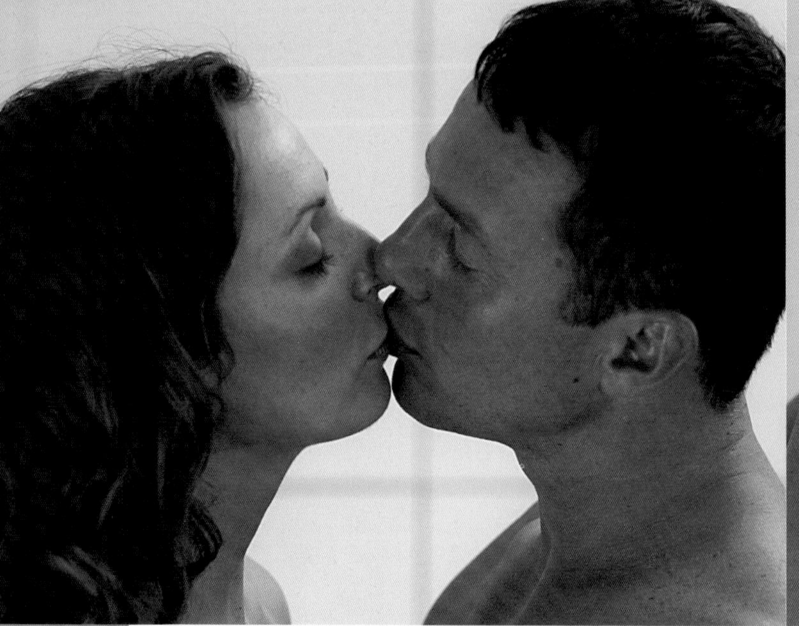

∧ THE STRAIGHT KISS: *"When the lips of two lovers are brought into direct contact with each other, it is called a 'straight' kiss." It is a gentle kiss that lovers often use in the earliest stage of their relationship.*

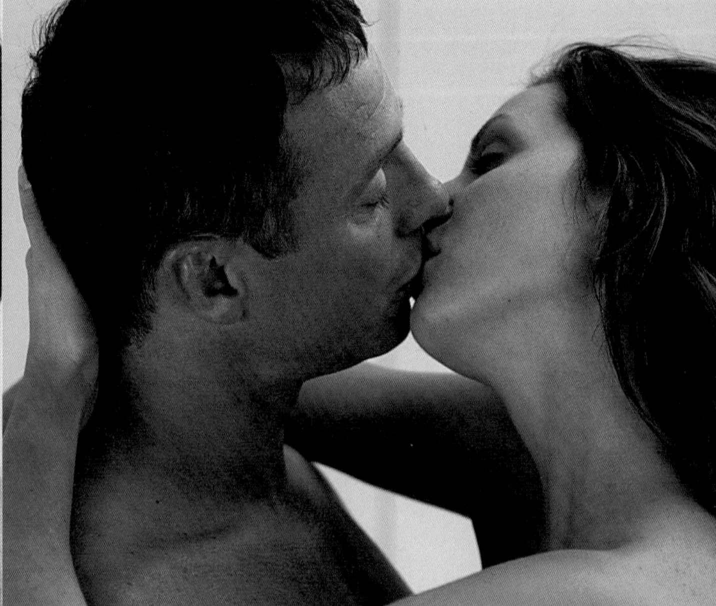

∧ THE BENT KISS: *"When the heads of two lovers are bent toward each other, and when so bent, kissing takes place, it is called a 'bent' kiss." This is the classic passionate kiss of intimate lovers.*

> *"Whatever things may be done by one of the lovers to the other, the same should be returned . . . if the woman kisses him he should kiss her in return . . ."* KSII:III

moderate, contracted, pressed, and soft, according to the different parts of the body which are kissed, for different kinds of kisses are appropriate for different parts of the body."

THE CHEMISTRY OF KISSING

Another area where Vatsyayana cannot be faulted is the timing of kisses, which he stresses is crucial to the success of a relationship. Because it is such an intimate act, it is always advisable to go too slowly rather than too quickly. Certainly few things are as unsavory in the mouth as an unexpected and unwelcome tongue, although during the height of arousal French kissing can be wonderfully passionate and a foretaste of more erotic things to come.

Kissing is a way of exploring whether or not there is any sexual chemistry, and as such can make or break a relationship. Keep the first kiss as affectionate as possible, no matter how turned on you are. Be sure of your partner's body language, and let this be your guide. Being a good lover is about being thoughtful, in tune, and affectionate. Needless to say, oral hygiene is crucial if you are to enjoy the close intimacy of a kiss—a kiss after one partner has indulged in a garlic feast can wilt the most promising of romances.

Biting

In the Kama Sutra, Vatsyayana dedicates an entire chapter to the subject of scratching and another to biting. Research has shown that women are more likely to bite during lovemaking, while men shy from biting or, indeed, being bitten. It has been suggested that it is more natural for men to express their passion through forceful bodily gestures rather than by biting.

In ancient India, when passions were aroused kisses turned into something harder and sharper—but even then Vatsyayana warns that scratching and biting are "not the usual thing except with those who are intensely passionate," and then only with "those to whom the practice is agreeable."

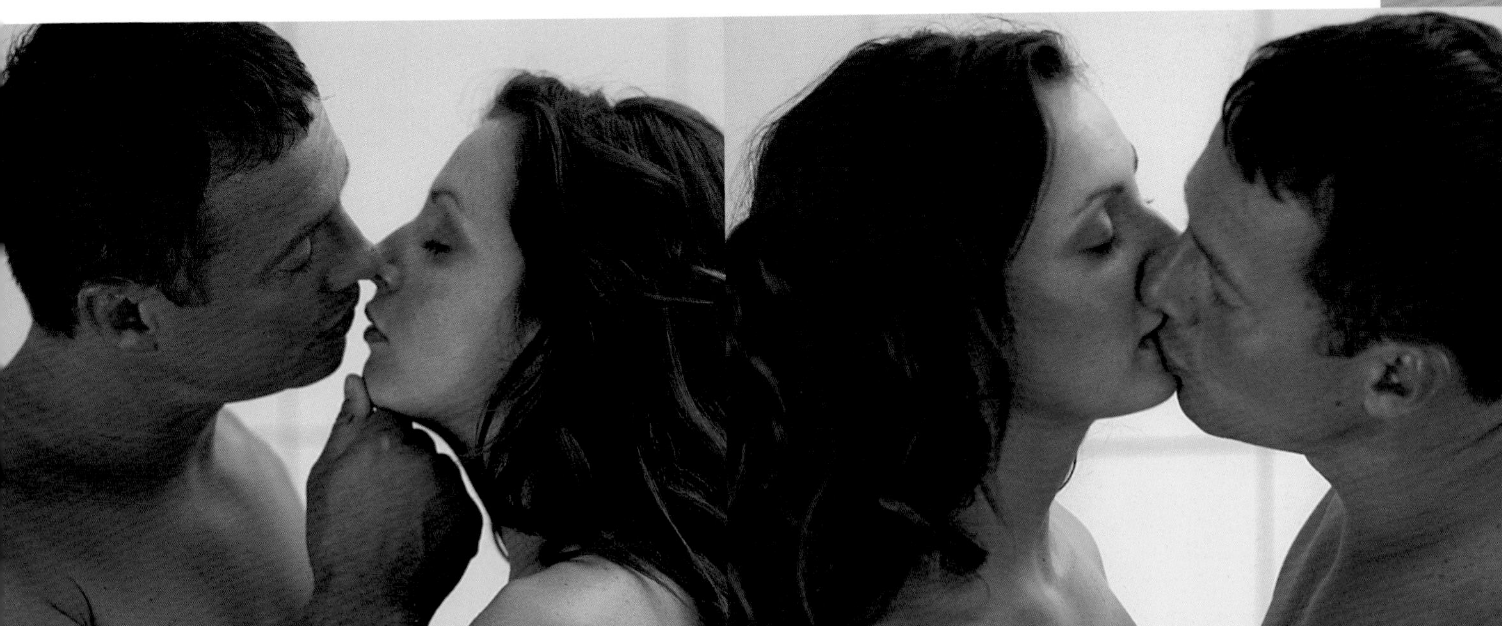

∧ THE TURNED KISS: *"When one of them turns up the face of the other by holding the head and chin, and then kissing, it is called a 'turned' kiss." This can be a tender expression of love or a subtle powerplay.*

∧ THE PRESSED KISS: *". . . when the lower lip is pressed with much force, it is called a 'pressed' kiss." This kiss usually occurs between mouth-to-mouth contact and the more intimate mouth-to-face contact* (see pg.22).

> *"When a lover coming home late at night kisses his beloved, who is asleep on her bed, in order to show her his desire, it is called a 'kiss that awakens.'"* KSII:III

> THIS WOMAN APPEARS *reluctant to be kissed; perhaps her lover has somehow hurt her feelings. Vatsyayana may have an explanation for this: "When a woman kisses her lover while he is engaged in business, or while he is quarrelling with her, or while he is looking at something else, so that his mind may be turned away, it is called a 'kiss that turns away.'"*

INDICATIVE KISSES

When two people become sexually attracted to each other, kissing clearly signals the different stages in their relationship (*see* pg.22–23). Kissing may begin as an affectionate peck on the cheek or a gentle brush of the lips, but if the chemistry is there, it will inevitably progress to become passionate and arousing. However, this transition needs to be treated with sensitivity. Let your partner's response dictate whether the kiss lingers with a light, soft contact of the lips or moves on to a more ardent embrace, vividly described by Vatsyayana as "the fighting of the tongues."

POWERFUL EMOTIONS

While our primary senses are sight and hearing, a kiss on the lips awakens and stimulates the secondary, more sensual senses of touch, taste, and smell. All three are invoked and heightened as we close our eyes and kiss our lover. This powerful combination produces intense feelings of emotion in both the giver and the receiver.

Embracing and kissing increase passion and are essential in foreplay. For a woman particularly, however, kissing is an essential part of all lovemaking, as it reassures her that she is loved as a person, not just for her body. So kissing should not be used as a precursor for sex and then neglected during the act itself. And it certainly should not be forgotten at the end of sexual intercourse. Sex should be punctuated with kisses: Like commas, tender kisses should appear at practically every natural breathing space. The passionate kiss is like an exclamation mark—though it can be used less sparingly than it should be in good written English—and can happily appear at the end of every sexual phrase. And the final period should be long and lingering.

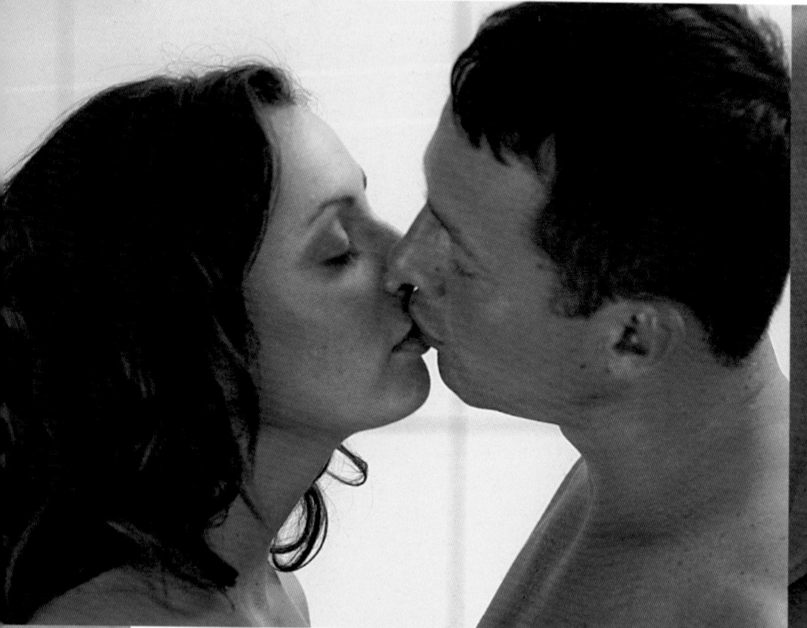

Λ KISS OF THE UPPER LIP: *"When a man kisses the upper lip of a woman, while she in return kisses his lower lip, it is called the 'kiss of the upper lip.'" This is the type of playful kissing that usual heralds more passionate making out.*

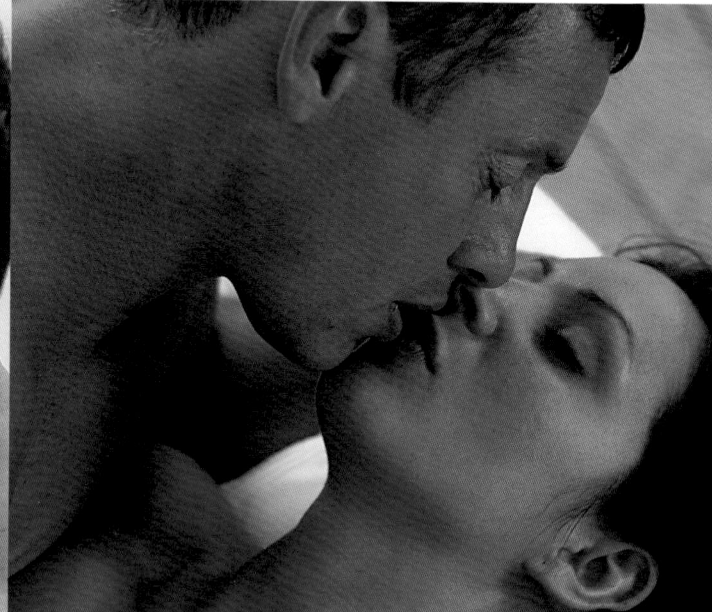

Λ THE CLASPING KISS: *"When one of them takes both the lips of the other between his or her own, it is called a 'clasping kiss.'" You certainly wouldn't greet your Aunt Ethel with this one.*

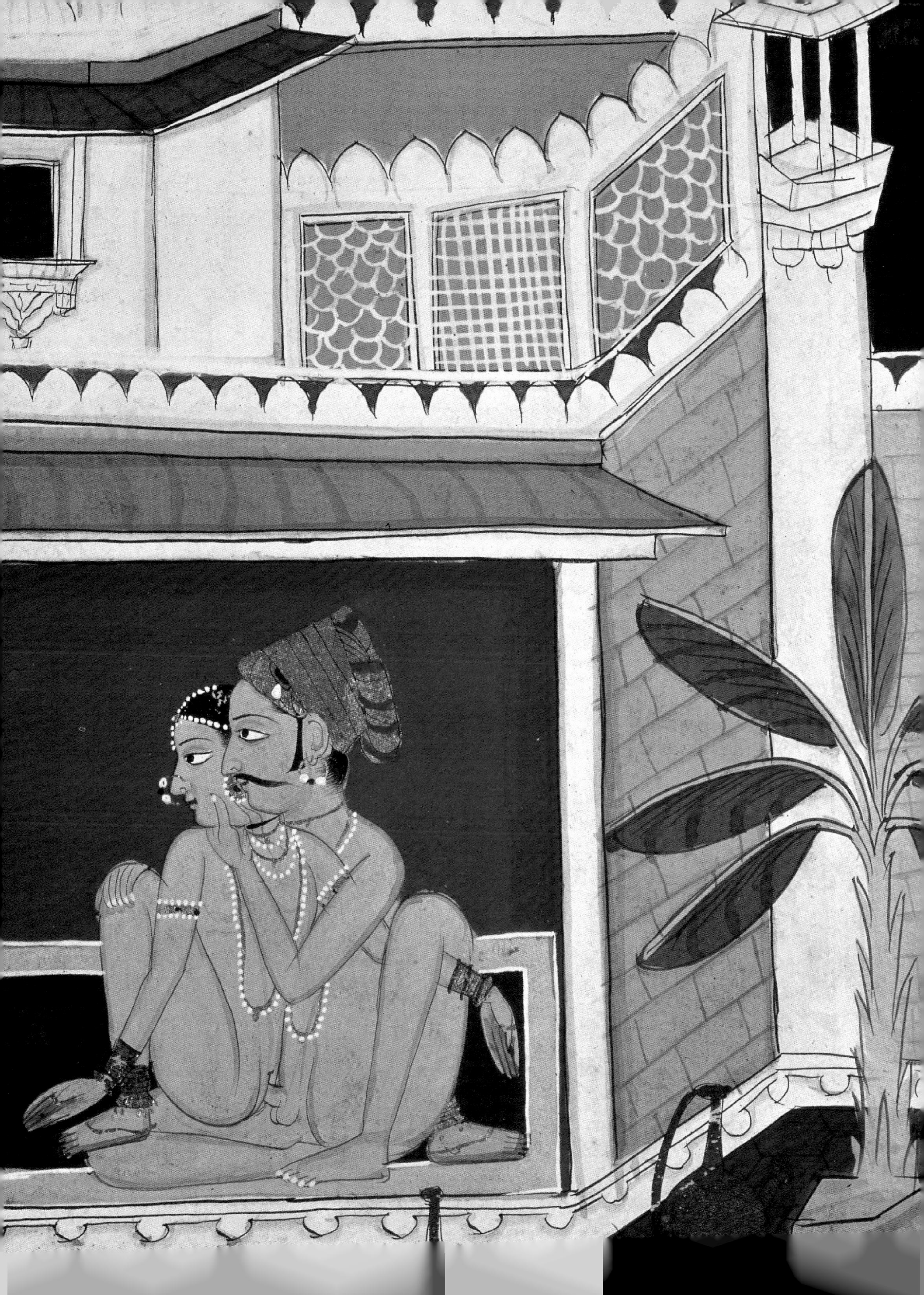

Oral sex

An entire chapter of the Kama Sutra is dedicated to oral sex. However, it is generally described as something practiced only by eunuchs and "unchaste and wanton" women. In his inimitable fashion, Vatsyayana divides oral sex into eight stages, beginning with "nominal congress" and culminating in "swallowing up." While variety is just as important today, much of the pleasure is actually in the anticipation.

THE ANTICIPATION

By kissing your lover all over from head to toe, moving in slowly toward the penis or the vagina, occasionally "accidentally" brushing your lips against the genitals, you can drive your lover wild with pleasure.

ORAL SEX FOR HER

Learn how your partner likes to be stimulated orally. Vatsyayana wrote that techniques for kissing the vagina "should be known from kissing the mouth." However, most women prefer slow, luxurious sweeps of the tongue to the rapid flicking action that many men take pride in. Your lover is the best teacher: All women have different responses, so let her guide you with words of encouragement and pelvic movements. She may show you that she wants you to be a little rougher by raising her hips to meet you or she may turn her pelvis away if you are too rough.

Arouse her through loving play before giving attention directly to the clitoral area. Stimulating the clitoris before she is aroused can cause discomfort. Concentrate on her vulva and her inner thighs, all the time caressing her thighs and buttocks. As she becomes more aroused the lips of her vulva will swell slightly. Gently part her lips and insert your tongue into her vagina. Vary your strokes at this stage and pay special attention to the area surrounding her clitoris. Suck very

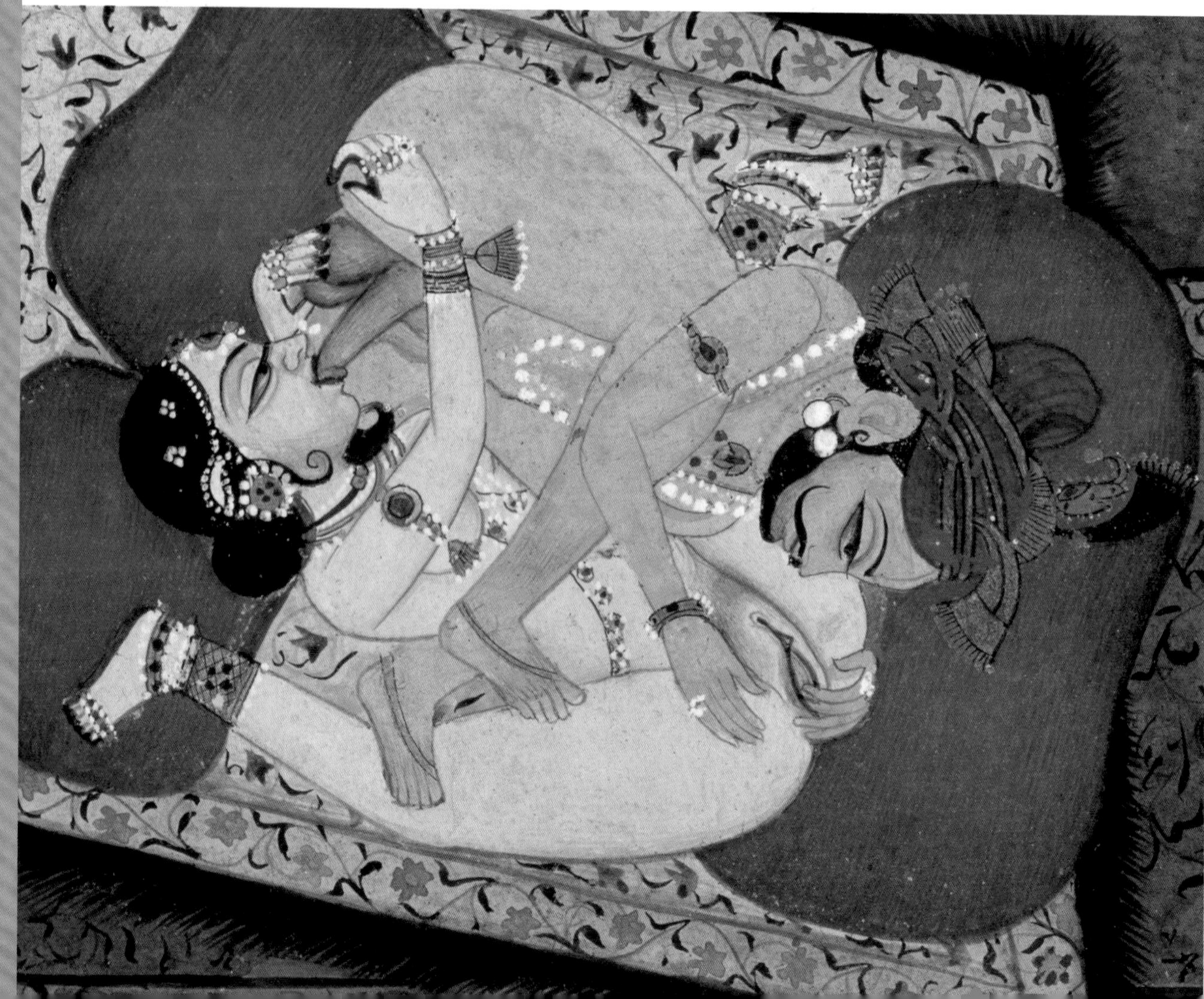

gently on her clitoris and flick your tongue from side to side. However, it is best to stick to one technique as she approaches her orgasm. Use up-and-down and circular sweeping motions with the flat of your tongue rather than the tip to give her maximum pleasure. Increase the speed and pressure a little but keep the rhythm regular and don't stop until she pushes you away or signals that she wants you to put your penis inside her. Some lucky women are multi-orgasmic and will want to continue with intercourse after reaching orgasm through oral sex. If it isn't obvious from her screams of delight, you will know she has had her orgasm when her clitoris becomes too sensitive to bear being touched.

ORAL SEX FOR HIM

There are many different positions that you can adopt to give oral sex, but men do find it very exciting when a woman kneels in front of them because it makes them feel powerful. Men also like to watch the proceedings, so be sure to leave a light on. Leave your own hands free to caress his thighs and buttocks or to squeeze his testicles gently.

Again, anticipation is everything: Tease him by licking and kissing the highly erogenous area around his thighs and abdomen; occasionally take his penis in your mouth but then move away again. When you are ready to take him in your mouth, don't concentrate solely on the head. Nibble and suck the

< VATSYAYANA *recognized the raw appeal of the 69 position, "Congress of the Crow," and warns, "For the sake of such things courtesans abandon men possessed of good qualities, liberal and clever, and become attached to low persons, such as slaves and elephant drivers." Who could blame them?*

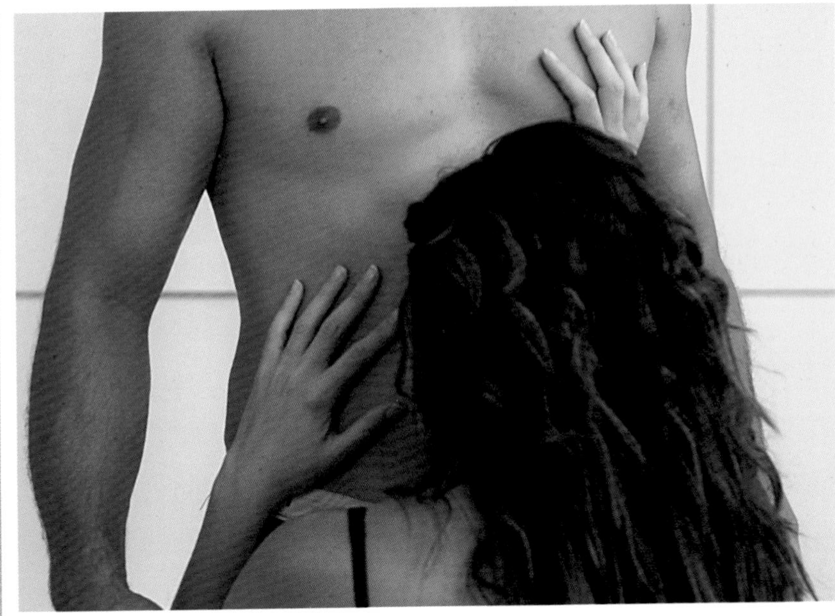

Λ NOWADAYS ORAL SEX *is toward the top of practically everybody's sexual wish list, and many people prefer it to intercourse. It is a foolproof way of arousing your lover to initiate sex and, if you reach your orgasm before your lover, it is a great way to bring him or her to orgasm.*

sides and underside of the shaft and grip the base of the penis tightly; flick your tongue from side to side across his frenulum (the strip of skin that connects the foreskin to the tip of the penis), and occasionally give his testicles a firm (but gentle) squeeze. Spend as much time as you like kissing and licking his testicles, delicately at first but later with long, sweeping motions of your tongue. For an interesting variation, give him an extra thrill by sucking a mint or a slice of lemon before oral sex. Or if you really feel like pampering him, take a mouthful of champagne before licking his testicles—it will send delightful tingling sensations through his entire body.

When you are ready to bring him to orgasm, slide your mouth over the end of his penis and as far down his shaft as you are comfortable. If he gets too carried away with his own thrusting and you start to gag, wrap your hand around the base of the shaft to limit penetration. Occasionally, swirl your tongue around the head of his penis and, once again, increase the pace and the pressure but maintain the rhythm as his climax approaches.

You can heighten the intensity of his orgasm by "peaking." Every time you sense he is reaching the point of no return, stop genital stimulation and concentrate on something else for a few moments. Go back to direct stimulation and repeat the process. His orgasm will be far more explosive as a result.

Climaxing during oral sex always raises the issue of to swallow or not to swallow. Many men love their partner to swallow their semen and the thought of it can greatly add to their excitement. If you don't like the taste, swallow it in one gulp as if it were an oyster, taking a large swig of that champagne to finish off. And, of course, if you really don't want to swallow, don't. It will more than compensate if you allow him to shoot his semen onto your breasts once in awhile. Whatever your preference, make sure you agree on matters beforehand.

Spontaneous sex

Your bodies somehow collide, you're kissing urgently, your hands are fumbling everywhere, pulling aside clothing—and you don't care whether you're on the kitchen table or joining the wildlife in the long grass. Spontaneous sex is when those amazing emotions, lust and desire, inflame all your senses and every ounce of you is driven inexorably to consummate your passion.

READY AND WILLING

". . . anything may take place at any time, for love does not care for time or order." So said Vatsyayana in the Kama Sutra. And it is its immediate and impulsive nature that makes all carried-away-in-the-moment sex so ravishingly spectacular. There's no planning involved, just someone pushing all the right buttons at once.

In the first, passionate days of a new romance, you literally can't wait to get your hands on your lover's body—and frequently don't. This is why elevators, supply closets, secluded open spaces and the back seat of the car are apt to witness scenes that will later make many of us blush with pleasurable recall. The moment is magical, when lust infuses every atom of your being, drenching your senses with an electrifying, erotic charge that's impossible to resist. Although you're almost out of control, engage in safe sex, and avoid being charged with obscene behavior in public or fired for "polishing" the boardroom table.

As the relationship progresses and you can manage to get through an entire afternoon without daydreaming of ravishing your other half, your propensity for "clothes-off-now" spontaneity diminishes. But just because your ardor may have cooled into a temperate love, it doesn't mean you can't still ignite your lover's passion as you have done previously.

Remind your partner how it felt to be desired like mad, in those sexually charged days together. Oddly, couples can become almost shy at expressing lust as the relationship matures. Monotony, not monogamy, is the problem; just break your sexual routine to rekindle the spark. Spontaneity, bizarrely, needs practice. The more often you both think of having abandoned sex, the more likely you are to end up smiling and in disarray after a surprise, supercharged encounter.

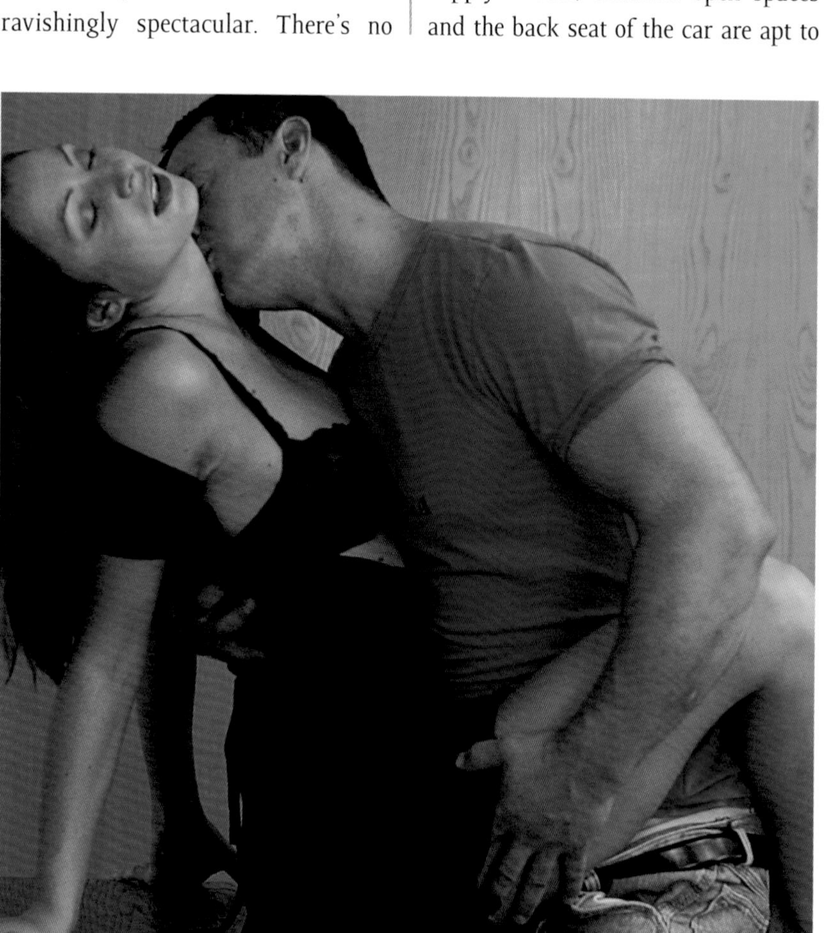

< ASTOUNDINGLY GOOD, *impulsive sex needn't be the preserve of new lovers, nor is it just about "quickie" sex. Intensity is the hallmark of passion: Block out everyday concerns and be prepared to lose control.*

> WHILE MUCH *of the Kama Sutra reflects on the various stages of courtship and seduction, satisfying, frenzied, mutual lust appears to have been more than acceptable.*

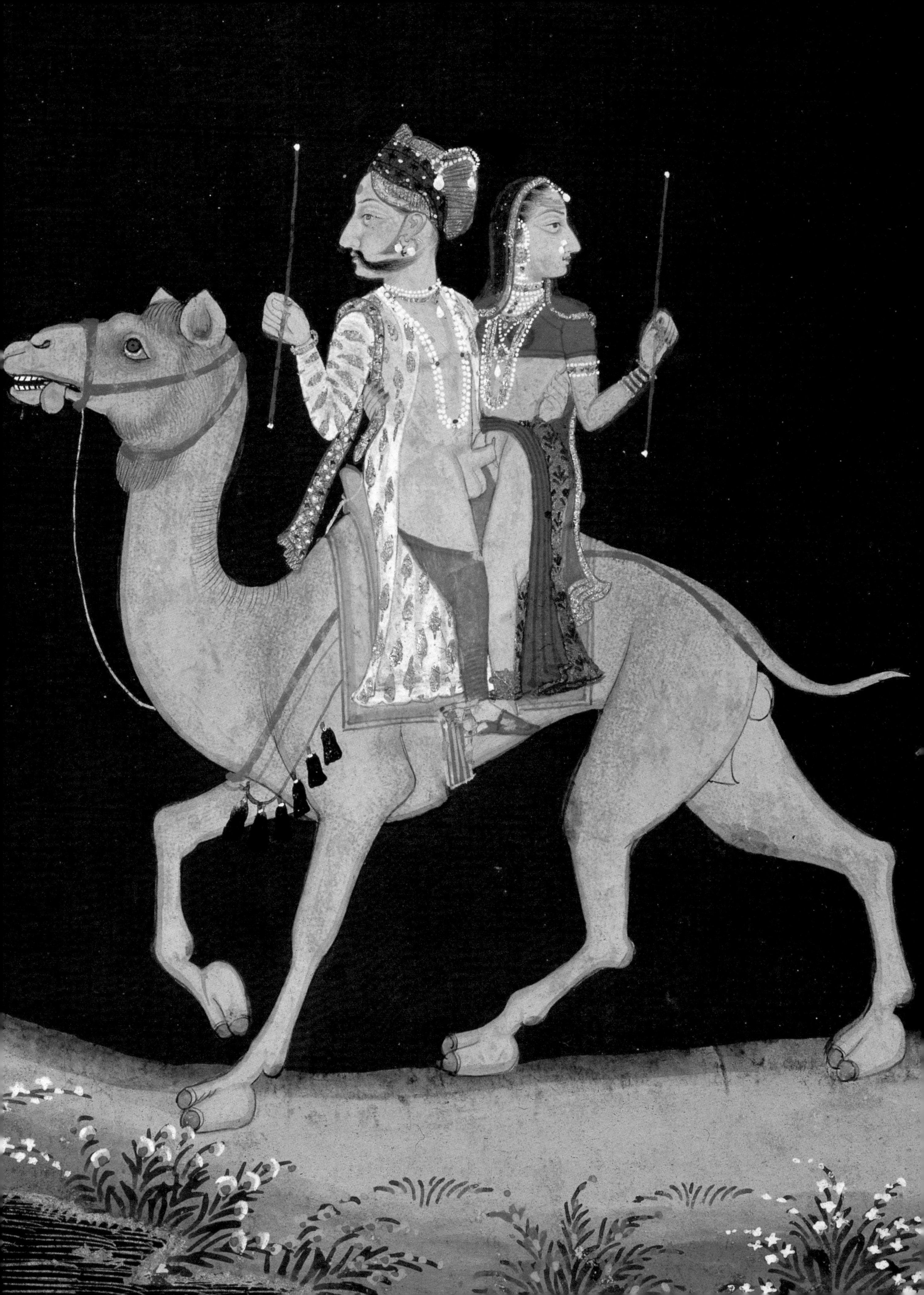

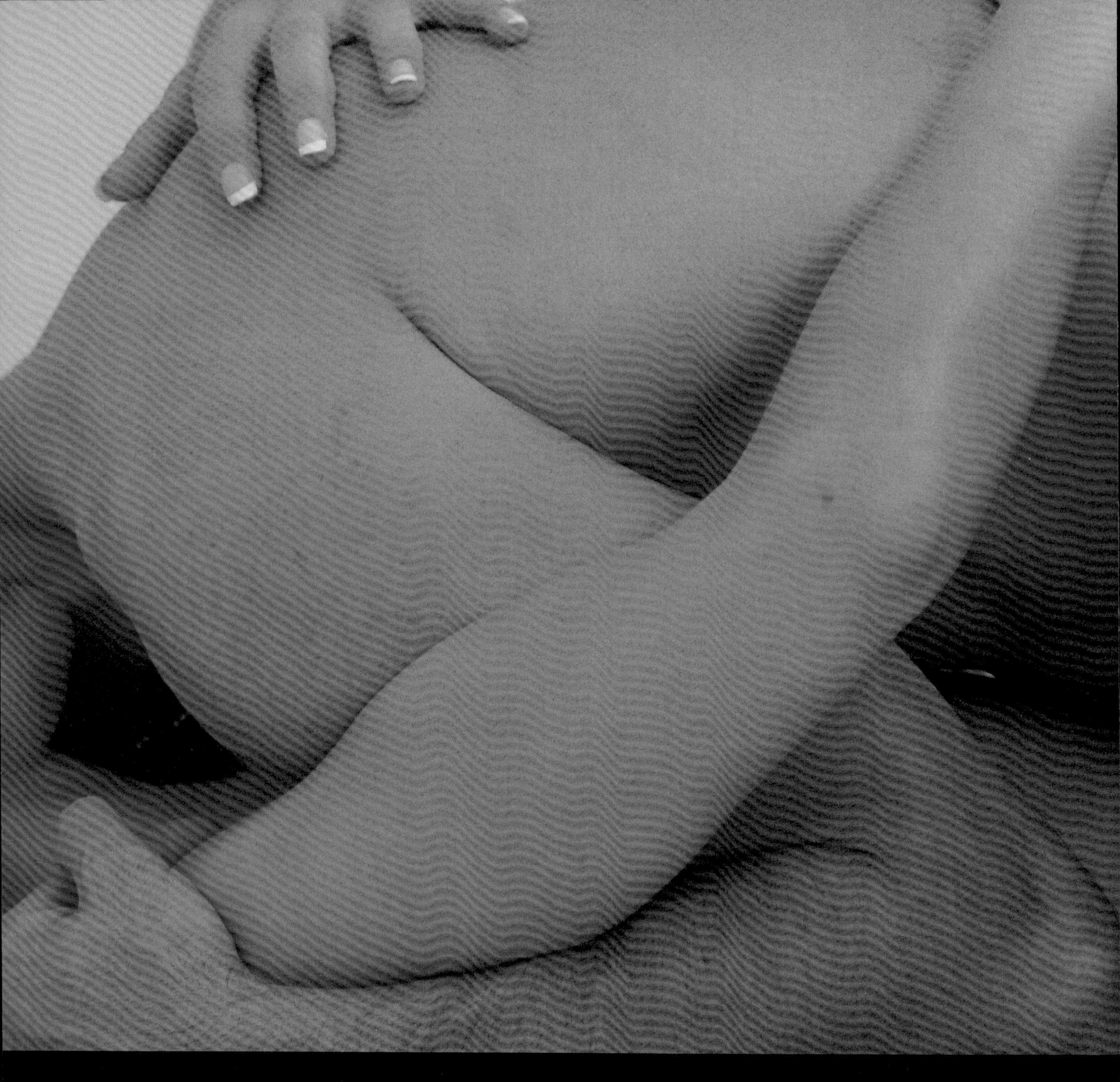

"When, a woman places one of her thighs across the thigh of her lover, it is called the Twining position."

KSII:VI

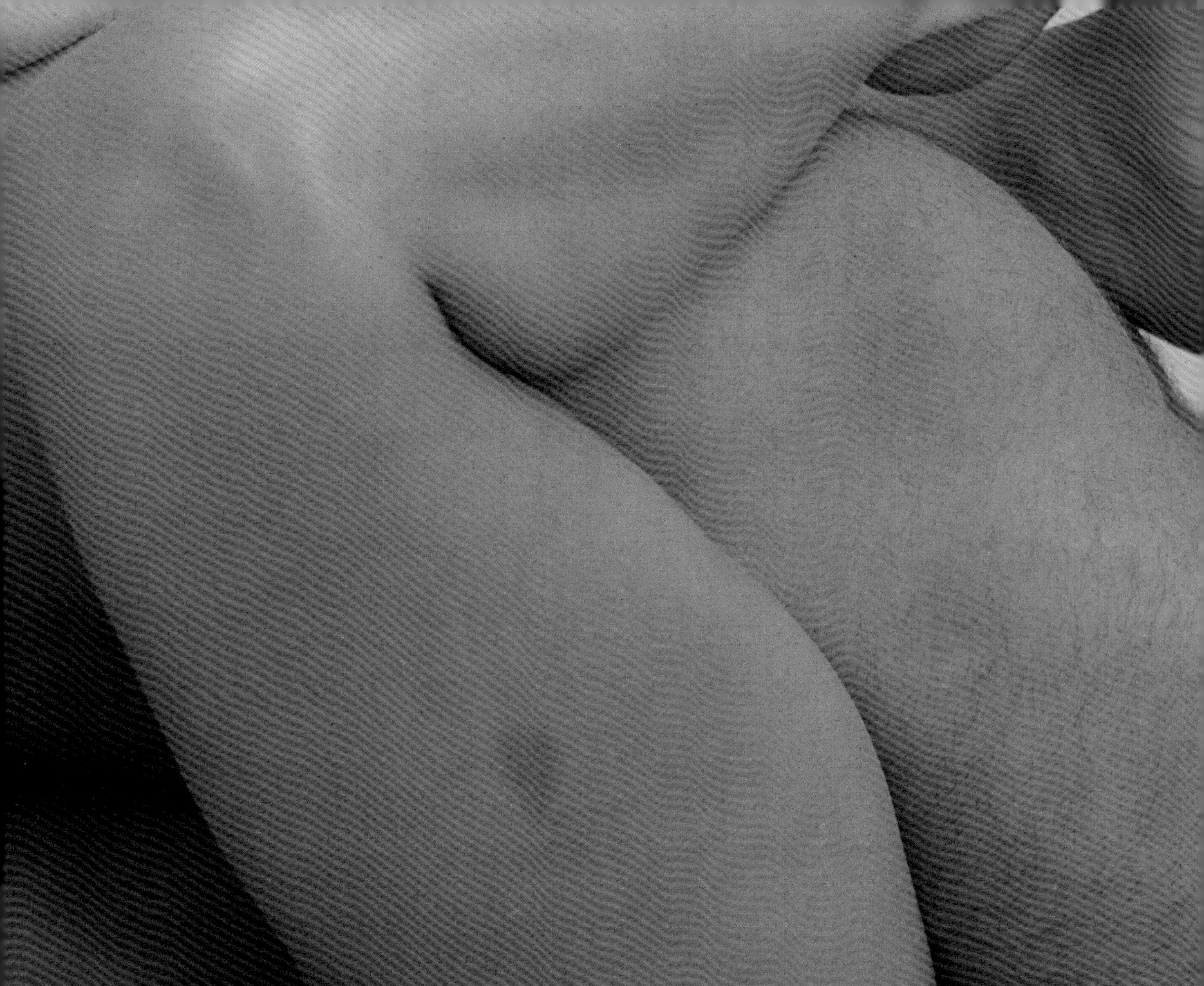

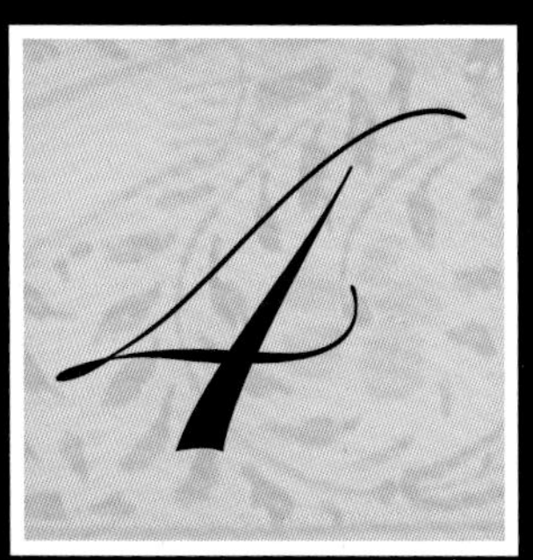

TWINING POSITIONS

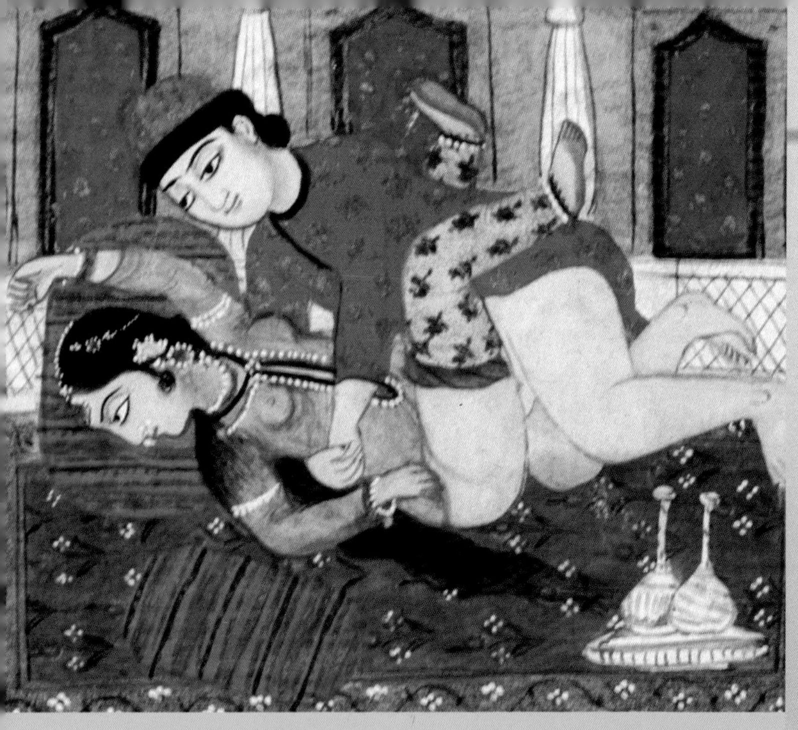

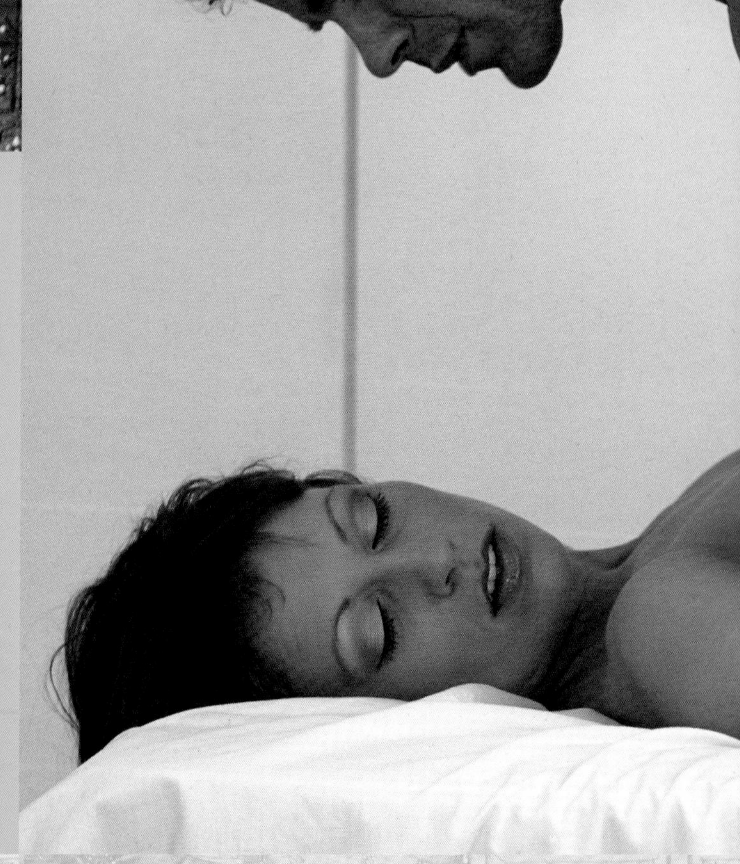

THE LOVEMAKING POSITIONS explored in this first sequence are an excellent way to begin your adventure into the Kama Sutra. They are very intimate, face-to-face positions with full front-of-the-body and eye contact. Plus, and it's a big plus, there is always the opportunity to roll around and get really lusty, exchanging active and passive roles, and building a potent sexual charge. A king-size bed is definitely a bonus.

CLASPING POSITION

SIDE-BY-SIDE CLASPING POSITION

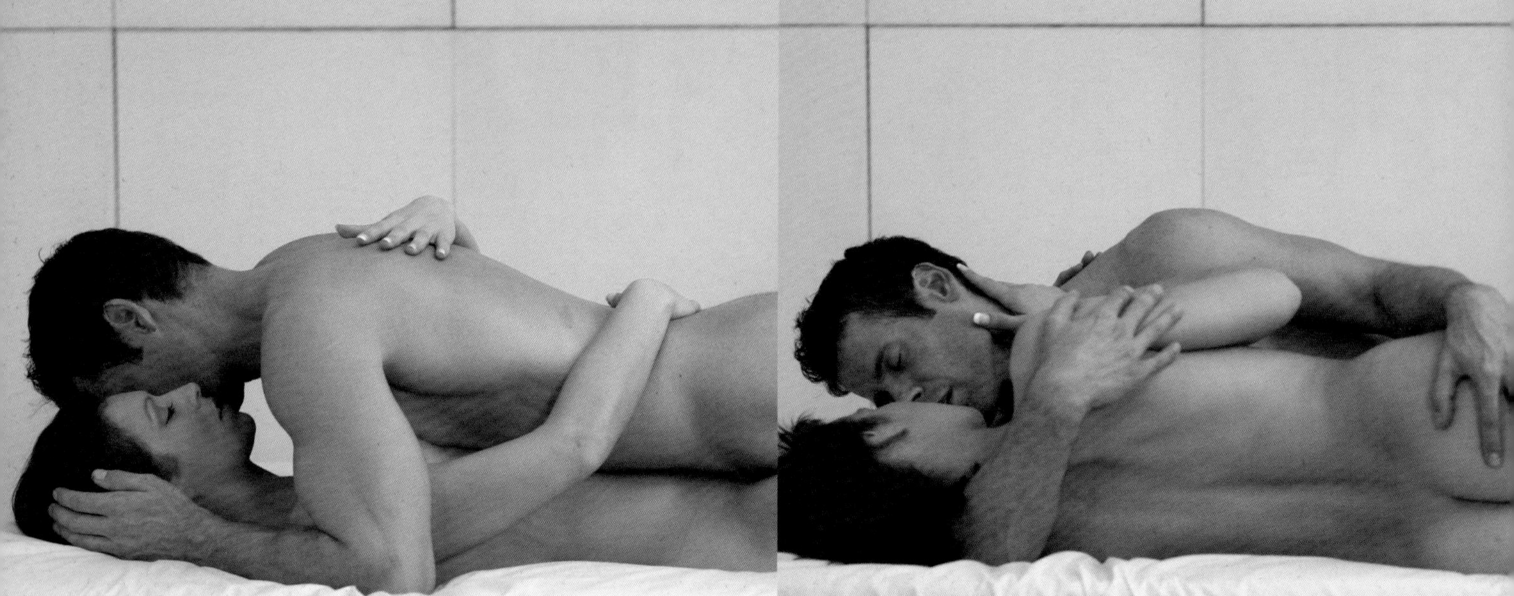

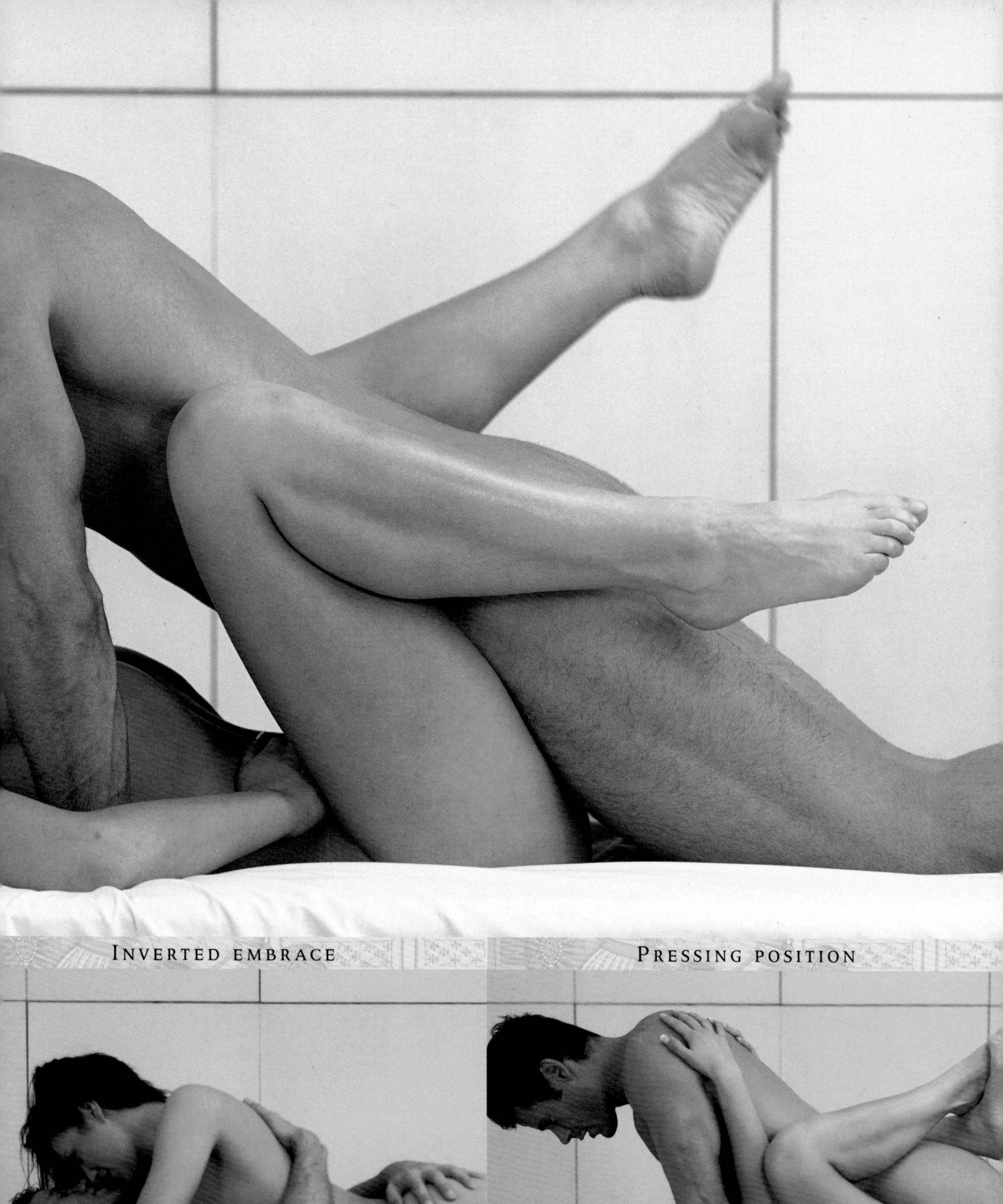

Inverted embrace

Pressing position

Clasping position

According to the Kama Sutra, "When the legs of both the male and female are stretched straight out over each other, it is called the Clasping position." Sounds very much like the ubiquitous Missionary position? It is! Nevertheless, it remains the ideal position to begin lovemaking because it allows you to exchange passionate and tender kisses, and it encourages passionate and tender words. The onus is definitely on the man to take the leading role, as the woman's movements are restricted.

V TAKE THE LEAD, *but take it slowly. Kiss her tenderly on her lips and neck and more intensely as she is aroused. Don't rush into full penetration. Even if she is ready, physically and emotionally, for you to enter her, she will love you to tantalize and tease her by gently slipping the tip of your penis into her vaginal opening without fully penetrating. However, remember that there is a fine line between tantalization and exasperation, so don't overdo it.*

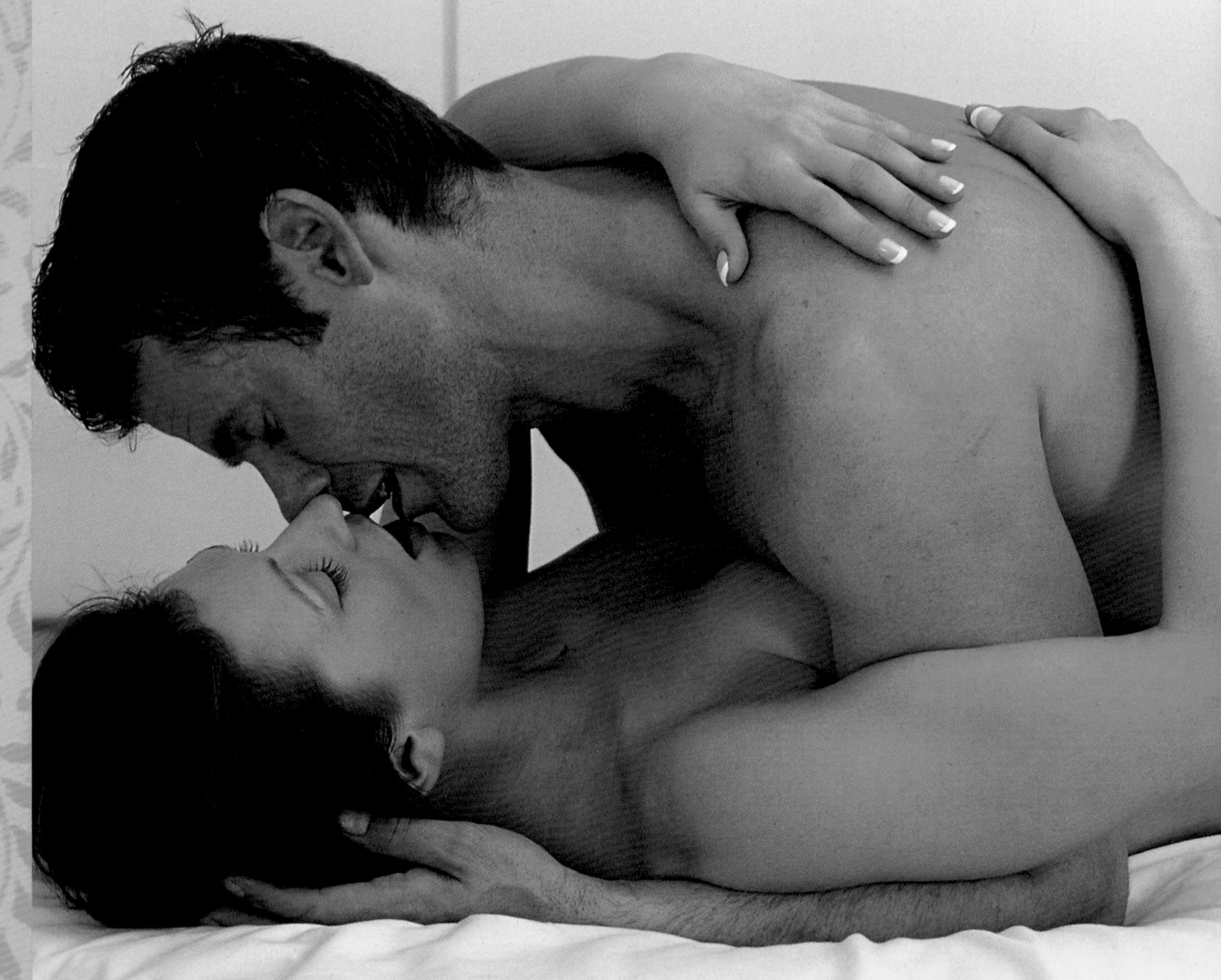

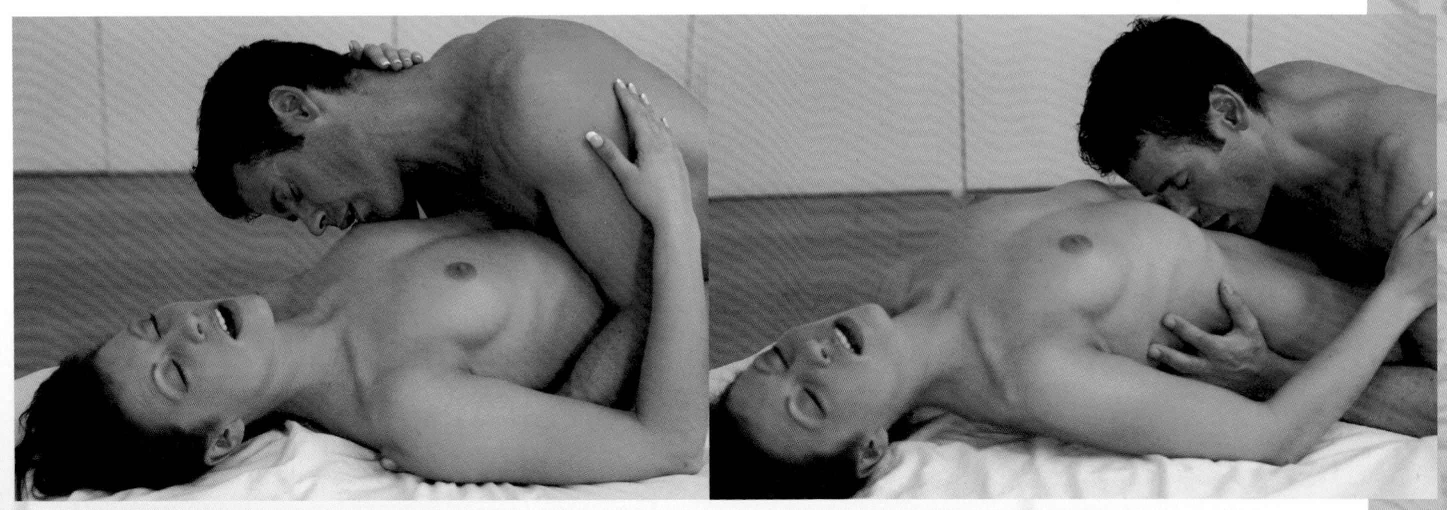

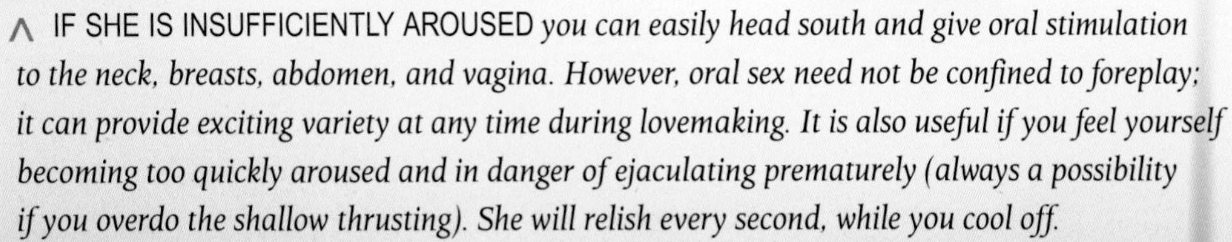

∧ IF SHE IS INSUFFICIENTLY AROUSED *you can easily head south and give oral stimulation to the neck, breasts, abdomen, and vagina. However, oral sex need not be confined to foreplay; it can provide exciting variety at any time during lovemaking. It is also useful if you feel yourself becoming too quickly aroused and in danger of ejaculating prematurely (always a possibility if you overdo the shallow thrusting). She will relish every second, while you cool off.*

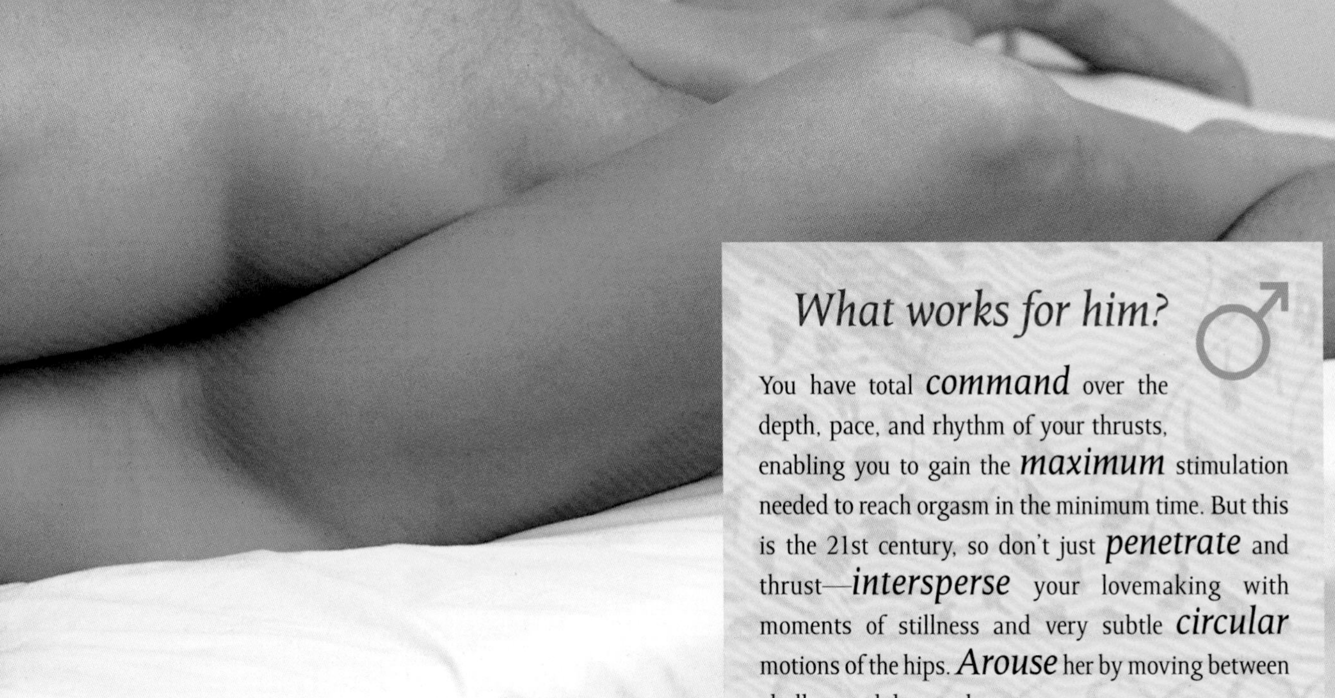

What works for him? ♂

You have total ***command*** over the depth, pace, and rhythm of your thrusts, enabling you to gain the ***maximum*** stimulation needed to reach orgasm in the minimum time. But this is the 21st century, so don't just ***penetrate*** and thrust—***intersperse*** your lovemaking with moments of stillness and very subtle ***circular*** motions of the hips. ***Arouse*** her by moving between shallow and deeper thrusts.

Side-by-side Clasping

Whole-body sensuality should not end just because sexual intercourse has begun. This is especially important to the woman, because every part of her body is highly sensitive to erotic touch. The Side-by-side Clasping position gives maximum body contact with increased scope for touching and feeling, so it's a firm favorite among romantics—that's just about everybody. It is a very gentle and loving position that you can return to whenever you want to express your feelings with tender kisses and soft caresses.

V FROM THE CLASPING *position he can roll over so that your hips turn with his and are free to join in the fun. There is an art to turning over without the penis slipping out of the vagina, especially if his penis is relatively small. However, you can help (and give your lover a sensational thrill) if you are able to squeeze the shaft of his penis by contracting your pelvic floor muscles (see the Mare's position, opposite).*

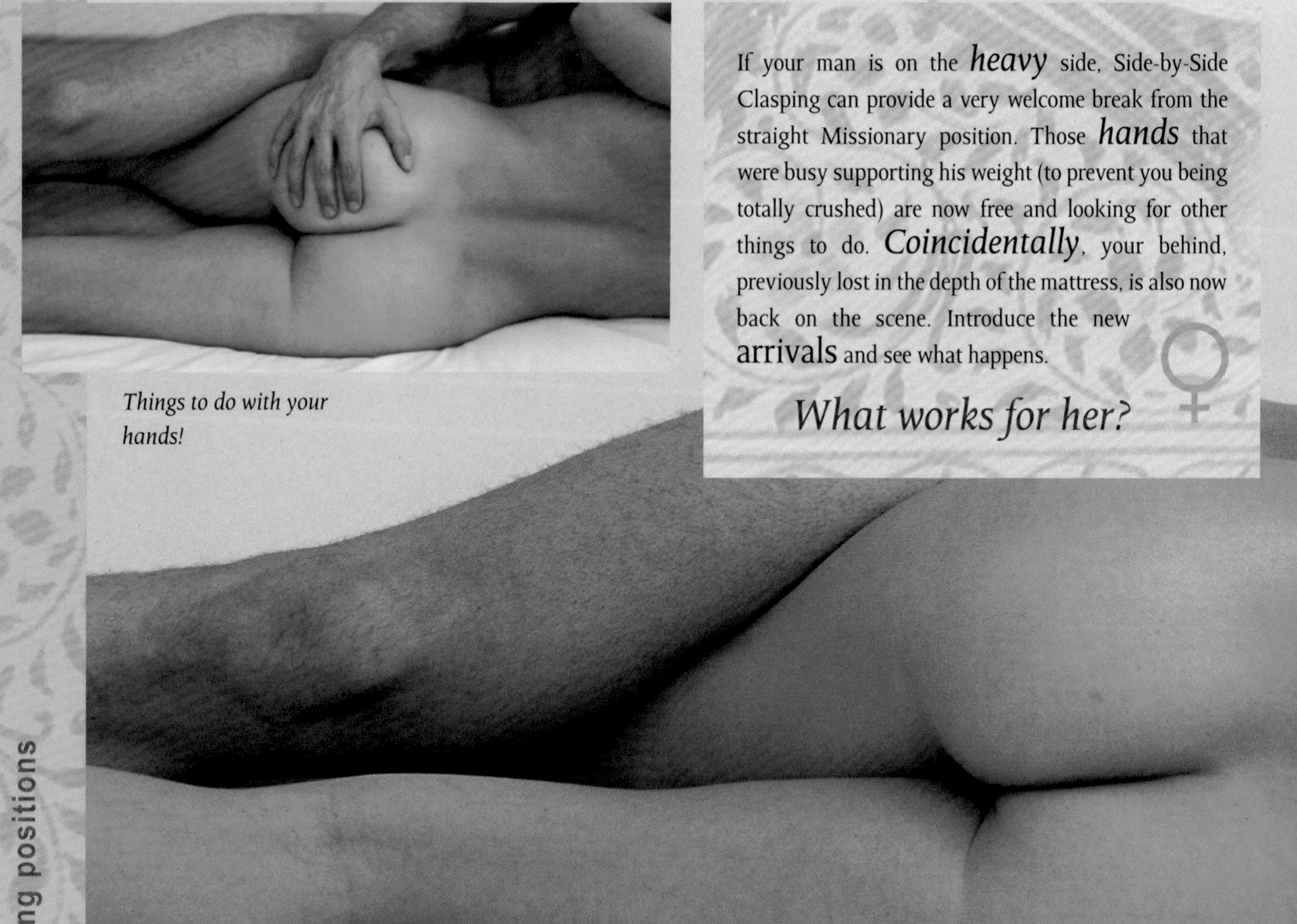

Things to do with your hands!

If your man is on the *heavy* side, Side-by-Side Clasping can provide a very welcome break from the straight Missionary position. Those *hands* that were busy supporting his weight (to prevent you being totally crushed) are now free and looking for other things to do. *Coincidentally*, your behind, previously lost in the depth of the mattress, is also now back on the scene. Introduce the new arrivals and see what happens.

What works for her?

The Mare's position

In the Kama Sutra, Clasping positions are recommended for low congress, when the penis is relatively small in relation to the vagina (*see* pg.28). In effect, they allow the woman to "clasp" the penis with her vagina using her pelvic floor muscles. This clasping action has its own name in the Kama Sutra: "When a woman forcibly holds in her yoni the lingam after it is in, it is called the Mare's position. This is learned by practice only . . ." So the Mare's position is not a position at all, but a technique that can be used comfortably and to great effect in a variety of squatting, kneeling, and supine positions.

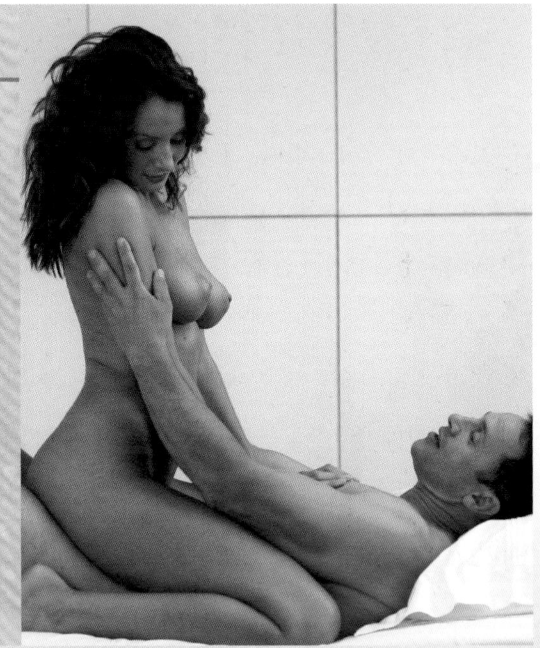

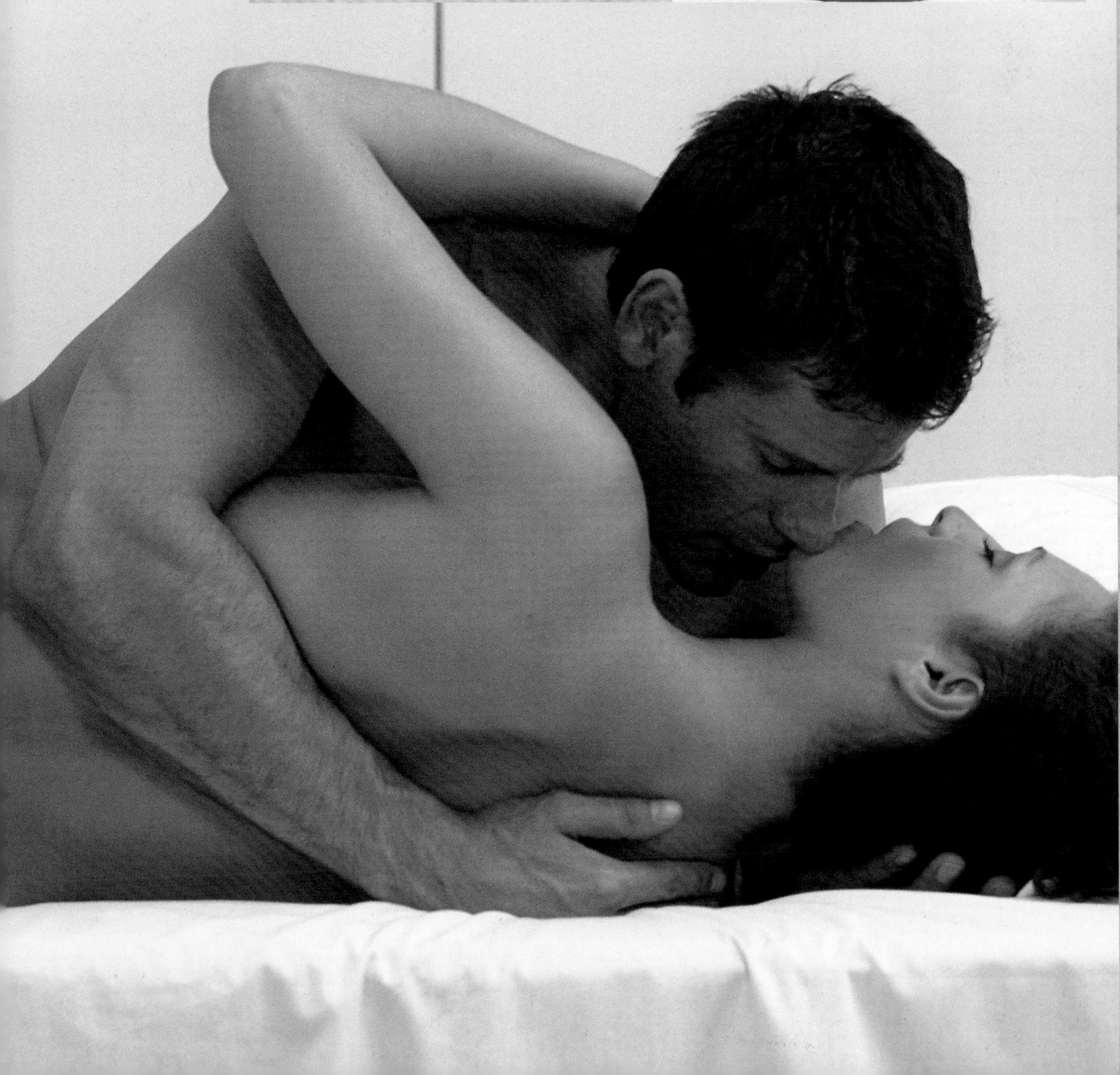

Inverted embrace

As you will no doubt have guessed, the Inverted embrace, which is described in the Ananga Ranga, is actually the Inverted Clasping position. So we still have the eye contact, the kisses, and the full front-of-body contact. But now the woman is in control. This reversal of roles enables you both to express new and exciting aspects of your sexuality.

∨ AFTER ROLLING *around with ever-increasing enthusiasm and energy, you may suddenly find yourself on top. Your first sensation upon arriving in the superior position will probably be the realization that you have regained full control of your hips, and you could be forgiven for wanting to test their 0–60 capability immediately. Don't. Slow and careful movements will help prevent the penis from slipping out while your bodies are adjusting to each other in this new position.*

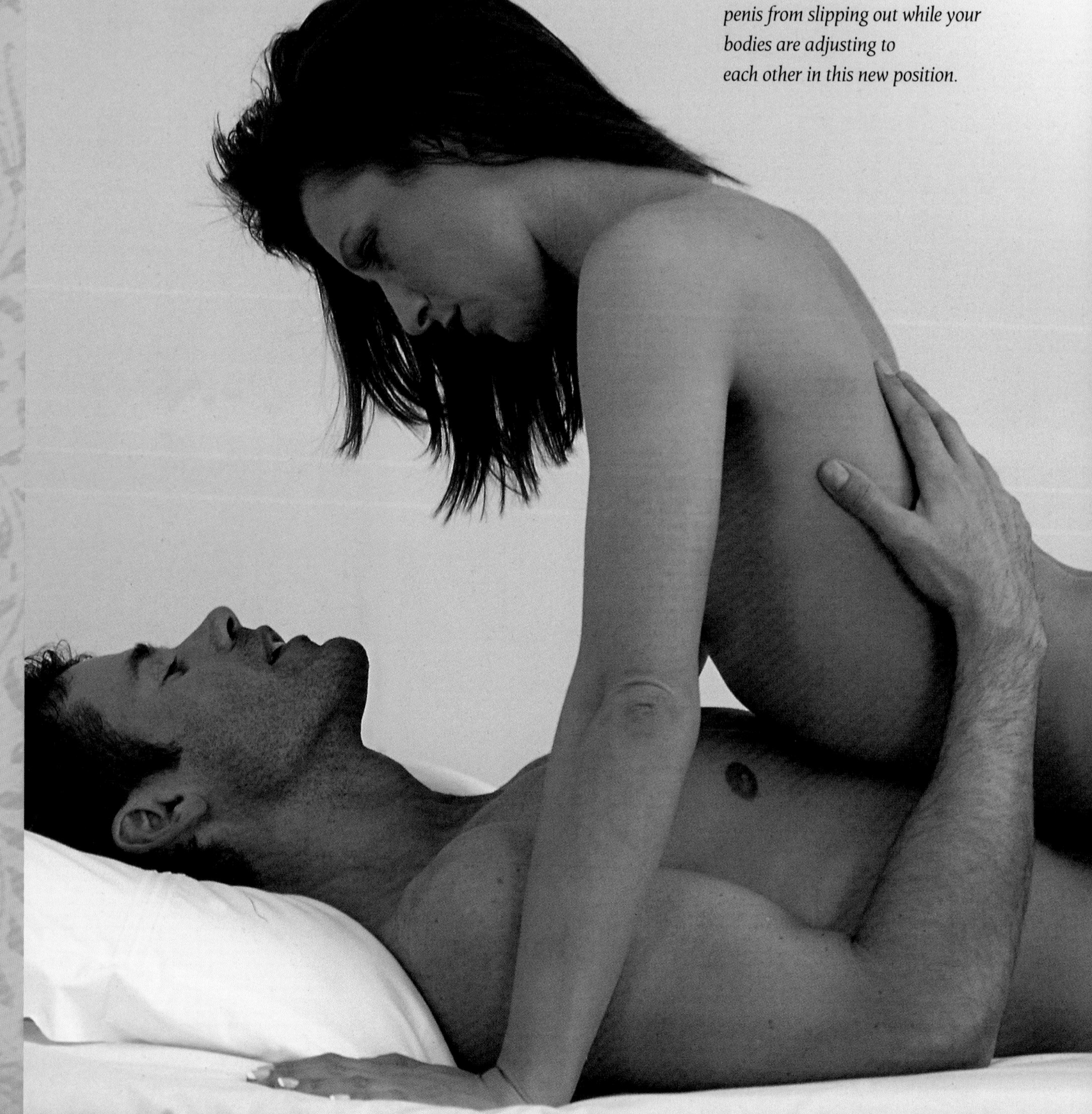

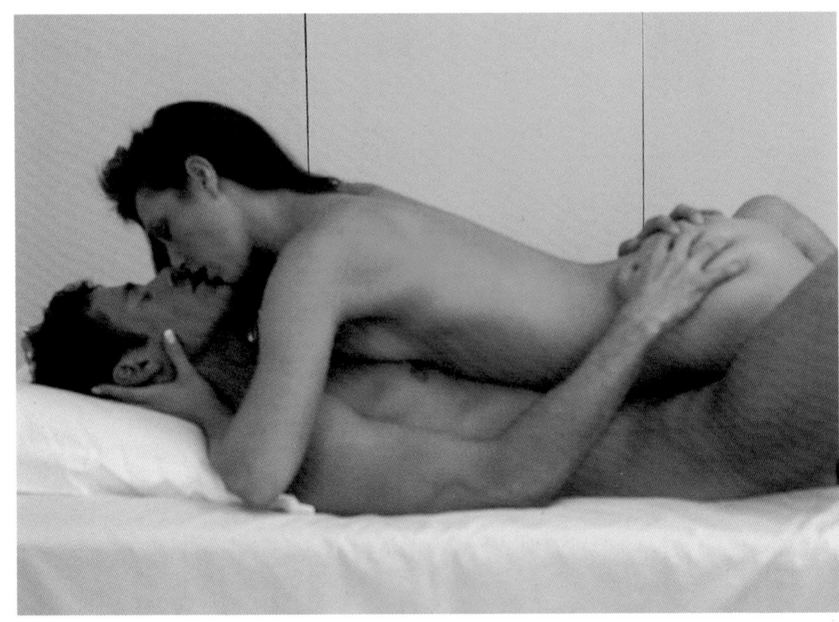

< YOU HAVE FULL CONTROL *of your hip movements, but if your partner is the dominant type he will immediately place his hands on your bottom in a subconscious attempt to retain control. There's no problem there: Most of us just love having our buttocks squeezed and fondled during sex! Even if your man is a bit intimidated at first, you should quickly be able to convince him that the Inverted embrace is a good idea by kissing him in the ways that you like to be kissed, nibbling his bottom lip, and kissing and licking the highly erogenous zones around his throat and ears.*

> IN THE CLASPING *position, the onus is definitely on the man to perform, which can be a disadvantage if he is feeling tired or stressed. If you sense this is the case, you can reverse roles and take over the reins even though you normally prefer him to dominate. Relax and enjoy the many opportunities for play; if you have long hair, use it to caress him, allowing it to brush beguilingly over his face and neck.*

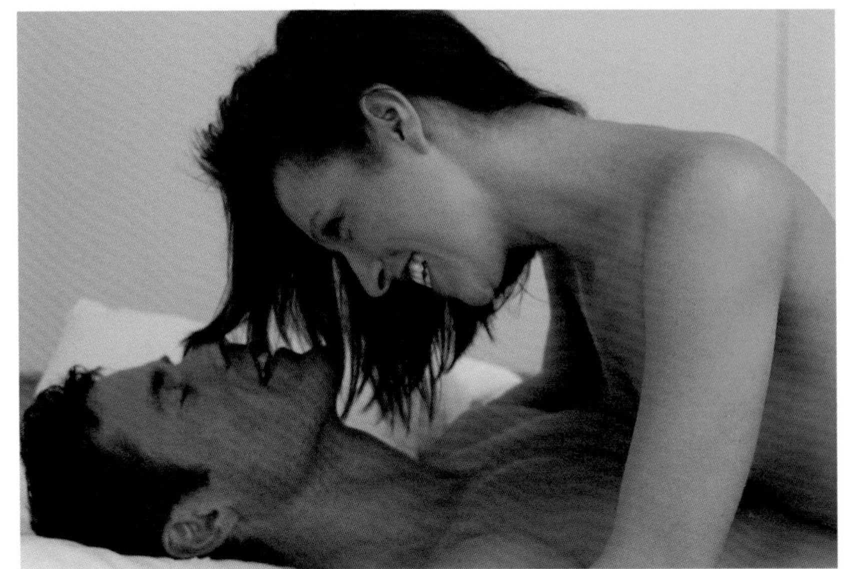

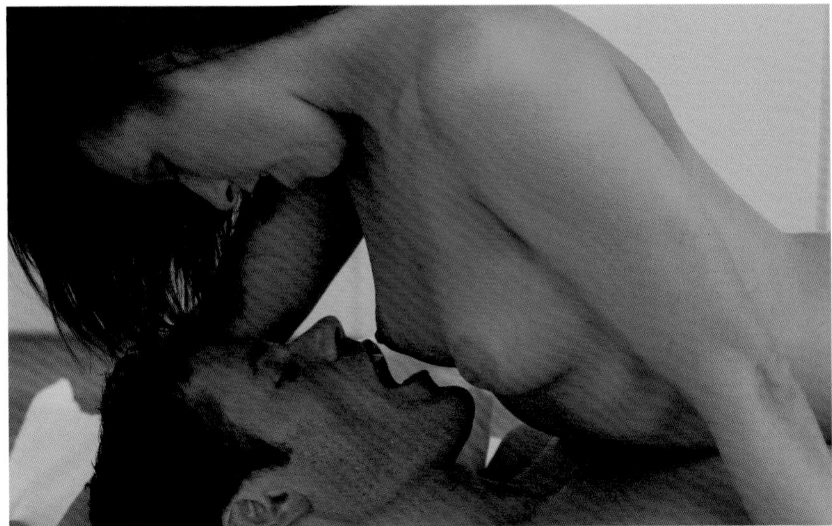

< HE WILL SOON FORGET *his stress as he focuses his attention on the sensual viewpoint offered by this position. Tease him by shimmying to maximize the sexy motion of your breasts. Proffer your nipples to his lips like exotic fruits and then move them just beyond his reach. When you feel that he has suffered enough of this tantalization (and before he sprains his neck), allow him full access to kiss and suck your nipples. Both of you will find this sensationally erotic.*

Role-reversal postures

The Ananga Ranga describes just three woman-on-top positions, collectively termed *purushayita-bandha*, or role-reversal postures. Such positions were generally frowned upon in Vatsyayana's day, and he advised that the woman should be "permitted" to go on top only if the man was tired or if the woman had not been satisfied by the lovemaking. Although women bridle at the idea of needing permission from men to do anything nowadays, Vatsyayana was actually very liberal for his time. Equally, it is certainly true that, even today, many men are still uncomfortable in this position because they feel that it compromises their masculinity. The female partner should patiently teach her lover the pleasure of sexual surrender.

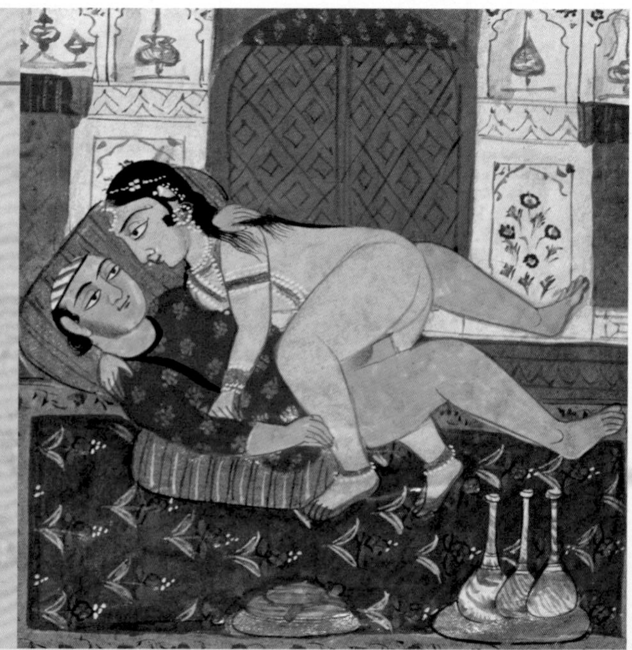

V GRIP YOUR VAGINA *and your thighs tightly around the penis and push your feet against his to allow a sensational grinding action against his pubic bone, which can stimulate your clitoris. Penetration is now deeper and you can kiss him more passionately to simulate what's going on below. Take his hands away from your body forcefully and hold them down. If he doesn't resist then he is certainly warming up to the idea of submission.*

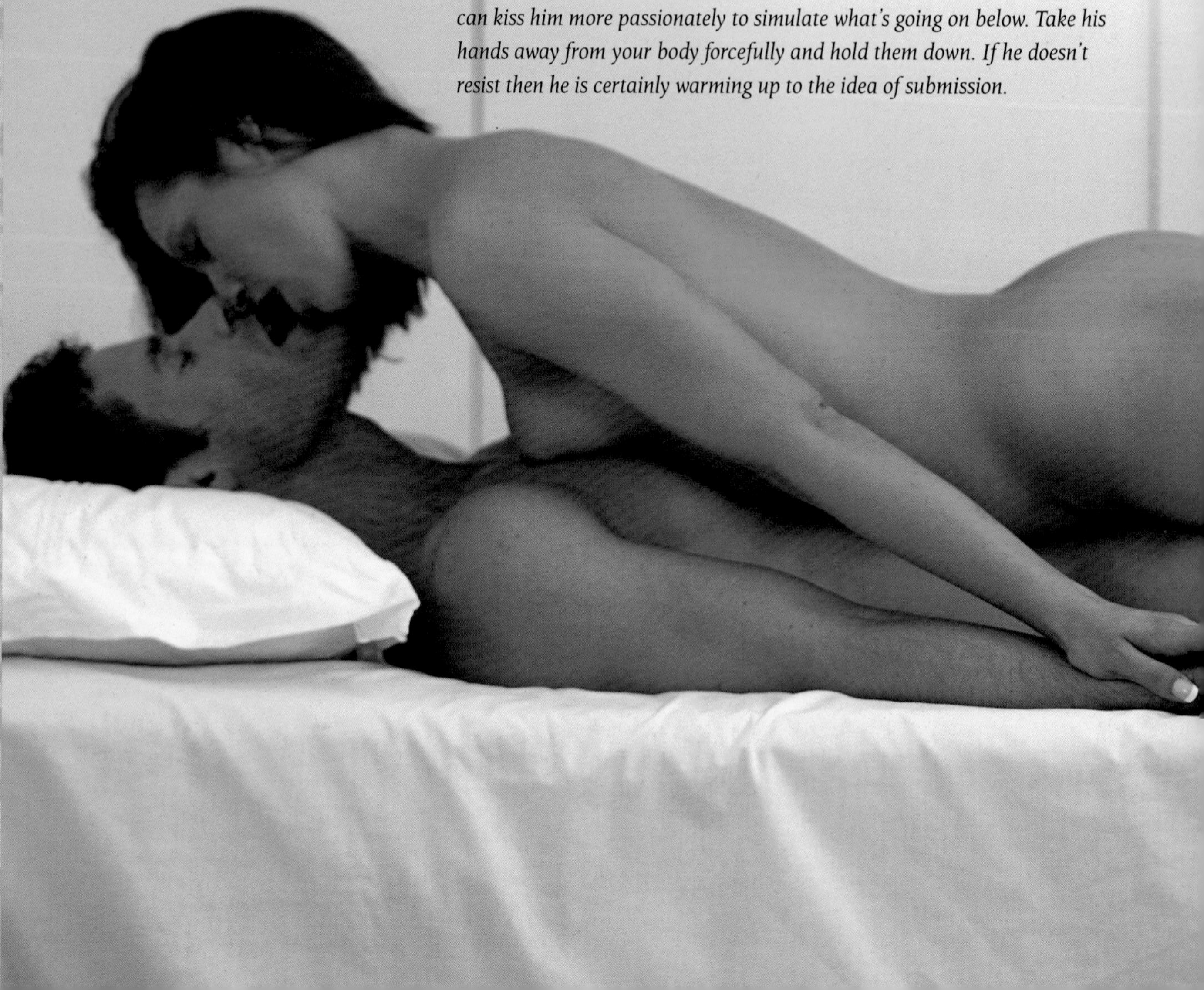

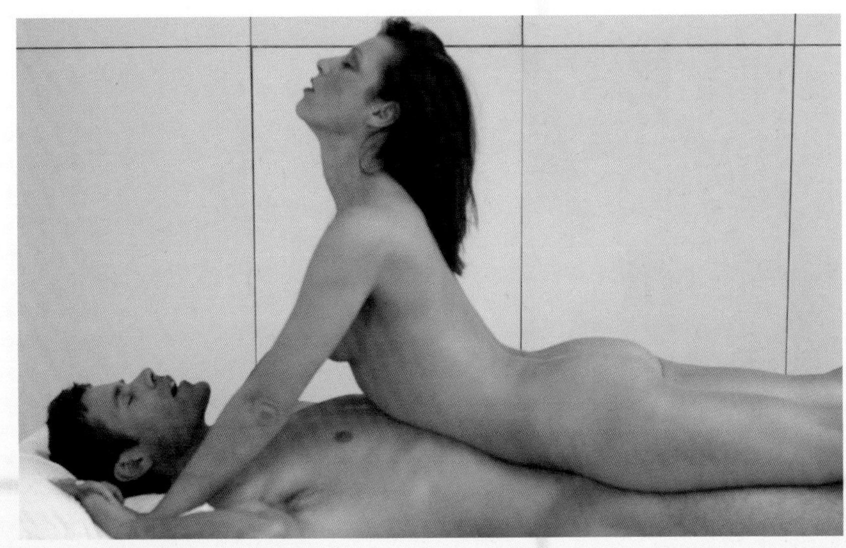

< SOME WOMEN SIMPLY *love to take the active role and cannot be satisfied sexually otherwise. Whether or not you are a dominatrix, it is time to put those hips to work and show him how it should be done: grind, wriggle, wiggle; here is the perfect opportunity to demonstrate exactly which movements work for you. Many men do love to be dominated. Hold down his hands and watch his reaction; it may be time to dust off the handcuffs and unleash that leather thong.*

> IF YOUR LOVER *is uncomfortable with the submissive role and loses his erection, you still hold an ace. Show him just how easy it is for you to move into manual and oral stimulation. Just pleasure him and show him how much you love his penis. Of course, another good reason for adding oral sex to your lovemaking is because you enjoy it and you enjoy making him happy—that, in itself, is a real turn on.*

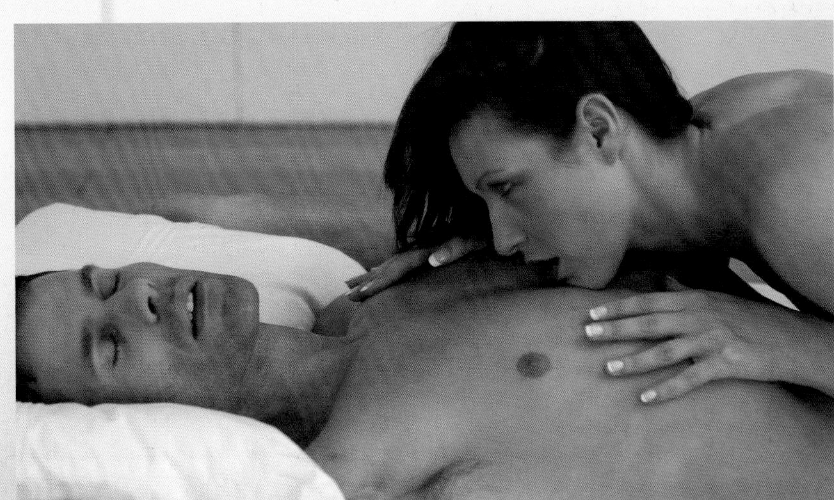

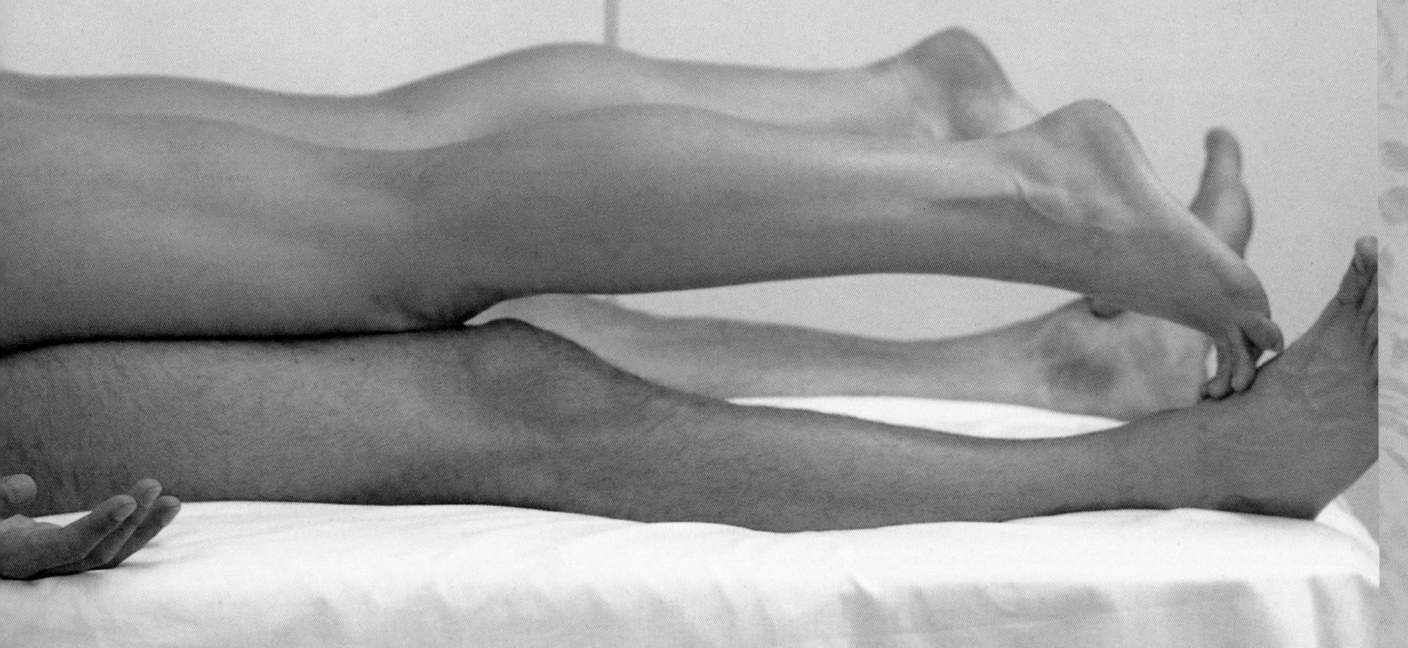

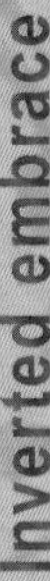

Pressing position

If you are both enjoying the woman-on-top position you may well want to take it further and try some of the more dominant squatting postures (*see* Chapter 9), taking full control of the depth and angle of the thrusts to bring yourself and your lover to a mind-melting orgasm. On the other hand, you may tire after a while and want him to take control again. There is, however, a middle way: The Pressing position enables the woman to be more involved in the action even though she is not the dominant partner.

V BY NOW *you will both be totally aroused and you may both be ready for some full-on, deep penetration. However, full penetration can create feelings of vulnerability as well as physical pleasure so, if your lover rushes headlong into thrusting, tell him that you want to remain still and enjoy the feeling of him inside you. You don't have to relinquish all control when he rolls back on top.*

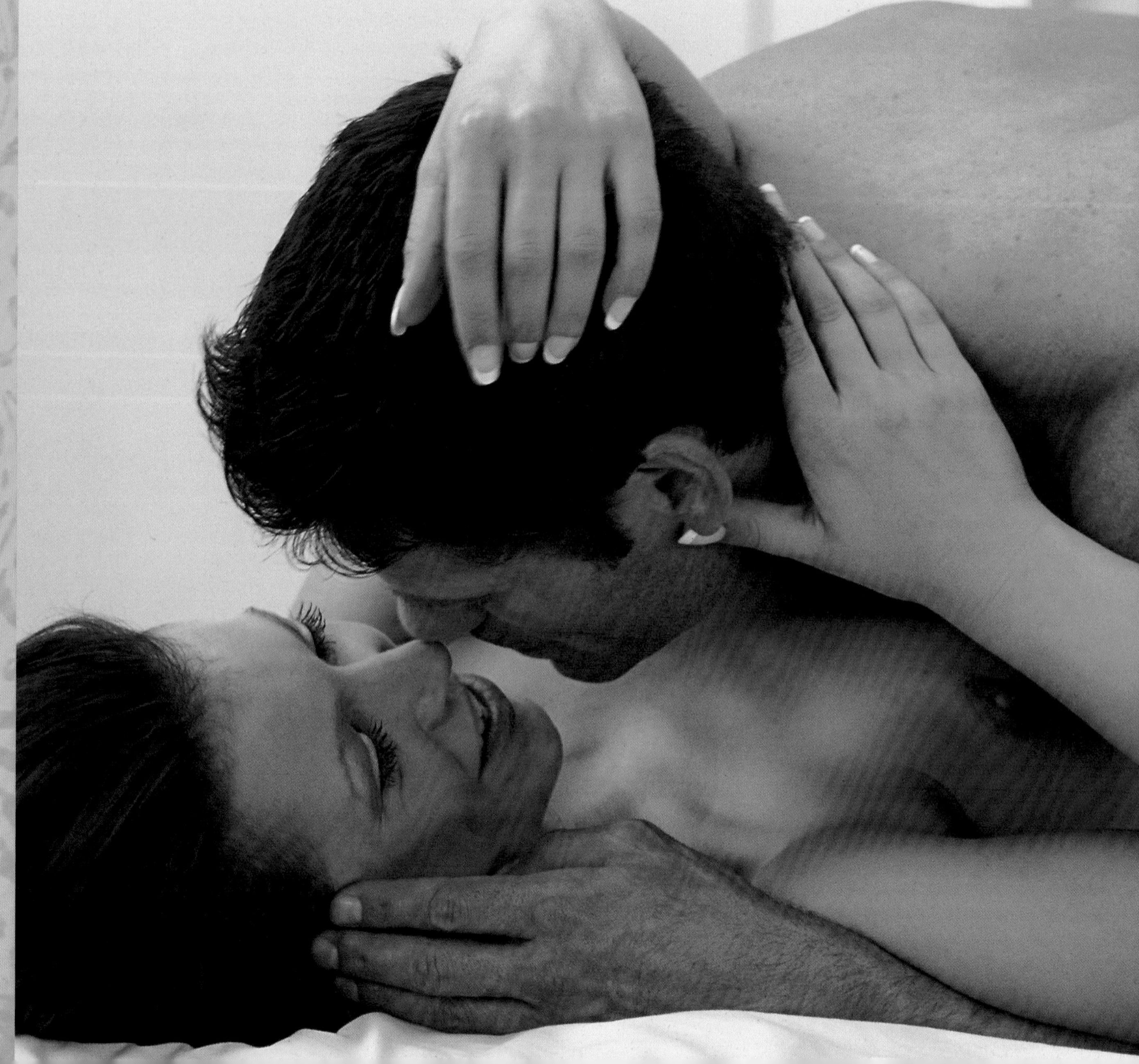

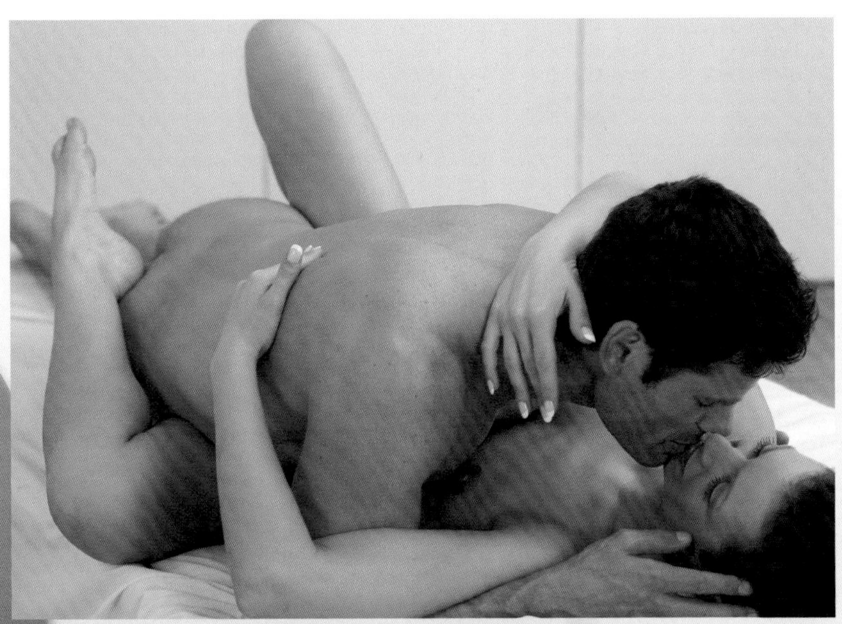

< THE KAMA SUTRA *states: "When a woman places one of her thighs across the thigh of her lover it is called the Twining position." This position is especially useful if your lover's actions have become mechanical and you sense that you are losing synchronicity and connectedness. Slow down once in awhile to stay in touch on an emotional level throughout intercourse. Allow the intimacy you feel to be expressed, silently or with words.*

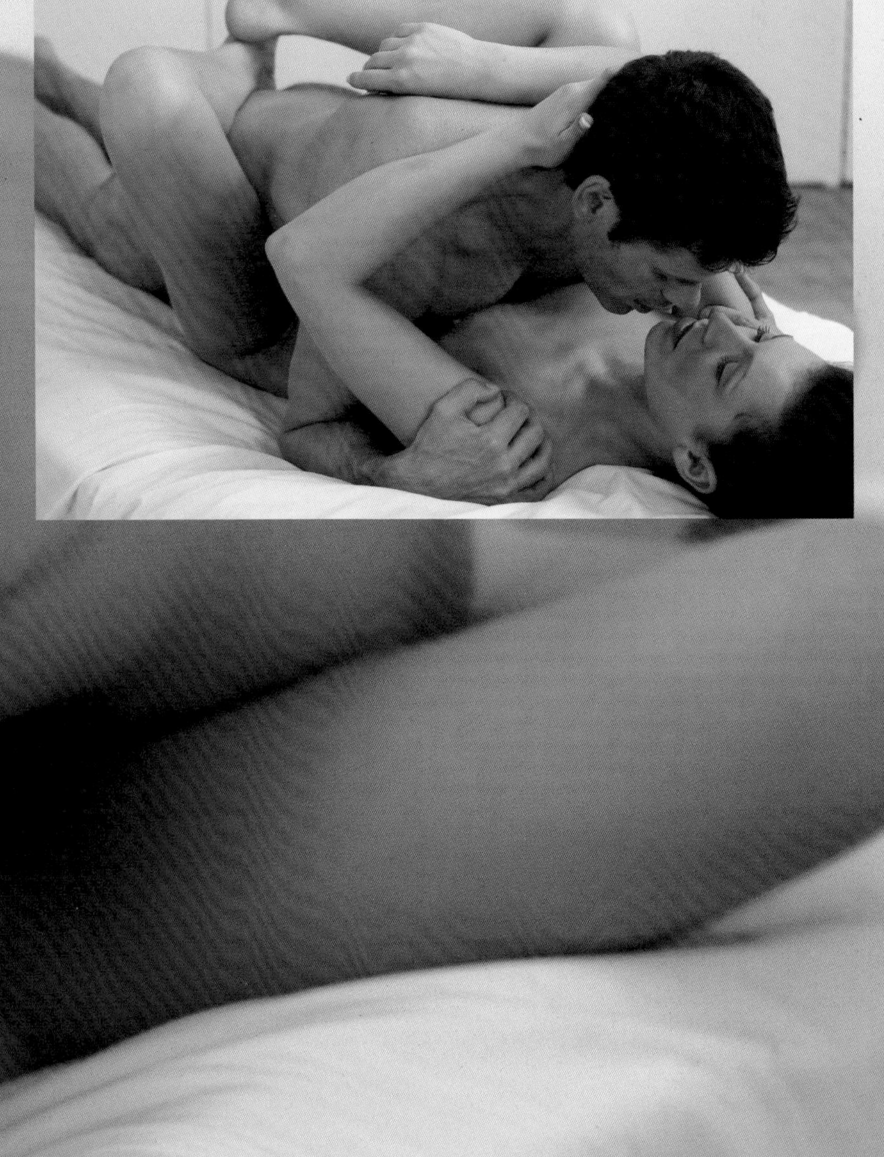

> USE YOUR ARMS *to pull him toward you and express your feeling with gentle kisses. When you are ready again for deeper penetration you can signal your desires and urge him on by wrapping your thighs around him and pulling him toward you. (The pressure of your foot on his buttocks is an added stimulation.) Vatsyayana called this the "Pressing position," and specified that it was the most natural progression from the Clasping position.*

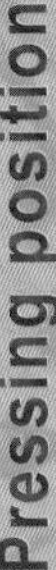

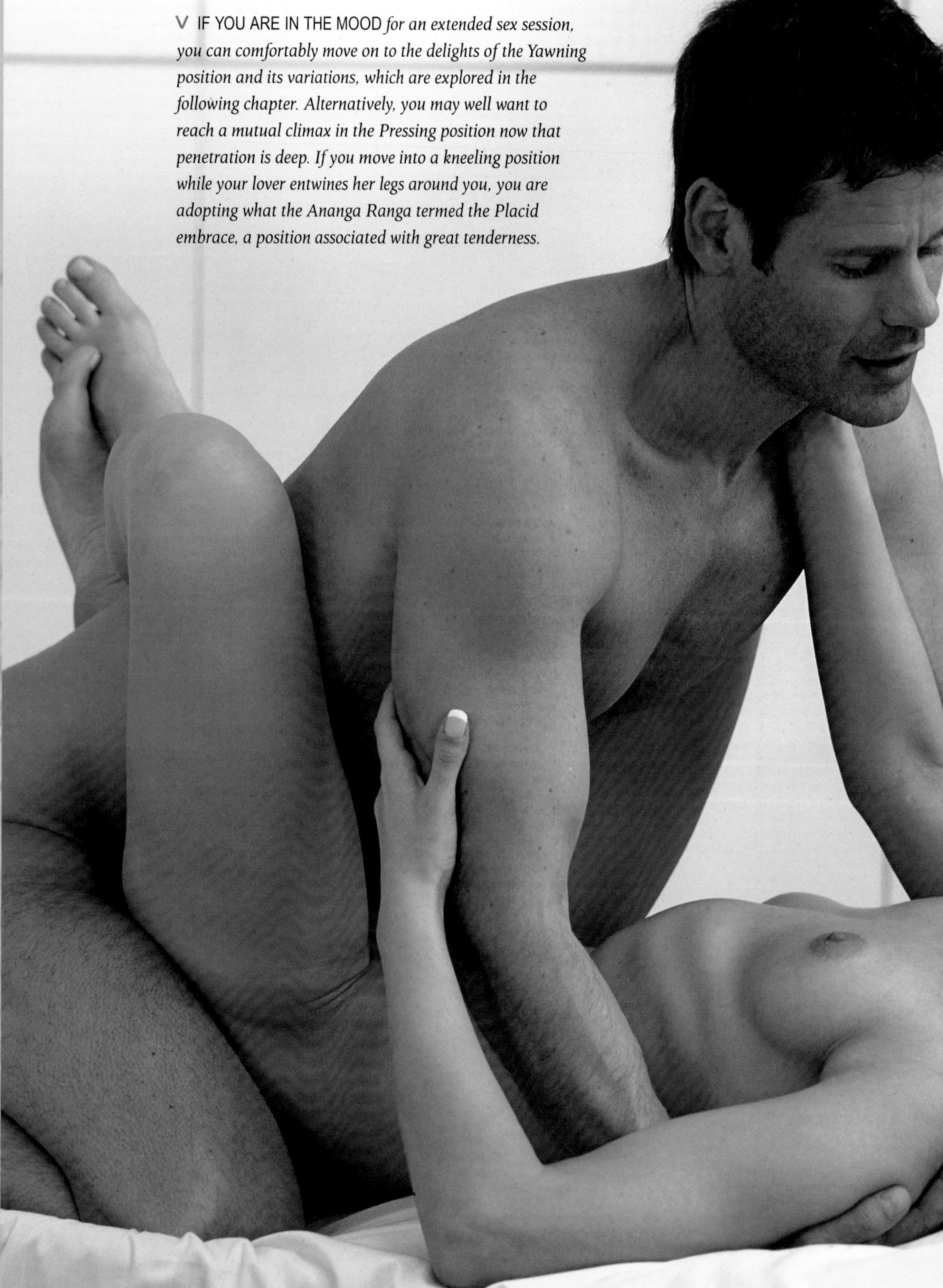

▼ IF YOU ARE IN THE MOOD *for an extended sex session, you can comfortably move on to the delights of the Yawning position and its variations, which are explored in the following chapter. Alternatively, you may well want to reach a mutual climax in the Pressing position now that penetration is deep. If you move into a kneeling position while your lover entwines her legs around you, you are adopting what the Ananga Ranga termed the Placid embrace, a position associated with great tenderness.*

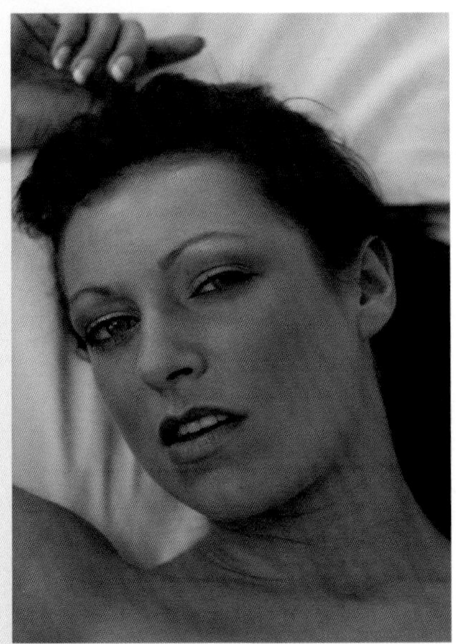

∧ OPENING YOUR EYES *enables you to watch and respond to your lover, and to silently express your own feelings of tenderness (or wantonness!). However, many lovers prefer to keep their eyes shut during sex. They find that closing their eyes allows them to reach a different level of sensuality because they are able to focus inward on each exquisite sensation. Strike a balance between the two so that you are more keenly aware of your own needs and those of your partner.*

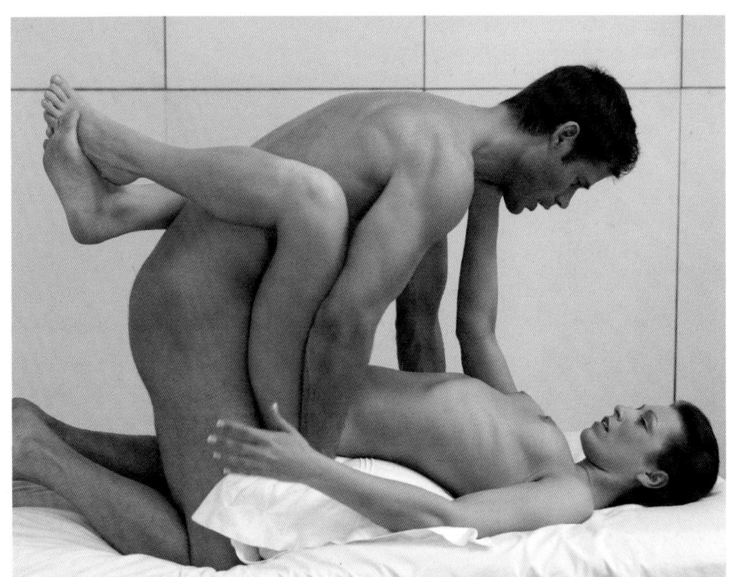

∧ VARY THE ANGLE *of penetration (and the resulting sensations) by putting your arms under your lover's hips and raising or lowering them. Be careful—raising them too far can put a strain on your partner's neck. It is a good idea to place a cushion or a pillow beneath the small of her back for extra support. The angle of her pelvis will enable your erect penis to put sustained pressure on the front wall of her vagina and G-spot, which can be extremely stimulating and can bring her to orgasm.*

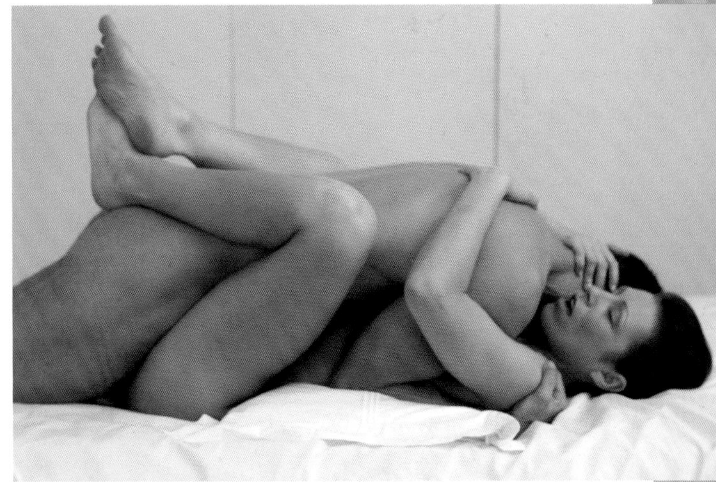

∧ VARYING THE WEIGHT *that you bear down upon your lover can also greatly alter the sensations and mood of your lovemaking. When your lover wraps both her legs around your body and draws you toward her, it is about as good as sex gets. By weaving herself around you she is expressing her desire to become one with you, to feel that ineffable sense of completeness that comes when making passionate love to someone you totally adore.*

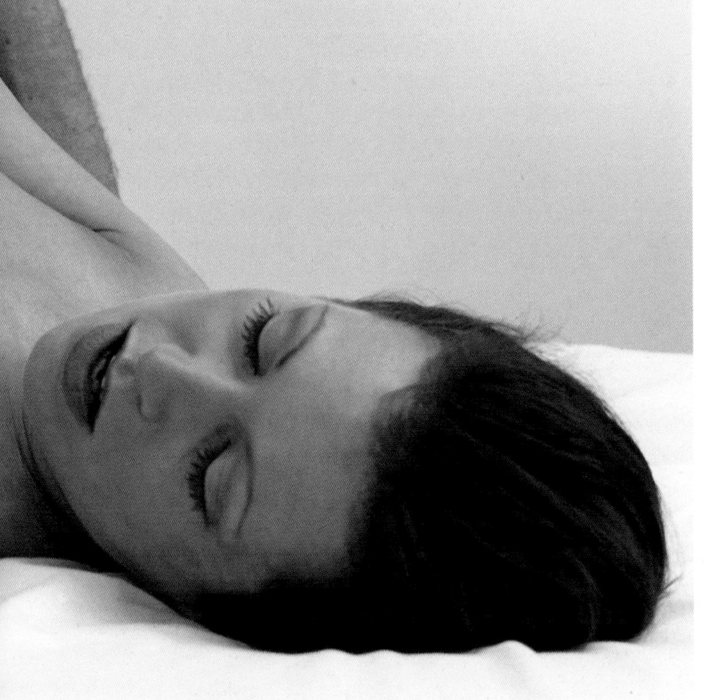

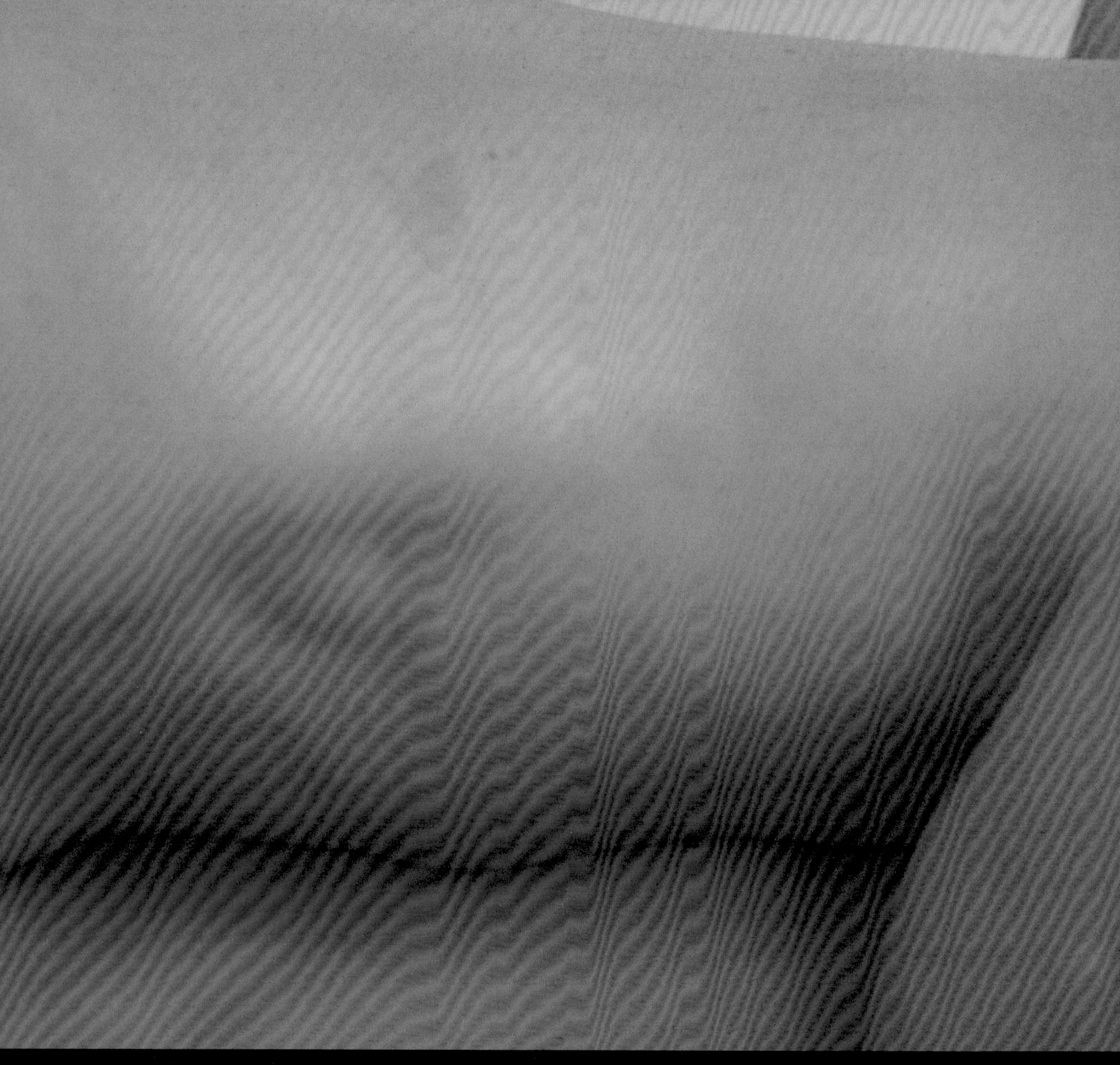

"On the occasion of a 'high congress' the Mrigi (Deer) woman should lie down in such a way as to widen her yoni . . ."
KSII:VI

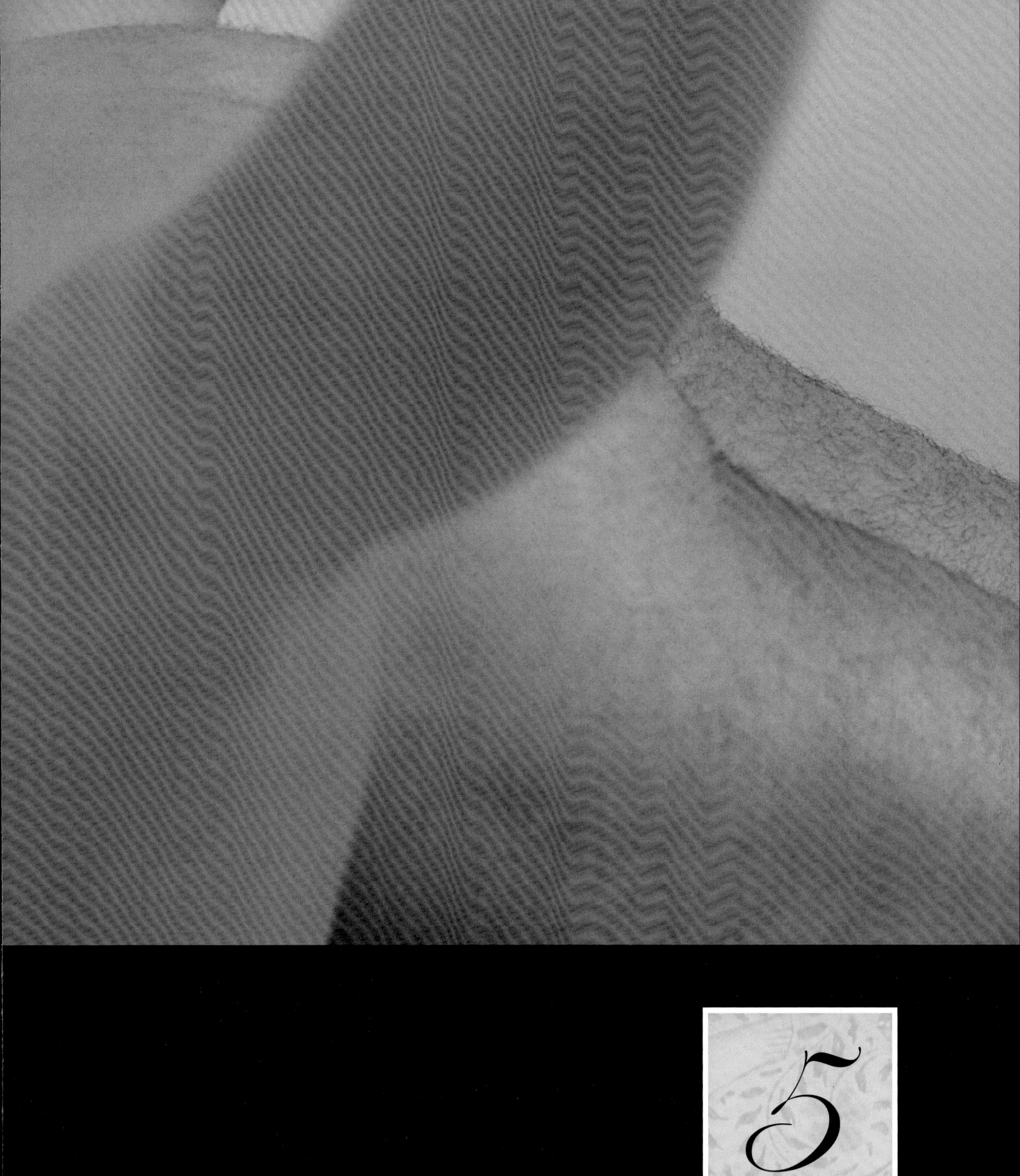
5

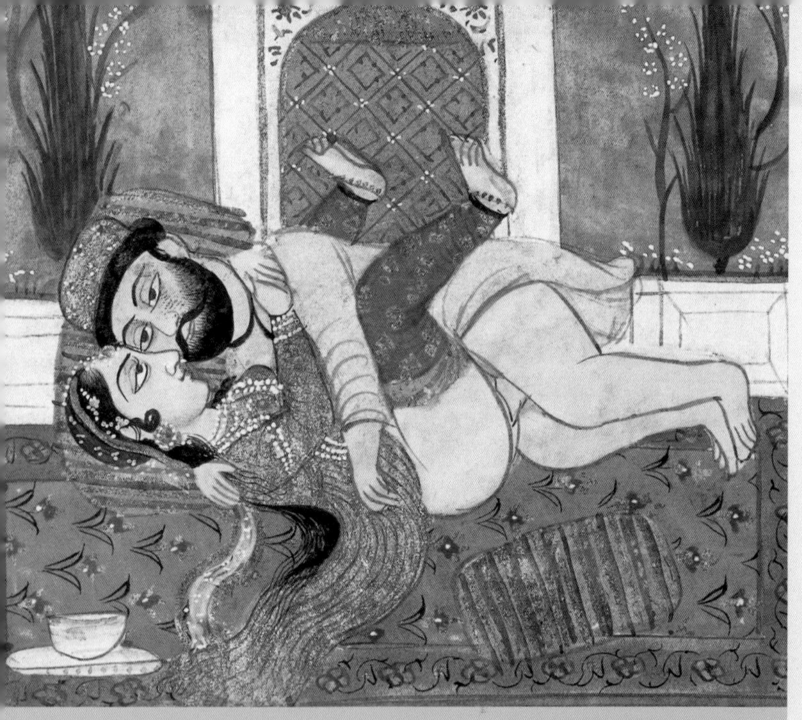

IN THESE positions the male assumes the more active role. However, the lovers remain face to face, which allows the intimacy and emotional exchange to continue. The Kama Sutra recommends these positions for "high congress," when the penis is large in relation to the vagina. The man must be careful not to thrust too hard or too soon, but must wait for signals from the woman that she is ready for deep penetration.

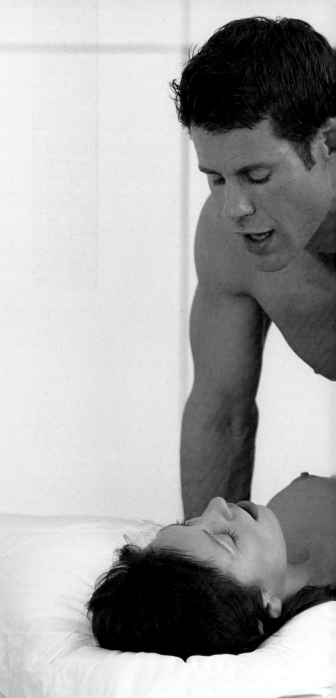

WIDELY OPENED POSITION

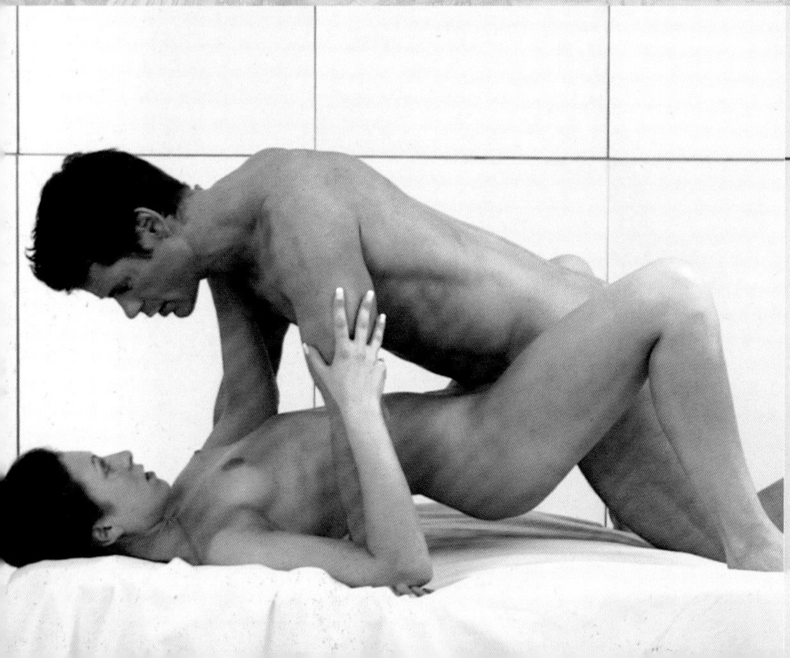

TURNING POSITION

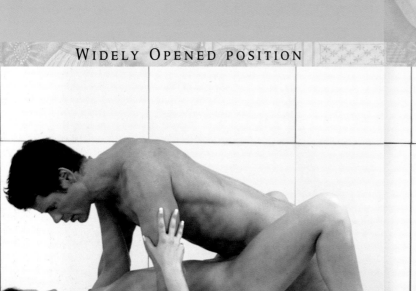

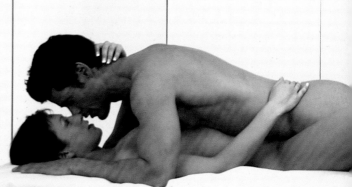

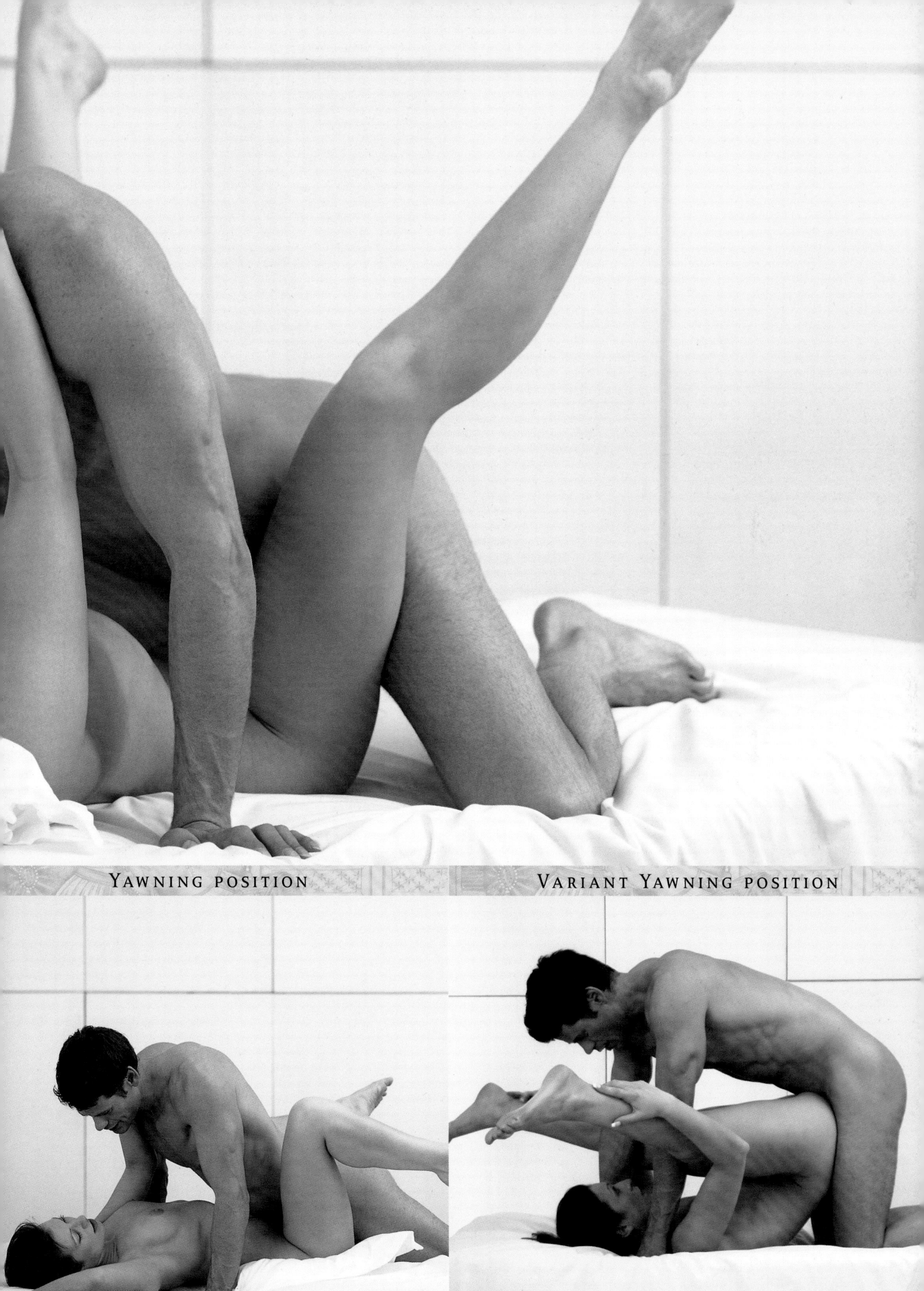

Yawning position

Variant Yawning position

Widely Opened position

According to the Kama Sutra, "When she lowers her head and raises her middle parts, it is called the Widely Opened position." Deep penetration is possible in this position, where the vagina is raised and open. However, it is a difficult pose for the woman to adopt for long, so the man can help by supporting her hips with his hands and pulling her toward him. The woman can then adjust the angle of her pelvis to maximize the friction on her clitoris by using her feet to tilt up and down (*see* insets, right).

> THIS POSITION *can follow very naturally after the Clasping position if both lovers are fully aroused. Kneel up and support your weight on your hands to allow your lover the freedom to raise her pelvis. Circle your pelvises slowly and sensuously. This can be a bit awkward, so if you lose synchronicity or begin to tire, take time out in the Clasping position (see below).*

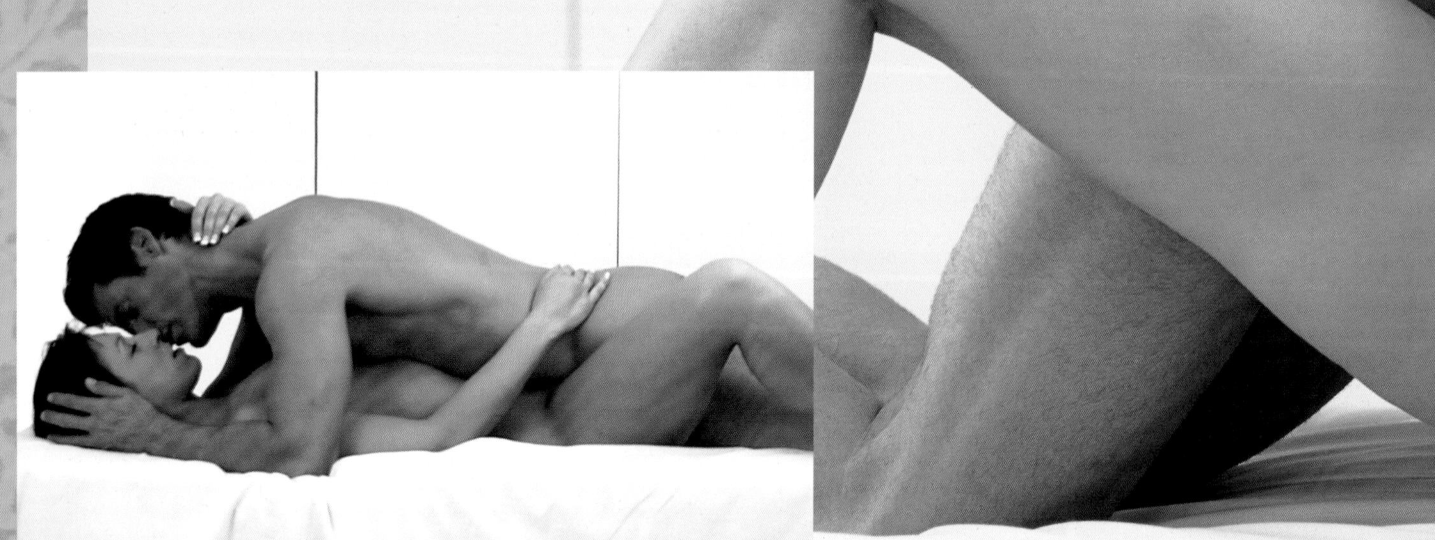

∧ RELAX *back into the Clasping position for restful interludes before returning to the raunch. It can be a time for you to reconnect, looking into each other's eyes, breathing together, and kissing tenderly. You can rest for as long as you like, enjoying the cozy full-body contact that the Clasping position allows. Just move your hips enough to keep his penis erect.*

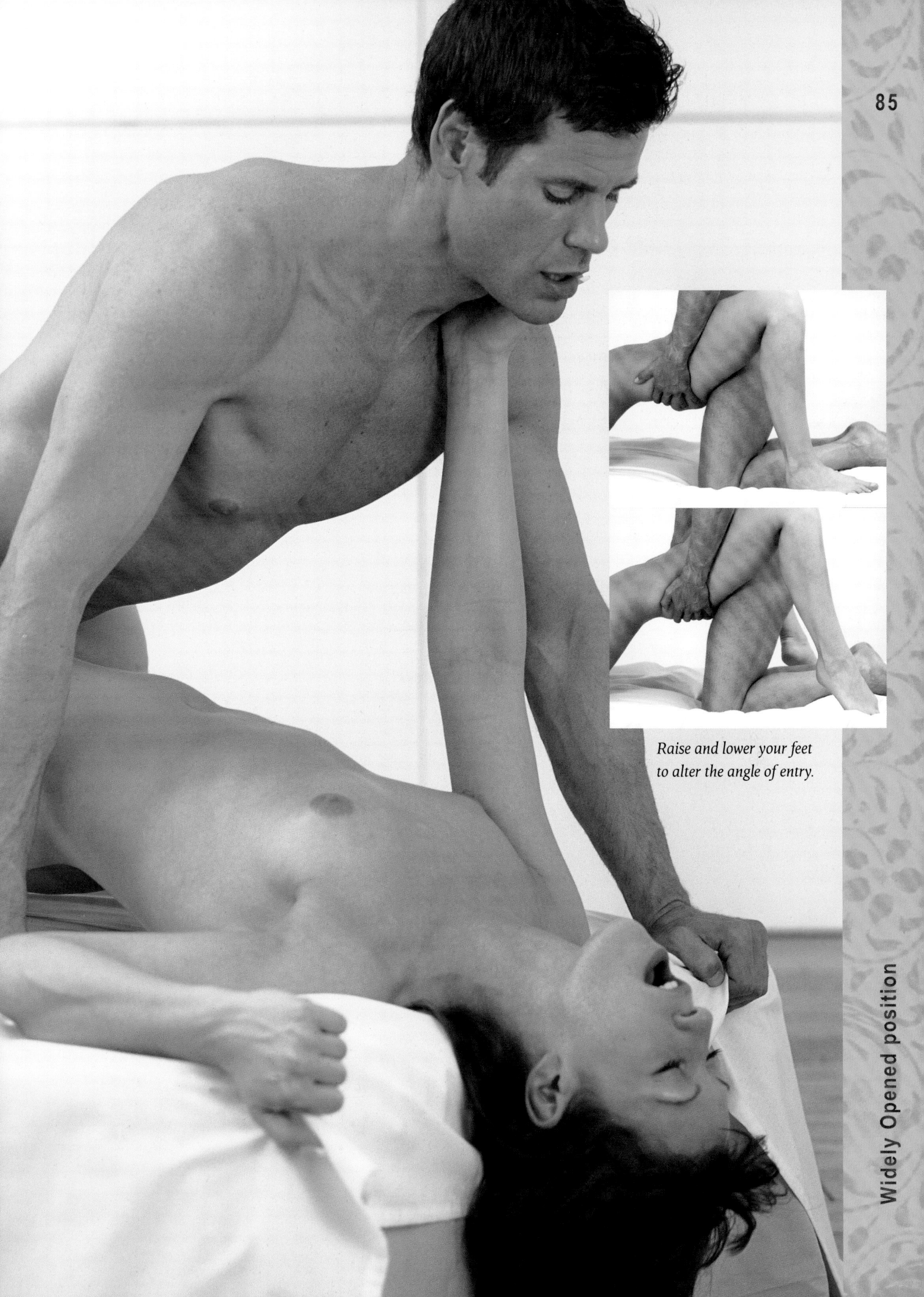

Raise and lower your feet to alter the angle of entry.

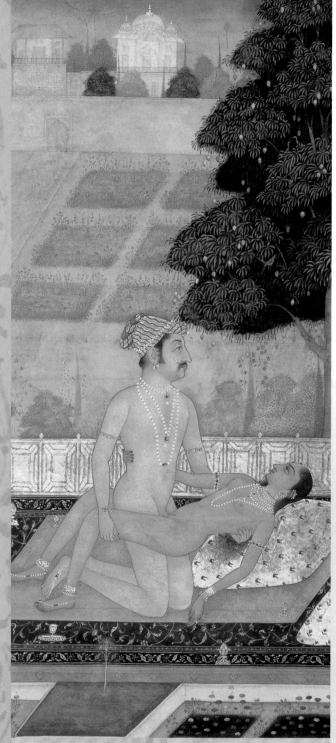

Widely Opened

This exquisite painting (c.1678–98) is called *The Private Pleasure of Emperor Jahangir*. The vessels for ointments that appear in the foreground suggest that the emperor has taken the Kama Sutra's advice seriously and is using lubricants. The image is a good example of the Widely Opened position, with the thoughtful emperor supporting his lover by placing one hand on her leg and the other beneath her back. A cushion is placed beneath her back for additional support and comfort.

> PLACE A PILLOW *or two beneath your lover's hips to increase her comfort. If you are not sure that she is receiving the stimulation she needs, support her hips with one hand and use the other to gently stroke her clitoris. Penetrate her more deeply as she is increasingly aroused. Rhythmic thrusting in the Widely Opened position can create intense vaginal sensations. When you sense that her arousal is beginning to peak, you can drive her wild by gently parting the cheeks of her buttocks, so that her anus is exposed and slightly stretched. Most women find this action intensely exciting.*

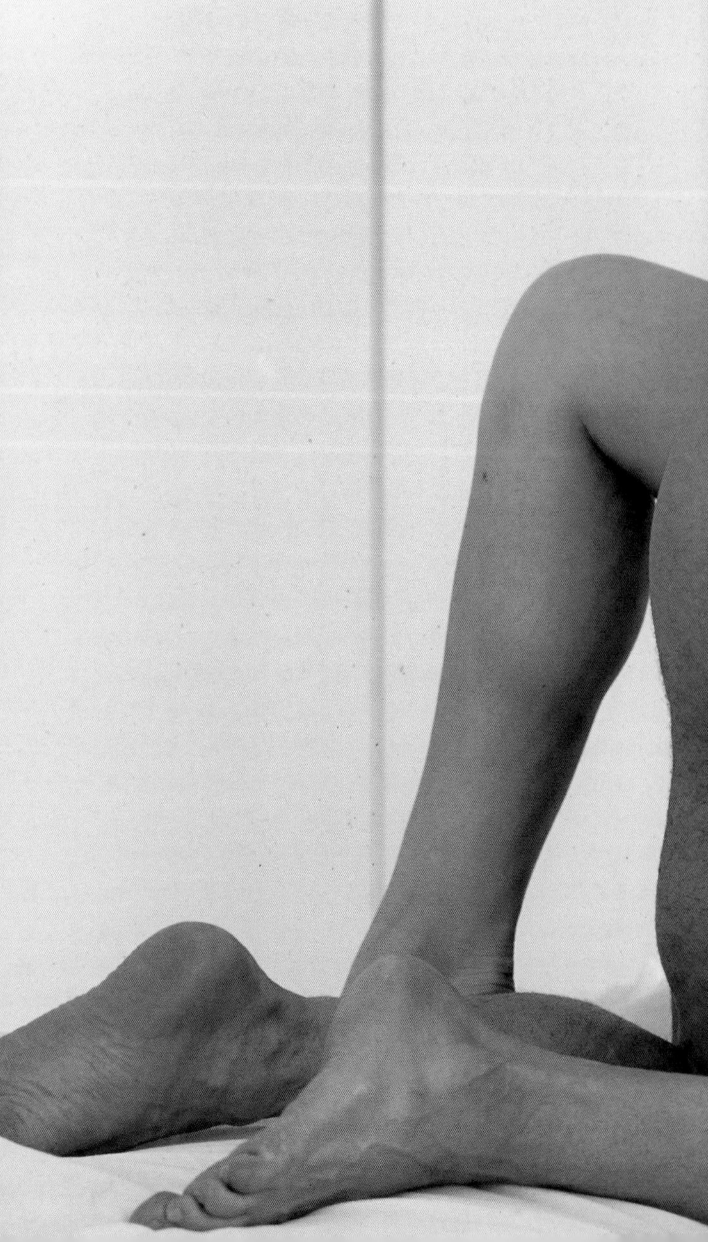

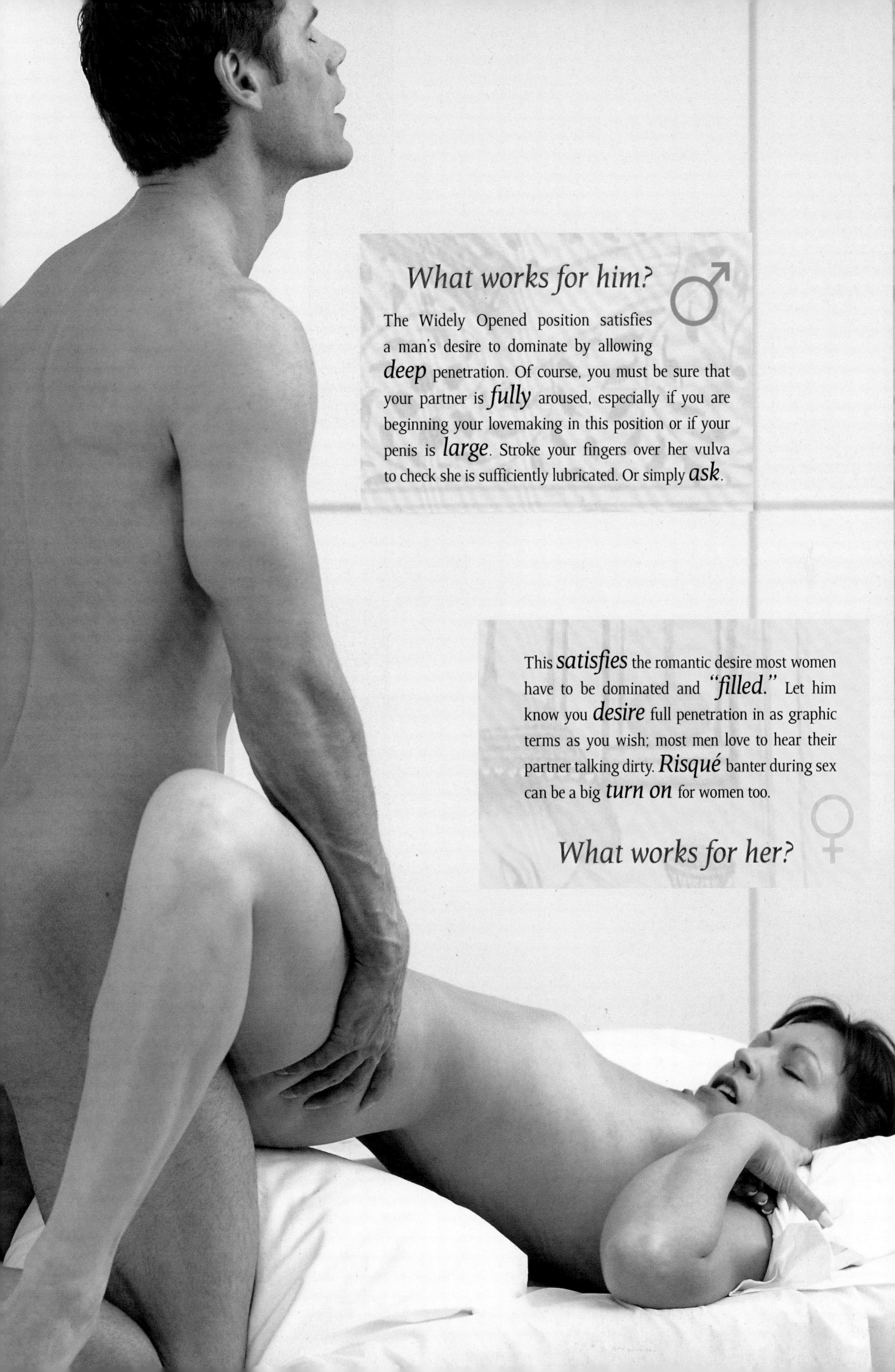

What works for him? ♂

The Widely Opened position satisfies a man's desire to dominate by allowing *deep* penetration. Of course, you must be sure that your partner is *fully* aroused, especially if you are beginning your lovemaking in this position or if your penis is *large*. Stroke your fingers over her vulva to check she is sufficiently lubricated. Or simply *ask*.

This *satisfies* the romantic desire most women have to be dominated and *"filled."* Let him know you *desire* full penetration in as graphic terms as you wish; most men love to hear their partner talking dirty. *Risqué* banter during sex can be a big *turn on* for women too.

What works for her? ♀

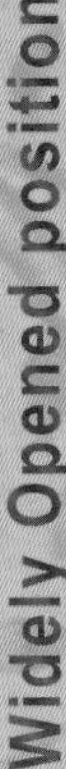

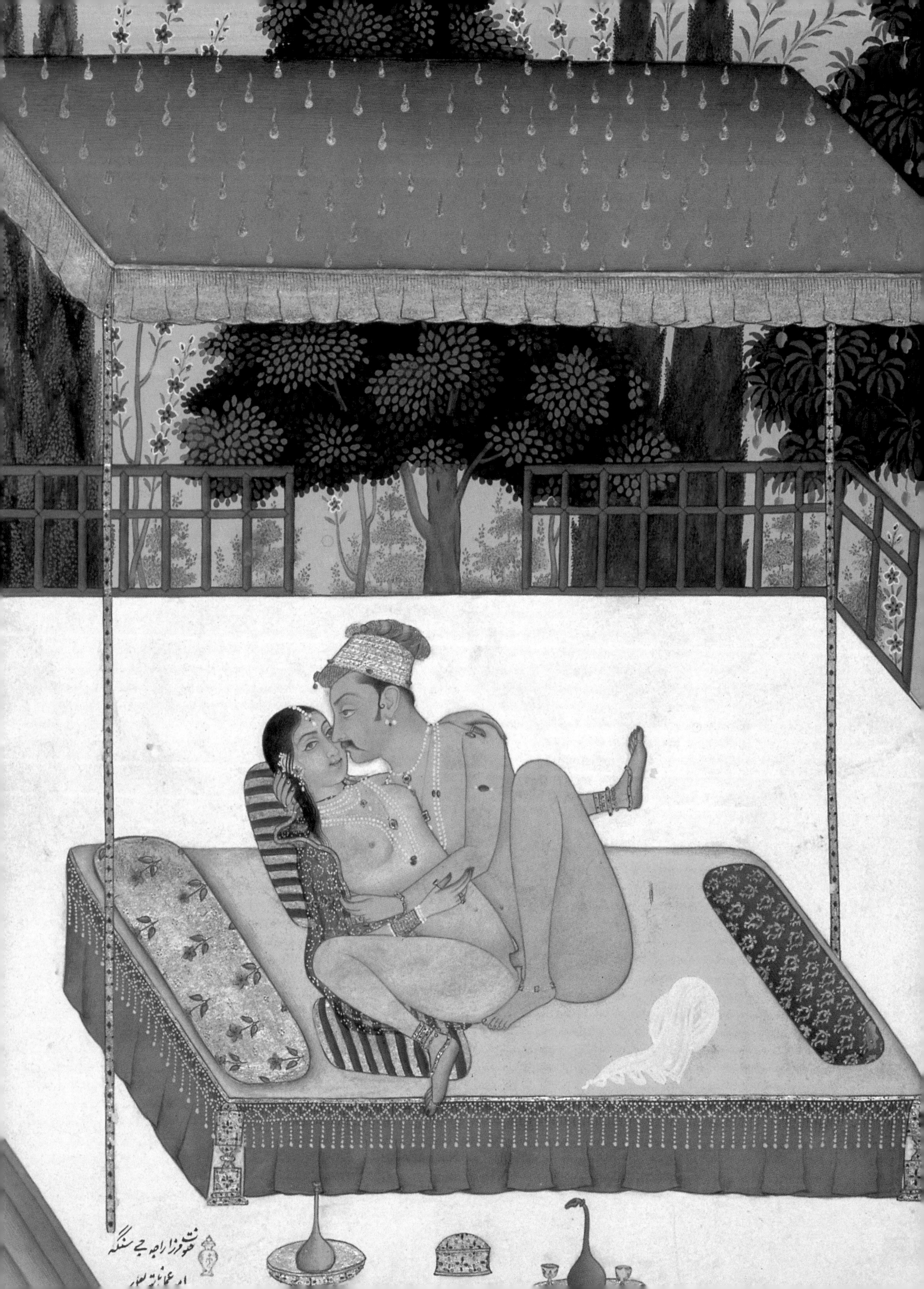
خلوت فزا راجه جی سنگه

> MEN ARE KNOWN *to be more highly responsive to visual stimulation, while women are more responsive to touch. However, watching the penis thrusting in and out of the vagina during sex can be highly erotic for both partners. By raising his torso off hers, both partners are able to enjoy this visual stimulation. For the man, having his lover watching in this way can make him feel very potent.*

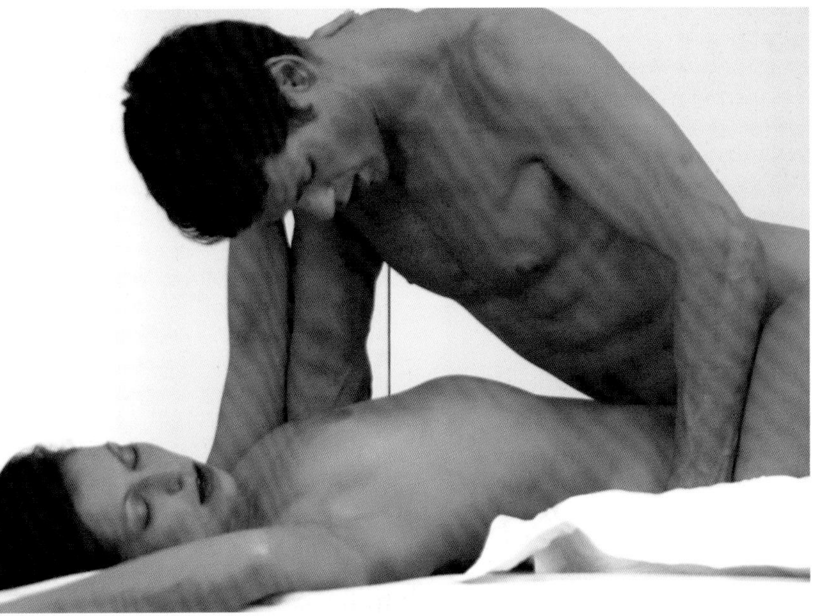

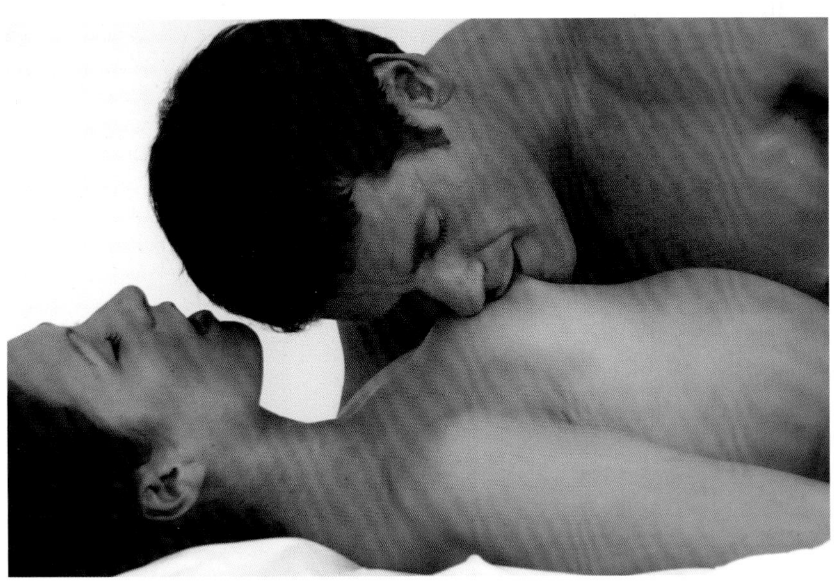

< CONTINUE TO CARESS *her body rather than focusing on your pelvic thrusts. Her breasts and nipples are easily accessible in this position. Suck, kiss, lick, and nibble her breasts until she is breathless with desire. When she is in such an aroused state the sensation of your lips on this highly erogenous area might easily trigger her orgasm. Your own pleasure will be heightened as you feel her nipples harden.*

> ALTER THE ANGLE *of your thrusting by shifting your weight to one side to create new and erotic sensations, using one arm to support yourself while the other caresses her thighs. It also allows your partner more freedom to move; she can rub her thigh against yours or stroke your back.*

< PILLOWS PLACED AT *either end of the bed enable these lovers to be flexible in their lovemaking. The "deer woman" has spread her legs widely so that her lover can penetrate her vagina deeply.*

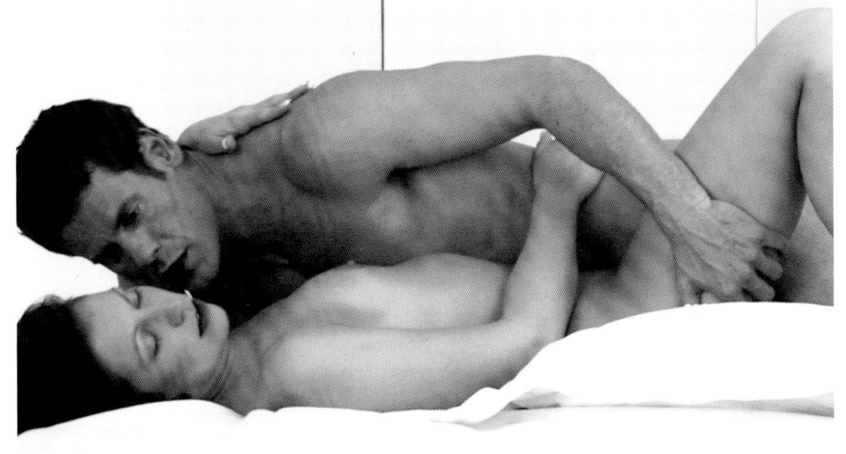

Turning position

Are you ready to try something really different? The Turning position definitely fits the bill. Vatsyayana says: "When a man, during congress, turns round, and enjoys the woman without leaving her, while she embraces him round the back all the time, it is called the Turning position, and is learned only by practice." If you were to try this during a one-night stand, your partner would have hysterics, or run a mile, or possibly both! As an experiment between lovers who know each other inside out and back to front (well, if you didn't before, you will now), it is a lot of fun and surprisingly erotic.

V THE KAMA SUTRA'S *"practice" recommendation is no joke. Although the Turning position starts from the familiar Clasping embrace, it soon turns into an acrobatic feat. Your lover will deserve a medal if he can go the full 360 degrees without his penis slipping out at least half-a-dozen times. At the halfway mark things start to get really interesting. You find yourself looking at him in a whole new light, and feel the most extraordinary sensations as his penis churns around, probing into every part of your vagina.*

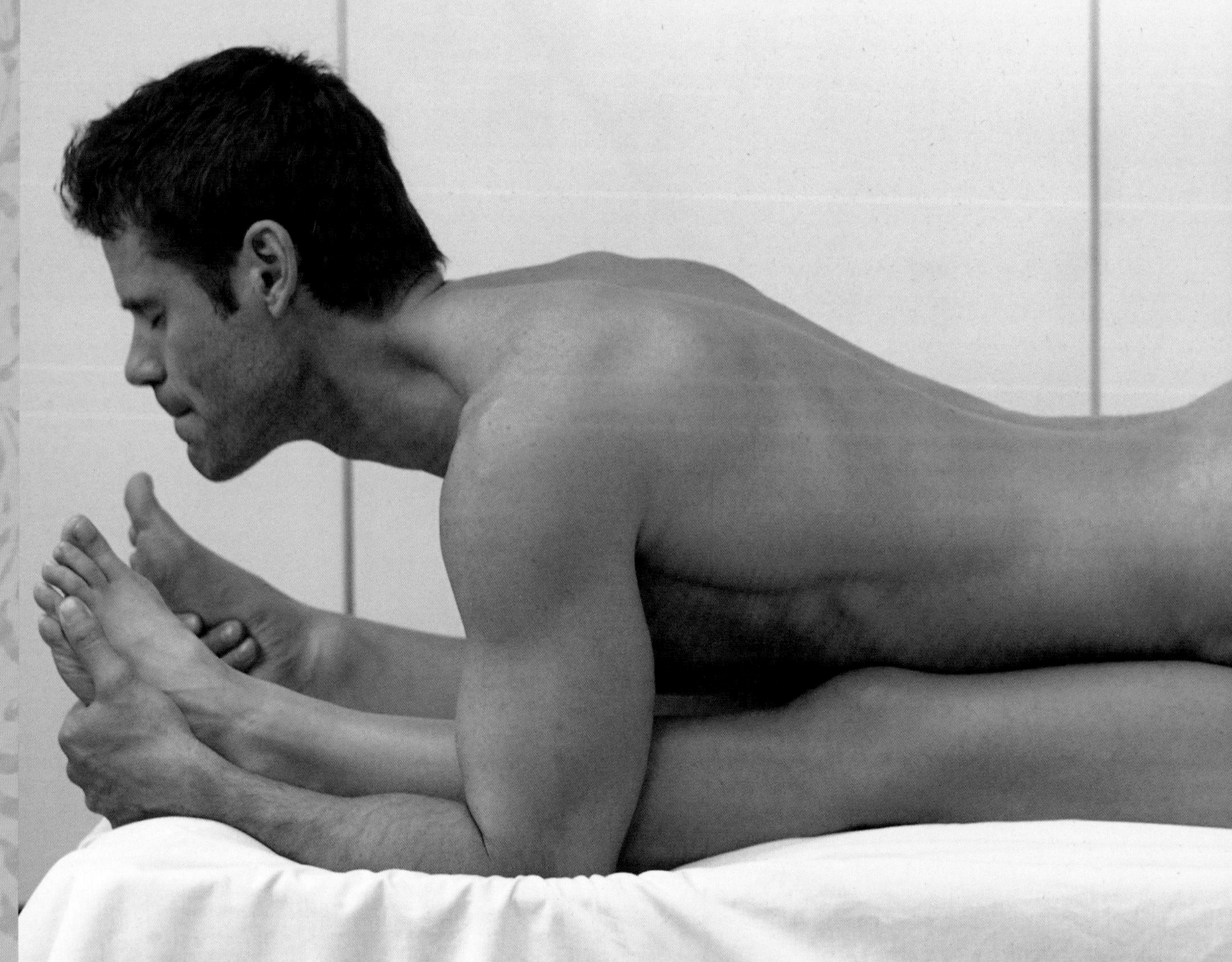

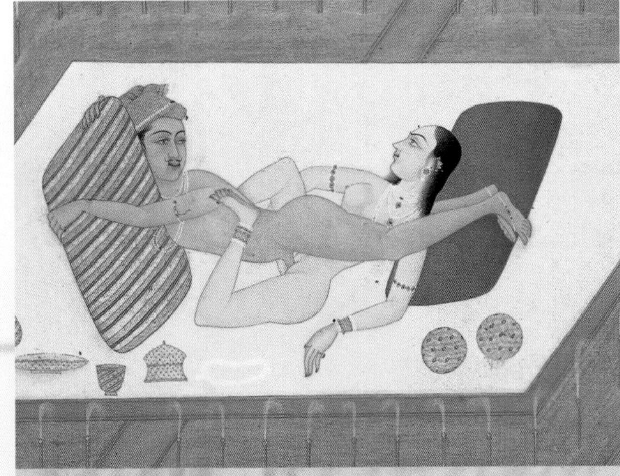

Turning

If you don't believe people really did this in ancient India or anywhere else, check out *The Private Pleasure of Kunwar Meghraj Ji* (*c.*1678–98), which depicts an interesting variation on the Turning theme. Kunwar and his lover seem to be very practiced in the art of Turning, continuing their conversation at 180 degrees when his penis must be bent at the most uncomfortable angle. His lover caresses his back with one very double-jointed leg. We can only speculate as to how Kunwar got his left leg into that position.

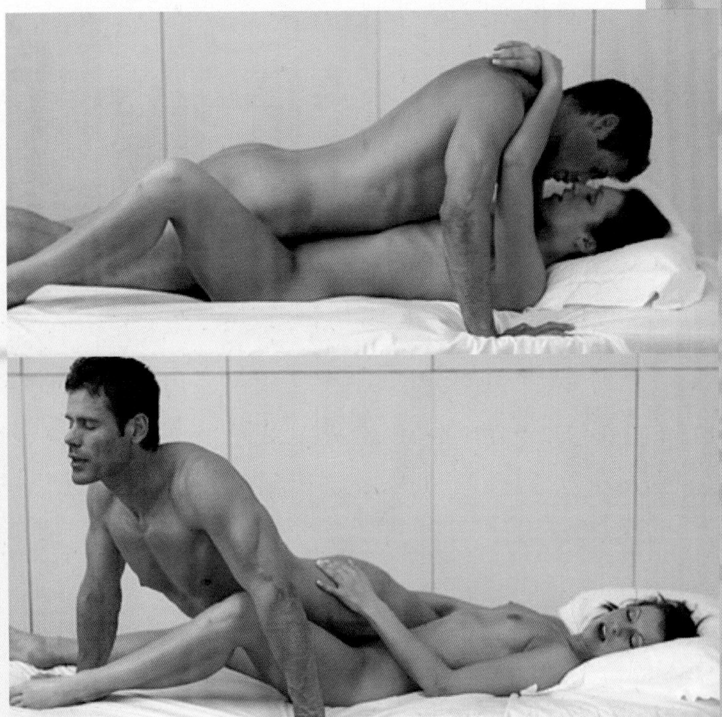

∧ IF OR WHEN *he completes the full circle, you can reward him with a passionate kiss and tell him all about which bits you like best. Ask him to do it again. And now that you know the ropes, take full advantage of the opportunity to squeeze and fondle that sexy behind. If you fancy taking a Turn yourself, switch roles and try the Top* (see pg.166).

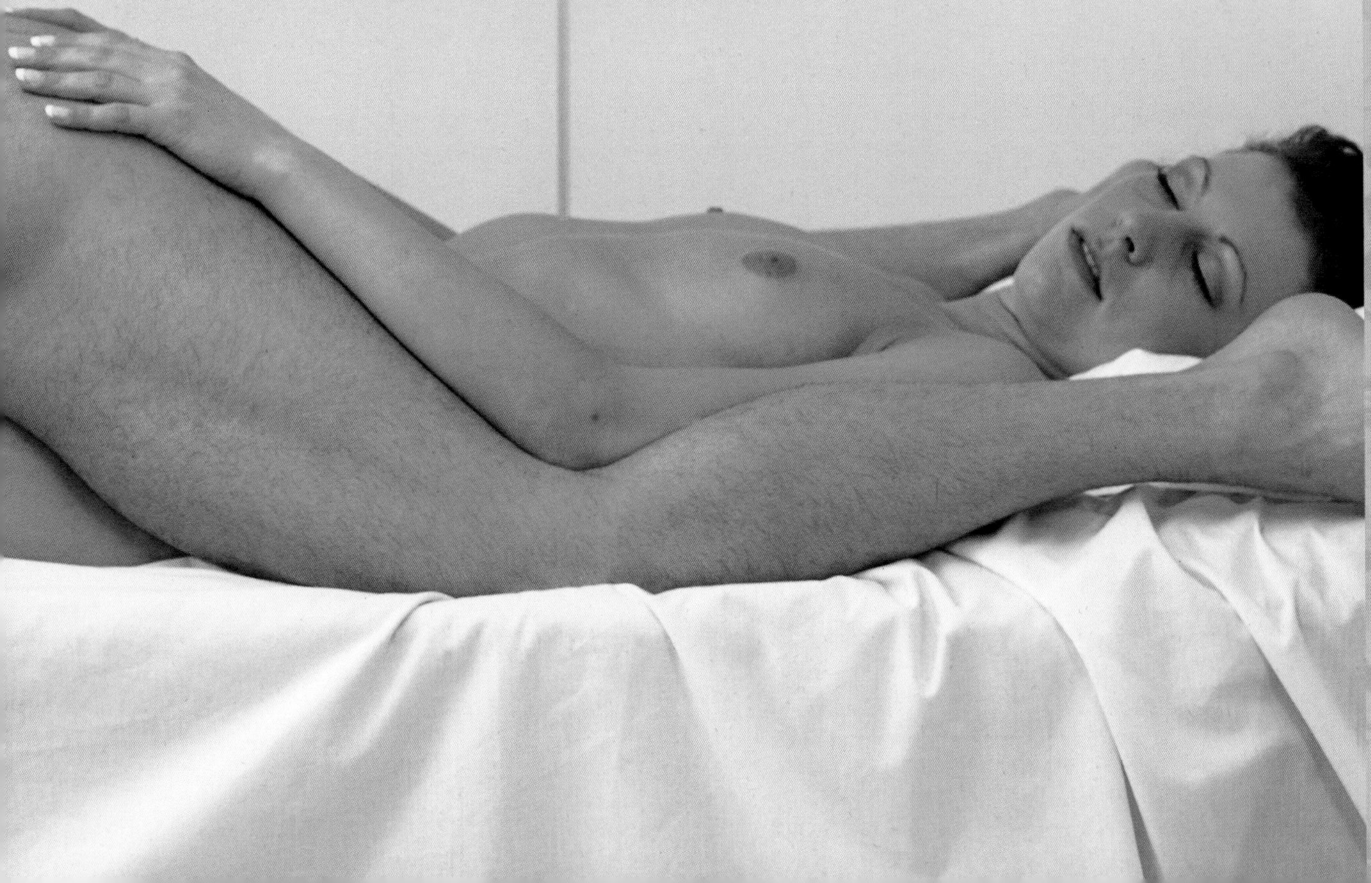

Yawning position

Nobody will blame you if you decide to skip the Turning position (*see* pg. 90–91) for now and move straight into the Yawning position, which follows very naturally from the Widely Opened. It is described as follows: "When she raises her thighs and keeps them wide apart and engages in congress, it is called the Yawning position." As one of the three positions that the Kama Sutra recommends for high congress (*see* pg.28), it allows maximum penetration. And by raising and lowering the legs, you create different and exciting sensations.

What works for him? ♂

This is the start of the really *raunchy* legs-in-the-air kind of sex. Wild and wonderful, it's the sort of sex where even if your bed caught *fire* you'd still have to think twice before leaving it. But unlike the relatively rough or detached raunchiness of the Pressed (*see* Chapter 9) and Animal positions (Chapter 8), you remain very *connected* with your lover and enjoy watching her expression change as you move *together* to new heights of excitement.

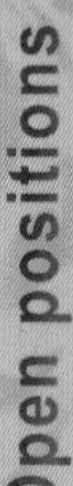

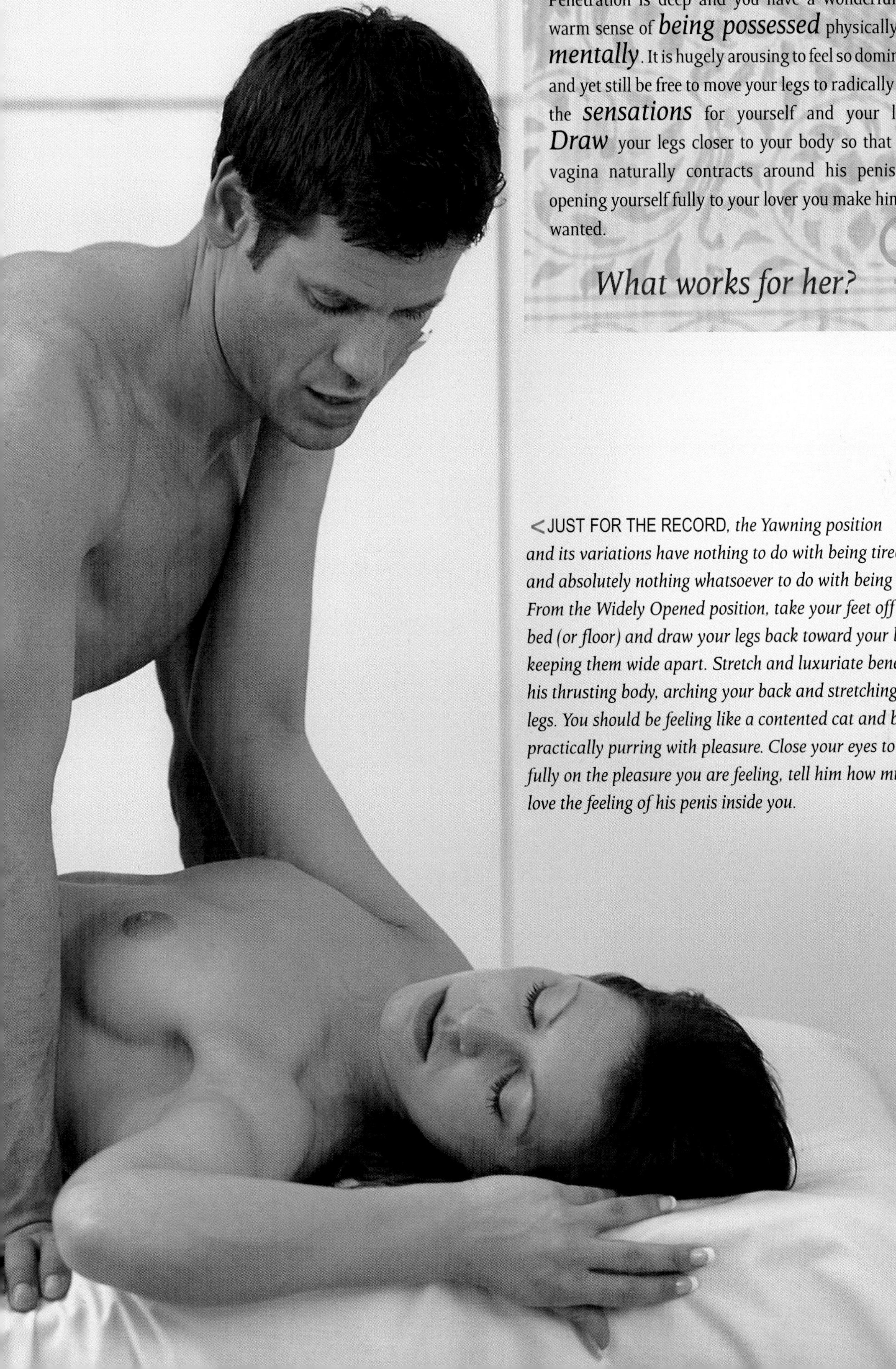

Penetration is deep and you have a wonderful and warm sense of ***being possessed*** physically and ***mentally***. It is hugely arousing to feel so dominated and yet still be free to move your legs to radically alter the **sensations** for yourself and your lover. **Draw** your legs closer to your body so that your vagina naturally contracts around his penis. By opening yourself fully to your lover you make him feel wanted.

What works for her? ♀

<JUST FOR THE RECORD, *the Yawning position and its variations have nothing to do with being tired and absolutely nothing whatsoever to do with being bored. From the Widely Opened position, take your feet off the bed (or floor) and draw your legs back toward your body, keeping them wide apart. Stretch and luxuriate beneath his thrusting body, arching your back and stretching your legs. You should be feeling like a contented cat and be practically purring with pleasure. Close your eyes to focus fully on the pleasure you are feeling, tell him how much you love the feeling of his penis inside you.*

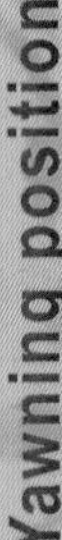

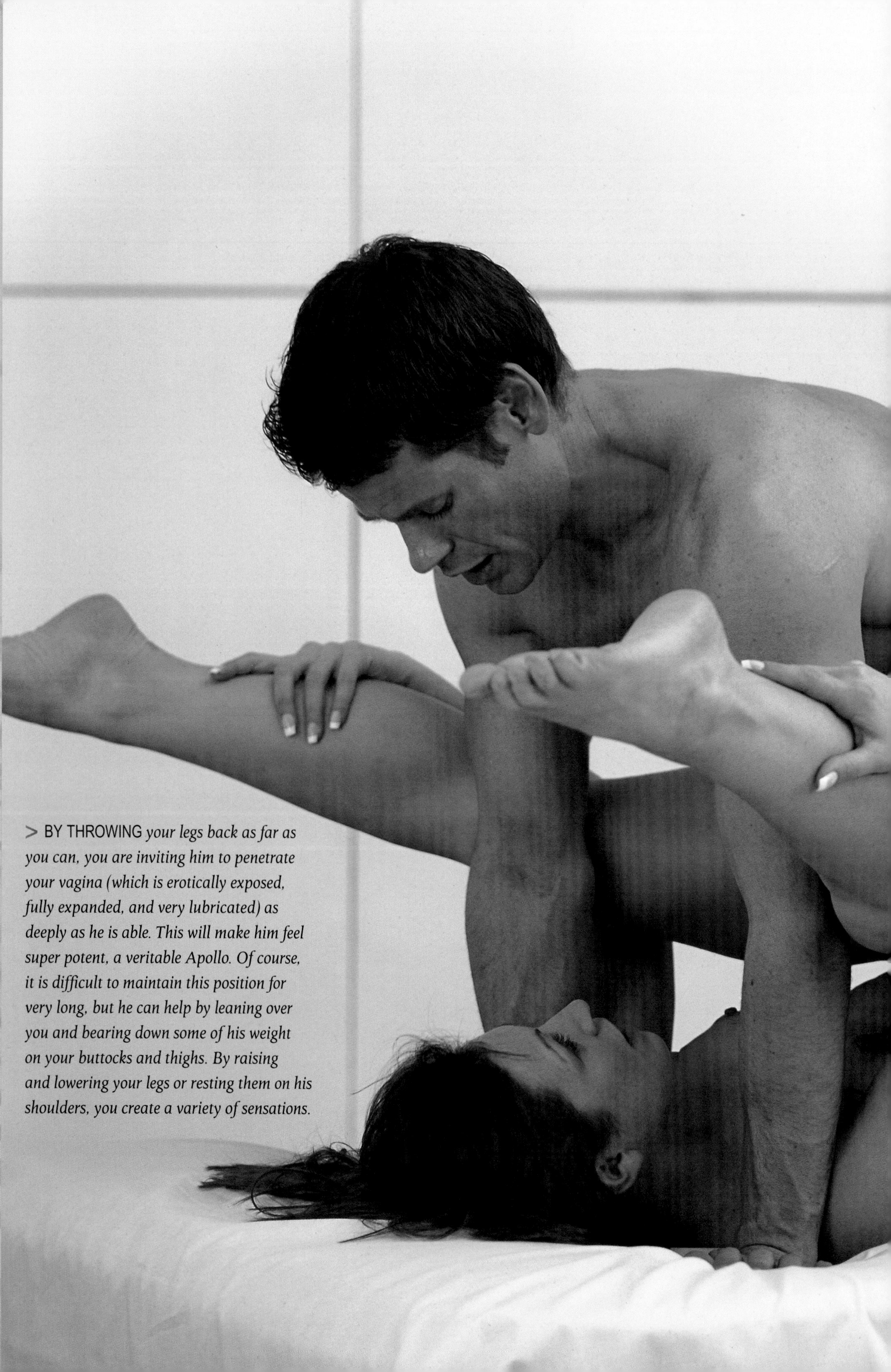

> BY THROWING *your legs back as far as you can, you are inviting him to penetrate your vagina (which is erotically exposed, fully expanded, and very lubricated) as deeply as he is able. This will make him feel super potent, a veritable Apollo. Of course, it is difficult to maintain this position for very long, but he can help by leaning over you and bearing down some of his weight on your buttocks and thighs. By raising and lowering your legs or resting them on his shoulders, you create a variety of sensations.*

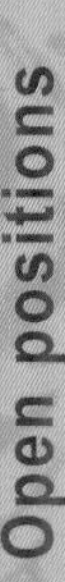

> AT FIRST GLANCE *there appears to be little difference between this pose and that of the main image, but there is a big difference. Because her legs are now inside your arms there is not the same sense of invitation and she feels totally at your mercy. As you lean forward, her legs are pushed toward her body. She will feel vulnerable and you may need to reassure her with loving words. Nevertheless, this position is actually more comfortable for her to maintain for long periods.*

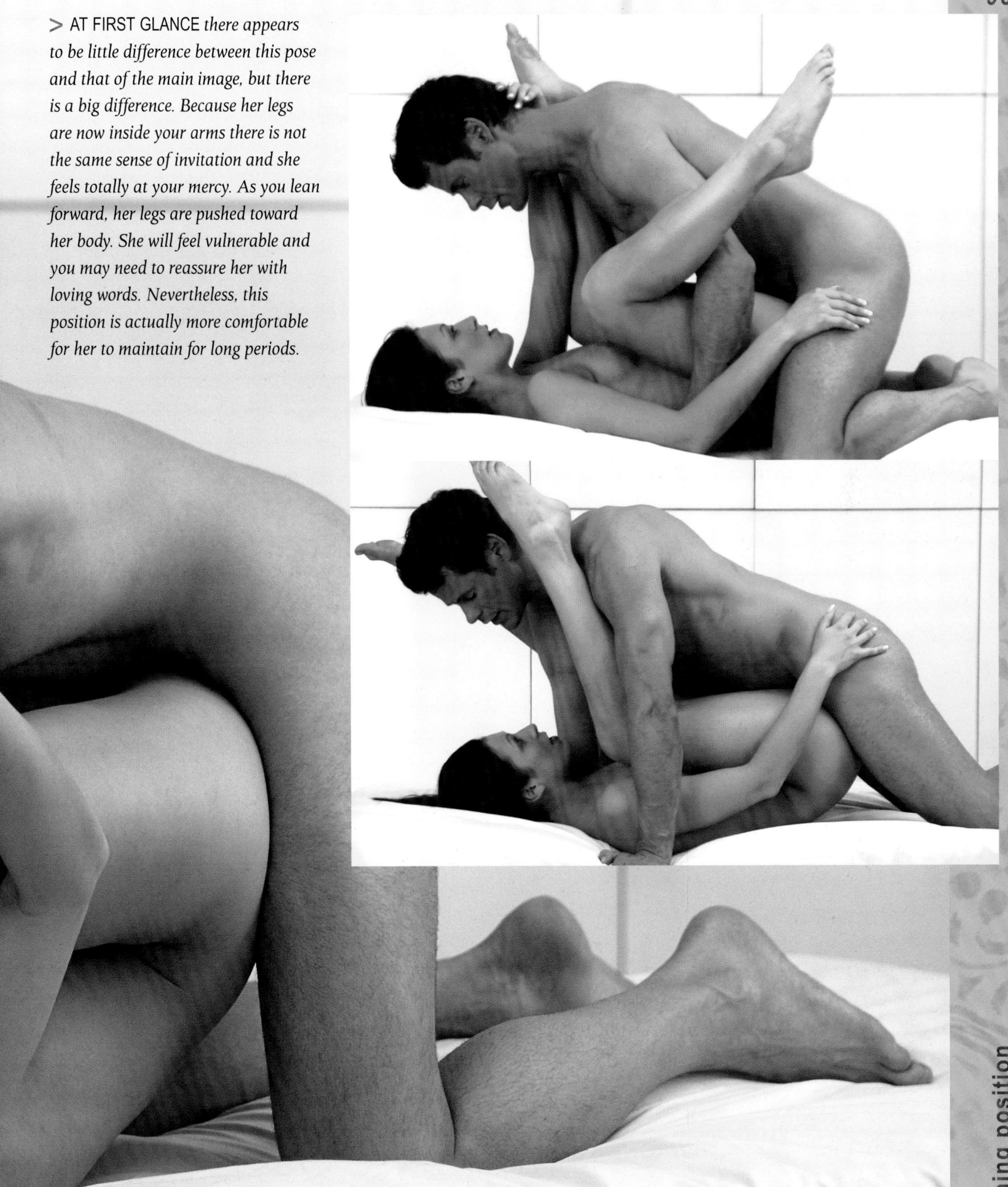

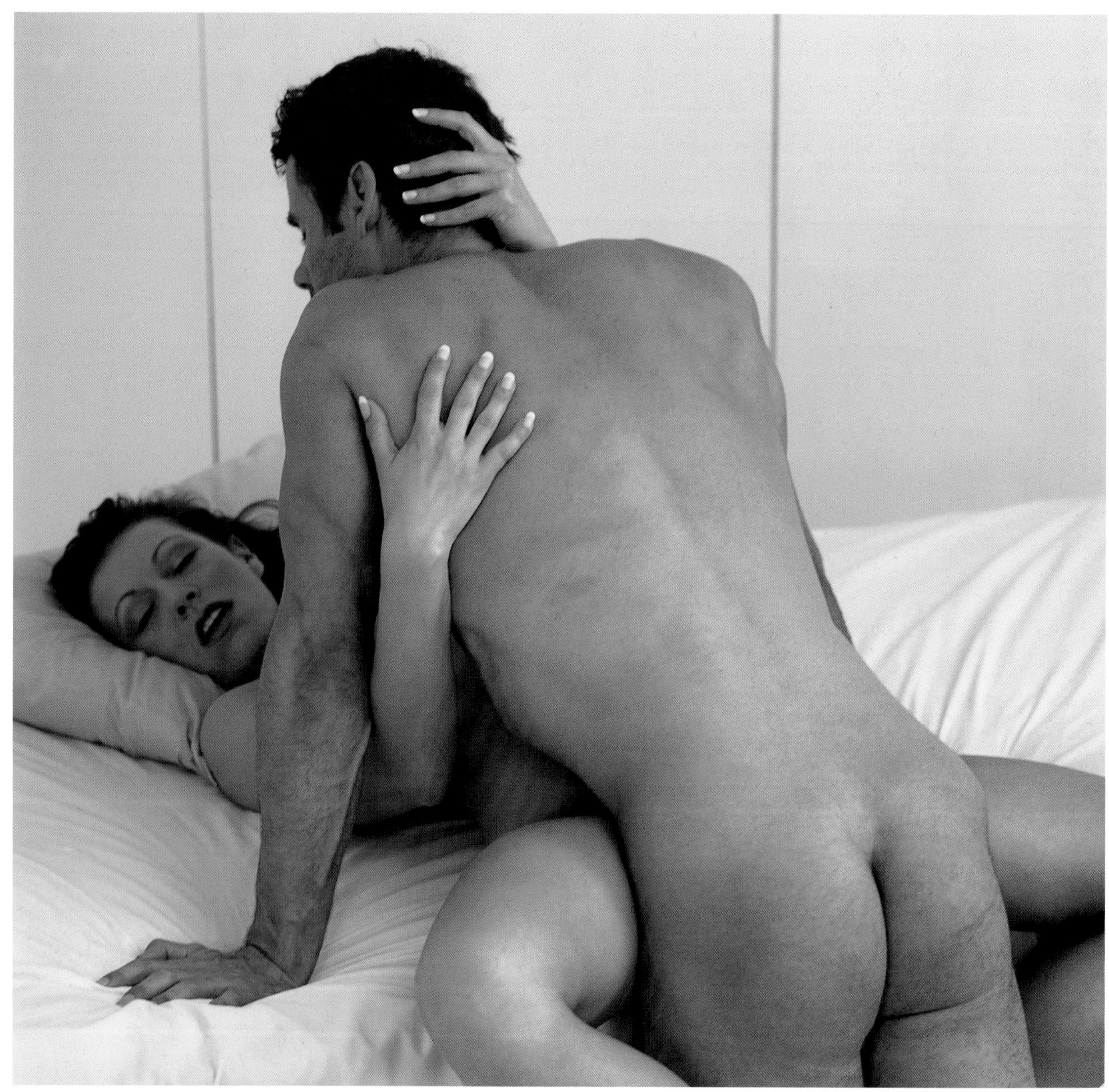

The Widely Opened position over the edge of the bed will feel wonderful after your acrobatics in the Yawning position. The *fullness* of his penis thrusting inside you can fill you with pleasure. As he *leans* over you it brings his pubic bone in close proximity to your vulva, giving your **clitoris** the stimulation it requires for you to reach orgasm. Enjoy the opportunity to let your **passive** nature come to the surface and surrender your body to your lover.

What works for her? ♀

∧ IF YOU ENJOYED *the packed and helpless feeling produced by the variant Yawning position* (see *pg.*95) *you may want to move straight into the Pressed positions* (see Chapter 7). *However, the Widely Opened position can be a wonderful position to culminate your lovemaking. As your orgasm builds up, tell him what you are feeling, or show him by stroking or scratching his back and pulling him toward you.*

> TELL HIM *that you are approaching your climax and then kiss him passionately as you abandon yourself to your orgasm. Focus on the supremely pleasurable sensation of his penis pulsating inside you as he too surrenders himself to his own exquisite release.*

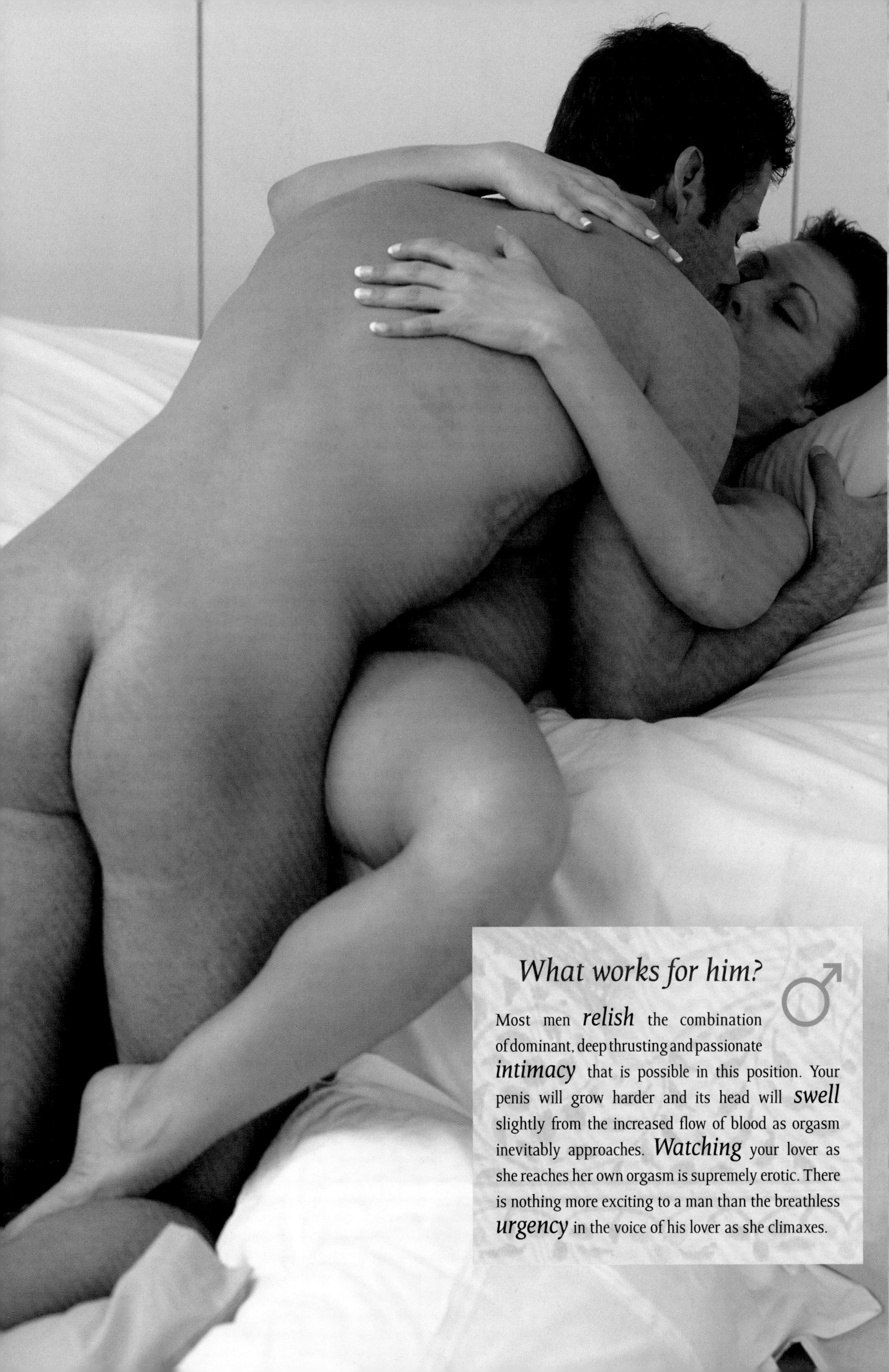

What works for him?

Most men ***relish*** the combination of dominant, deep thrusting and passionate ***intimacy*** that is possible in this position. Your penis will grow harder and its head will ***swell*** slightly from the increased flow of blood as orgasm inevitably approaches. ***Watching*** your lover as she reaches her own orgasm is supremely erotic. There is nothing more exciting to a man than the breathless ***urgency*** in the voice of his lover as she climaxes.

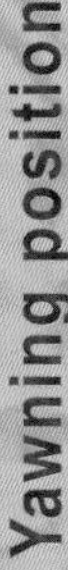

A Private Pleasure

There is something very exciting about adopting the Yawning position while the man enters you from a standing posture. This is a very submissive position from the woman's point of view and always feels impromptu and deliciously wicked. To get yourselves into this position, you will usually have to use a table in the kitchen or dining room or a desk—which may go a long way towards explaining its "forbidden" power. Curiously, it can be more erotic still when both partners remain partially dressed.

> IN THIS PAINTING, The Private Pleasure of Prince Muhammad Shah, *the prince apparently doubles as the local fakir and has put his powers to a practical use by causing the couch to levitate to just the right height for sex!*

V THE YAWNING *position is only a small step away from the exciting Pressed positions (*see Chapter 7*), where the woman places her foot on her lover's chest to constrict her vagina.*

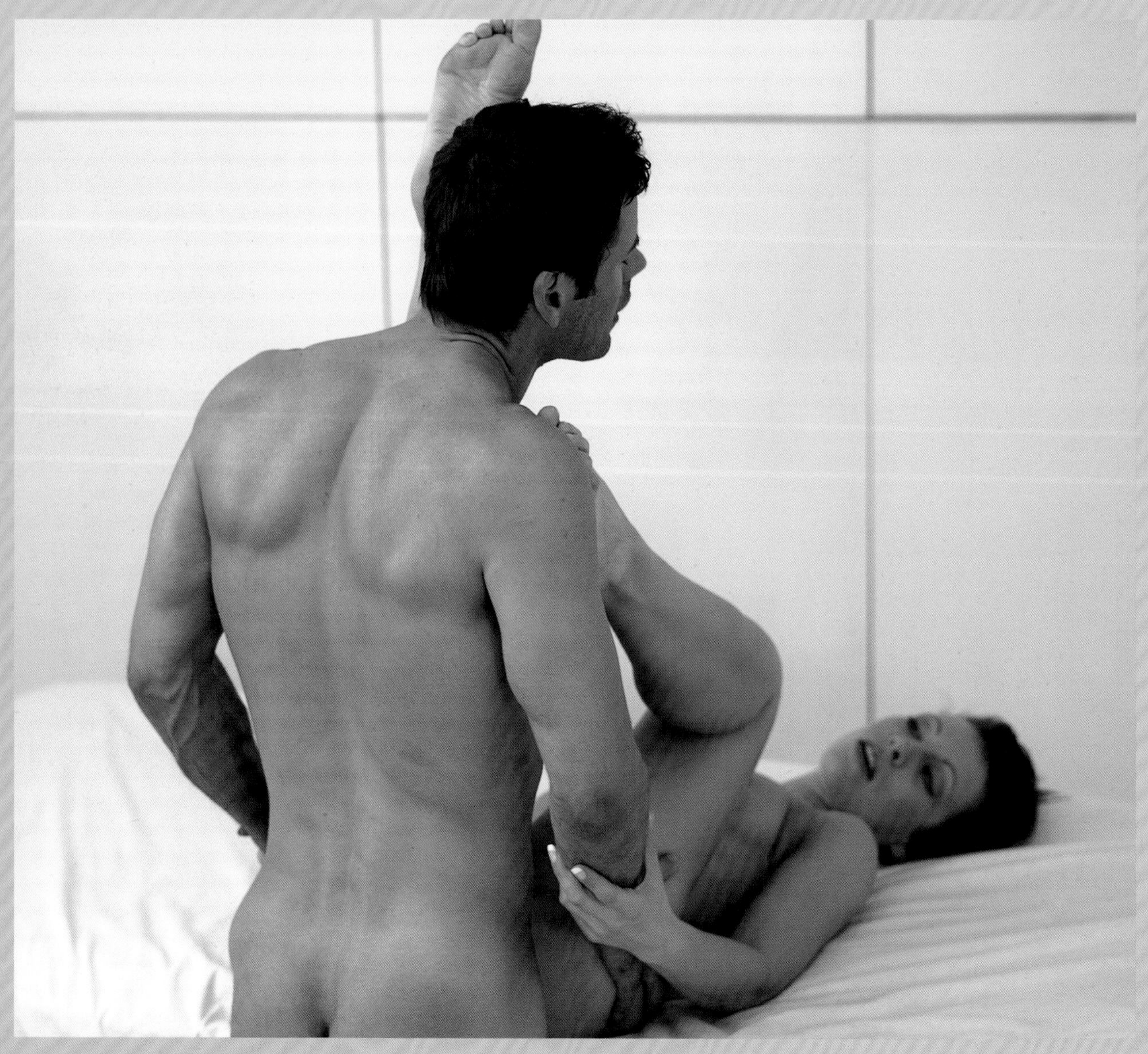

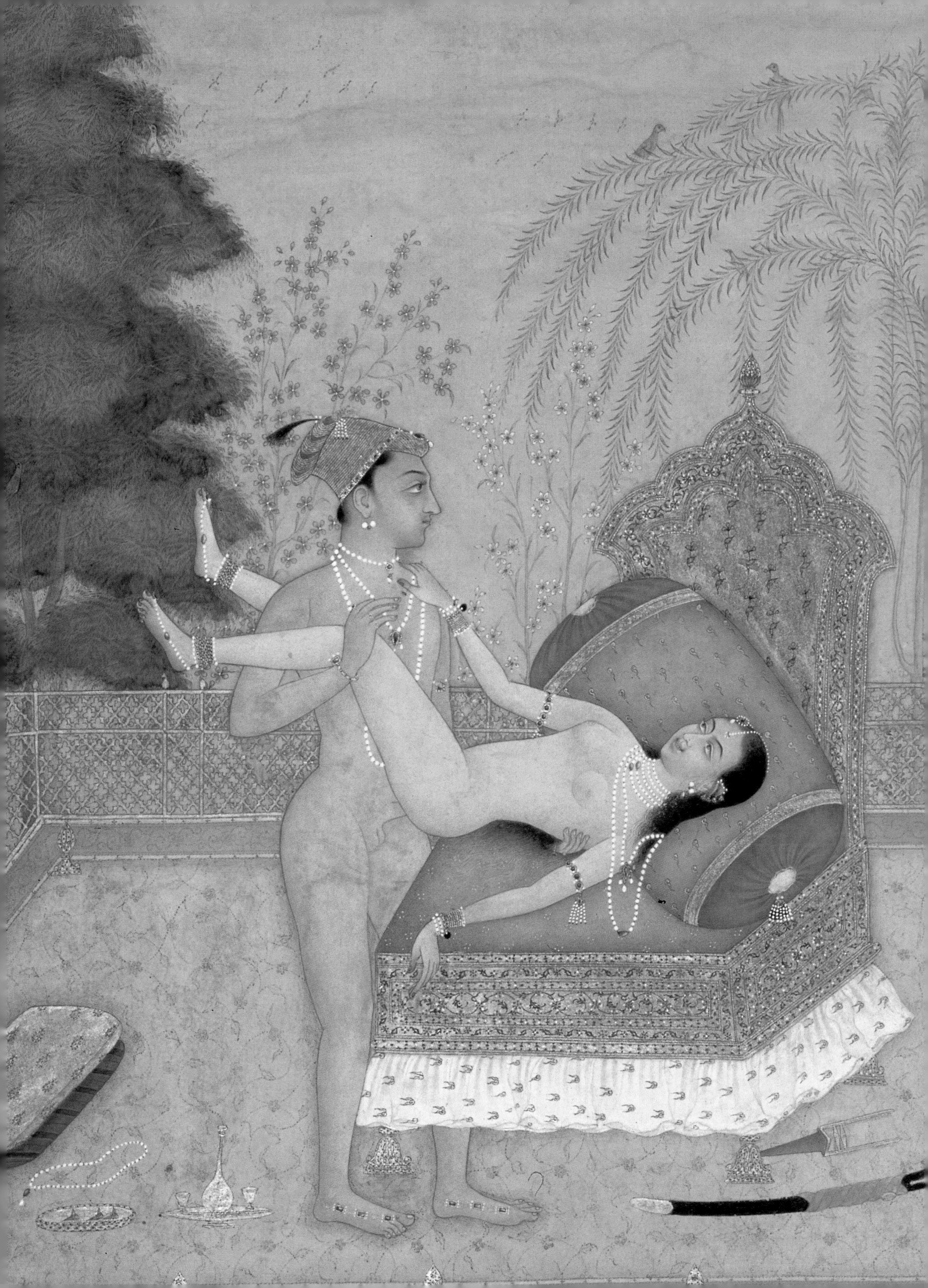

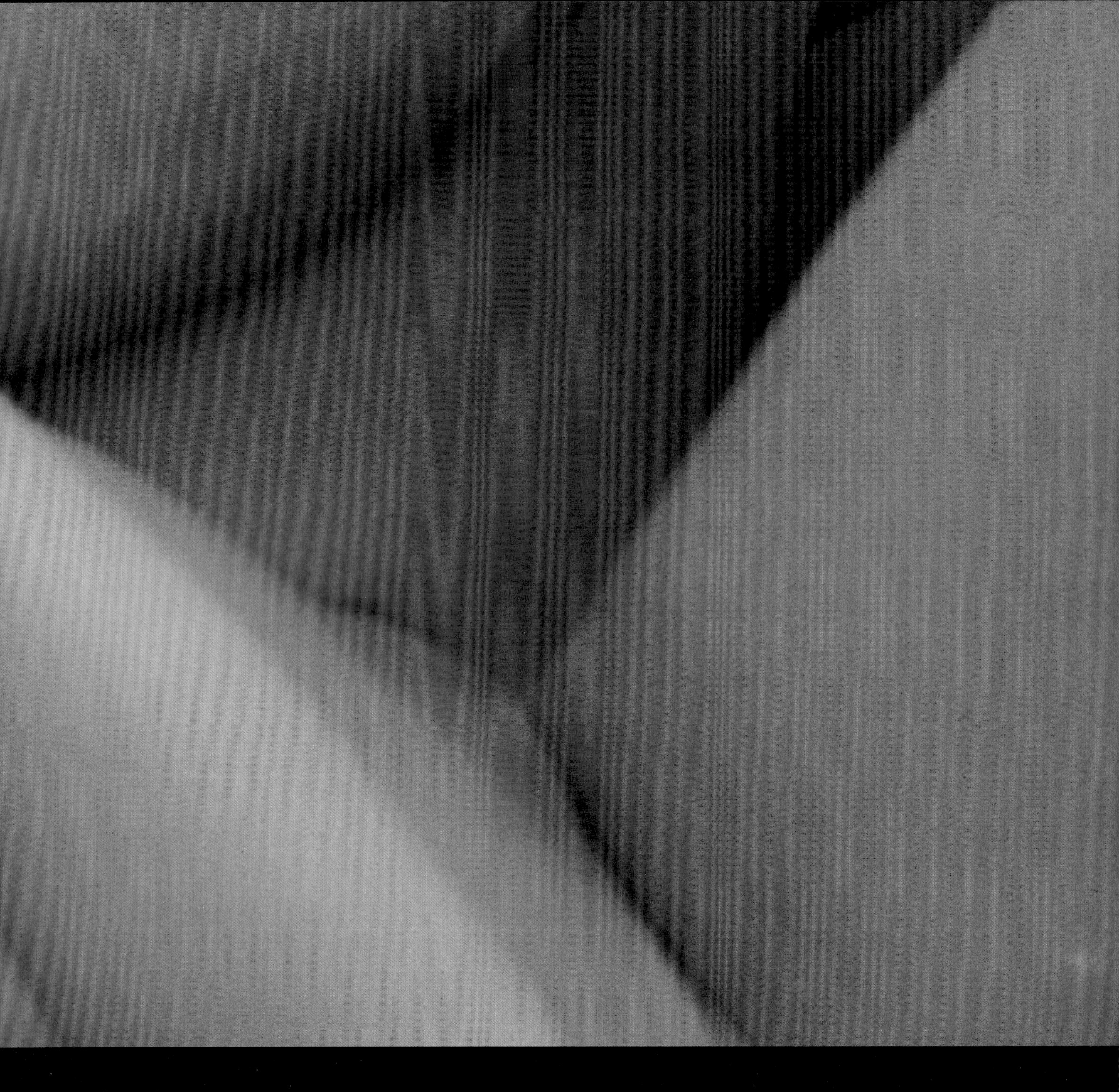

"When the female raises both of her thighs straight up, it is called the Rising position."
KSII:VI

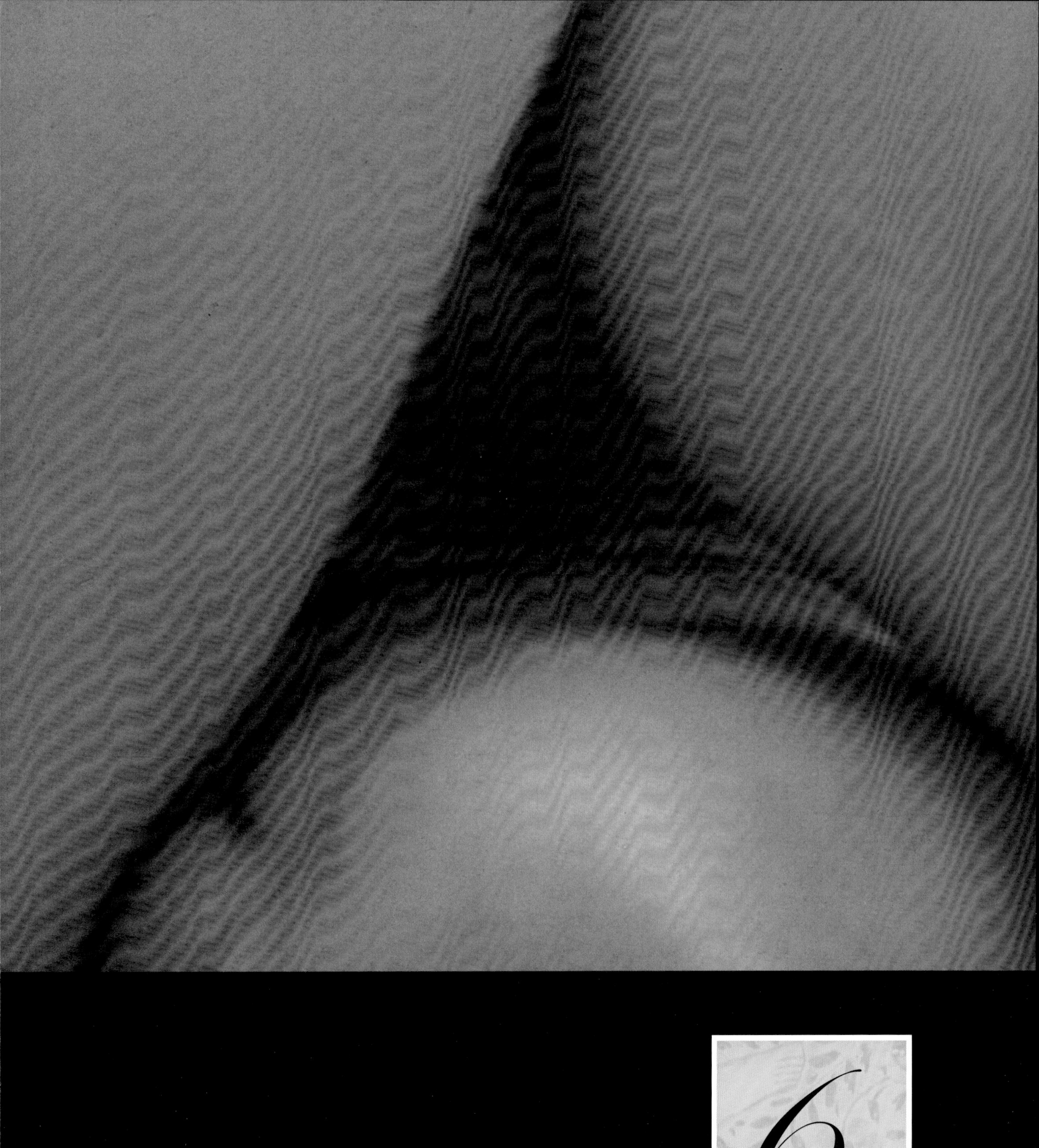

6

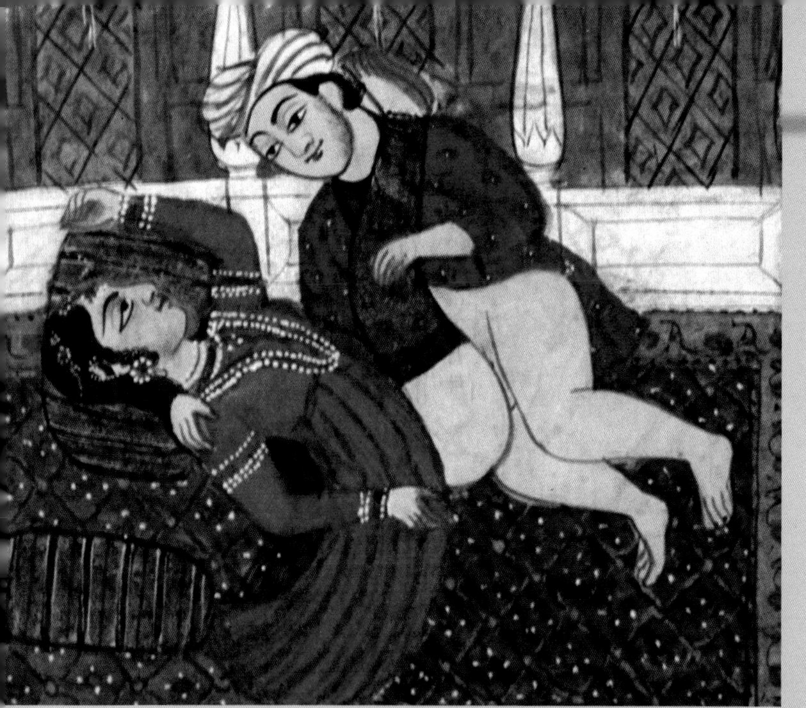

THESE POSITIONS are good for older men (because of the intense friction), and for women who want full-on, deeper than deep penetration. For her, there's something hugely erotic about throwing your legs over your partner's shoulders in a gesture as helpless as it is abandoned—especially since you're safe in the knowledge that you'll be using your thighs and vaginal muscles to thrill him.

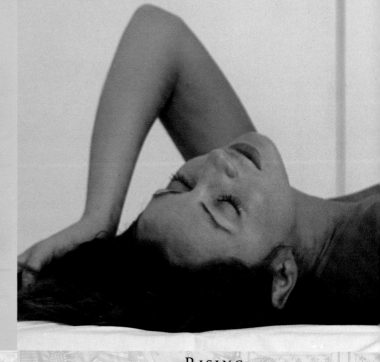

SPLITTING OF A BAMBOO

RISING

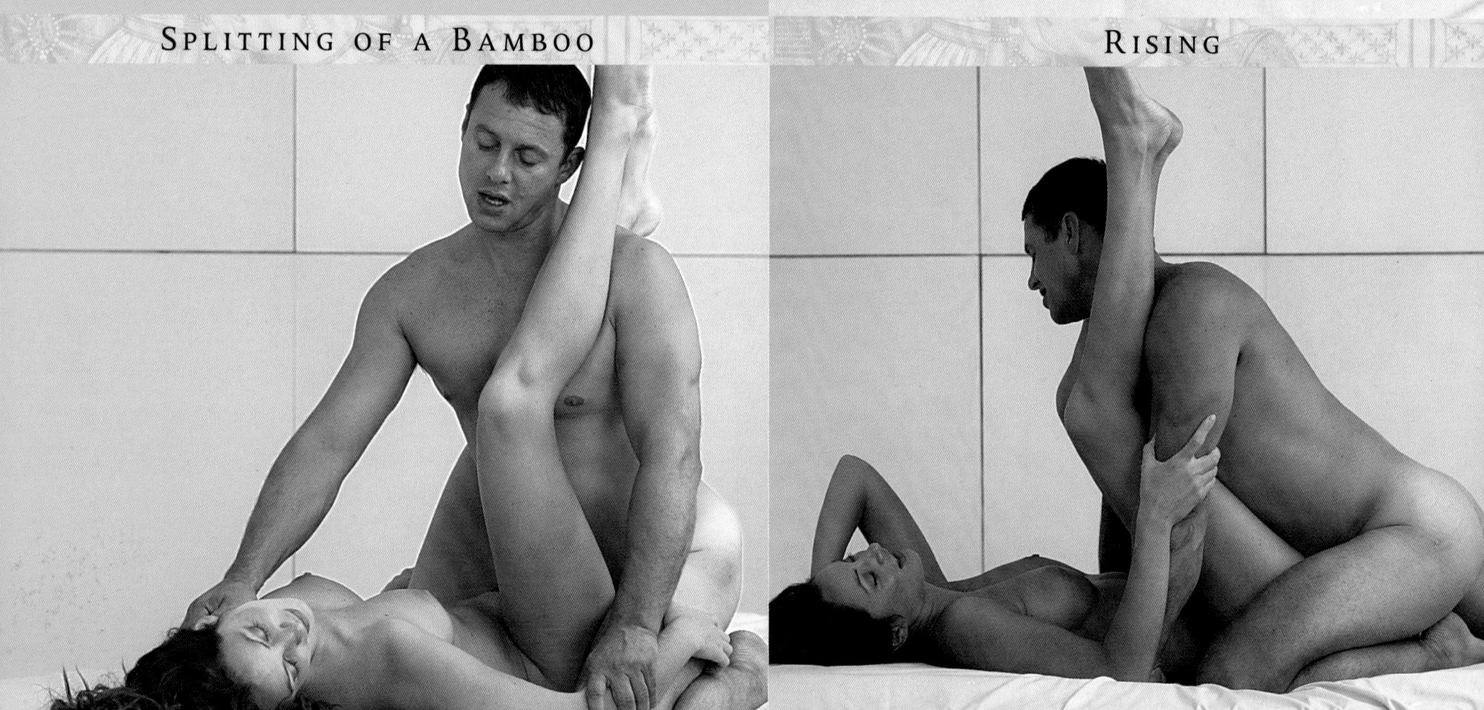

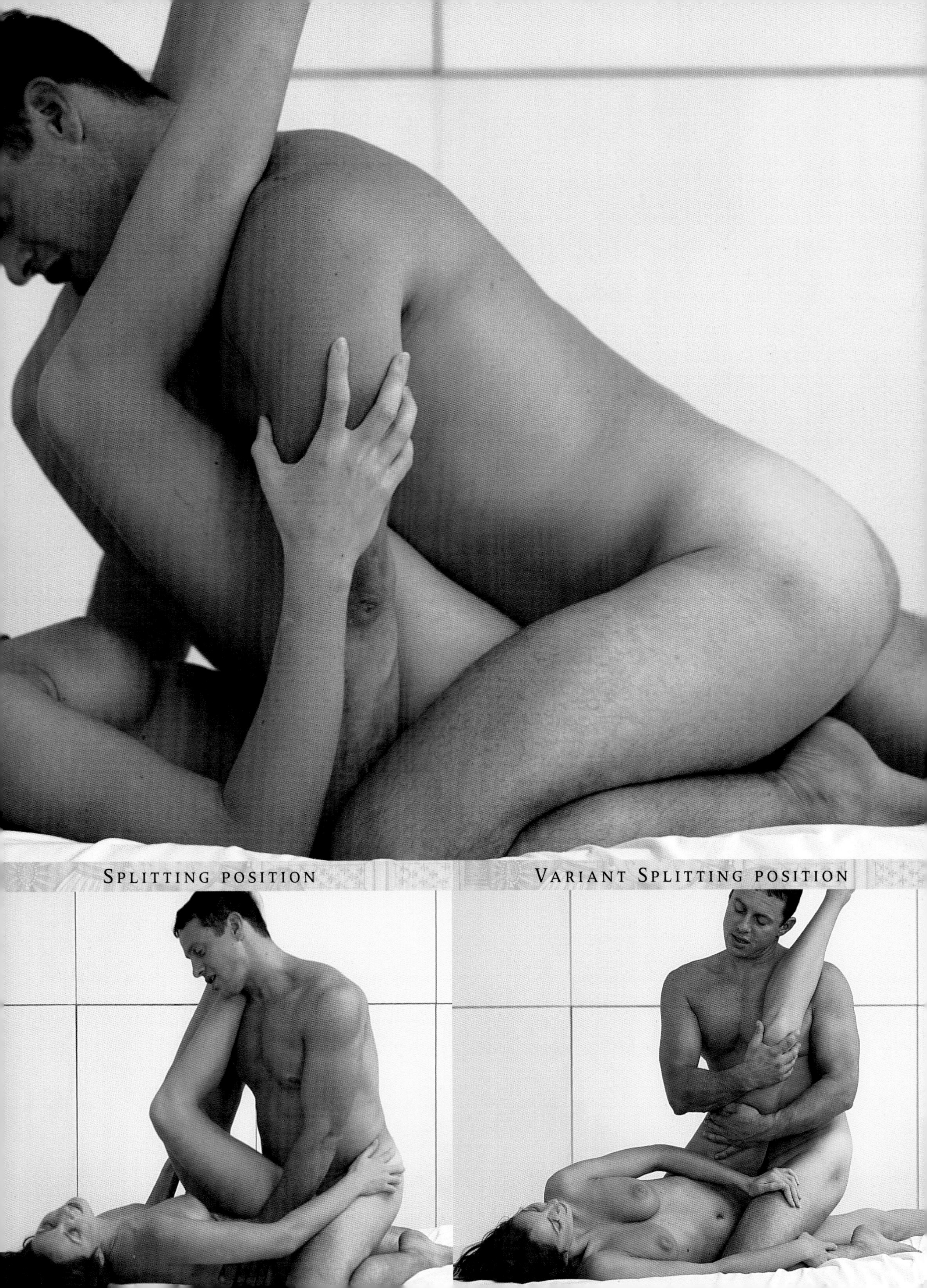

Splitting position

Variant Splitting position

Splitting of a Bamboo

This exotically named position is easy to move into from the Yawning position (*see* pg.92). She needs to be very supple for this to work well, as her legs will play a starring role. Wait until you know each other well before you try this out, as the windmilling legs and the strange but wonderful sensations may put a new lover off his stride. Make sure that she's at the peak of arousal, as the vaginal canal needs to expand to accept the depth of penetration that this position enables.

> USE YOUR LEGS *to help your vagina squeeze his penis while he thrusts (you may want to emphasize the role of your legs by wearing stockings and garter belt). Just raise one leg onto his shoulder, then lower it; raise the other leg, then lower it. Repeat as desired. Some believe that this is impossible, but it is worth trying.*

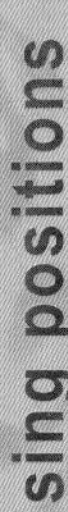

Fixing of a Nail

Home improvement will never be the same again once you have mastered this variation on Splitting of a Bamboo. Instead of putting her leg on your shoulder, she places her heel on your forehead, as if she were hammering a nail in. This may be particularly erotic for foot fetishists, or you might want her to try it when that slingback won't come off and you'd rather know where the spike is. Whatever the reason, this is a little bit of home improvement that's not a chore.

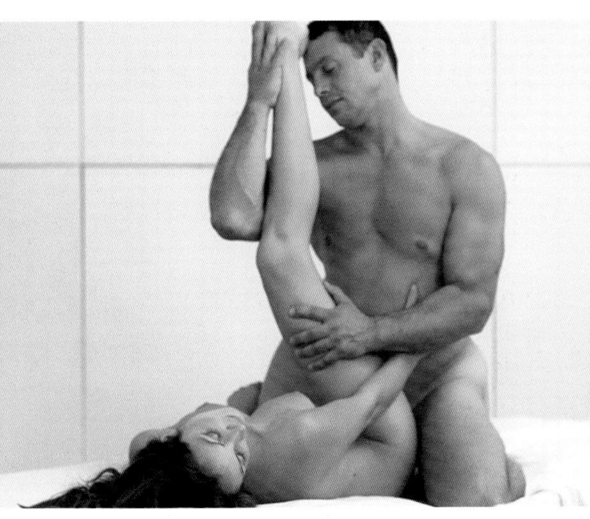

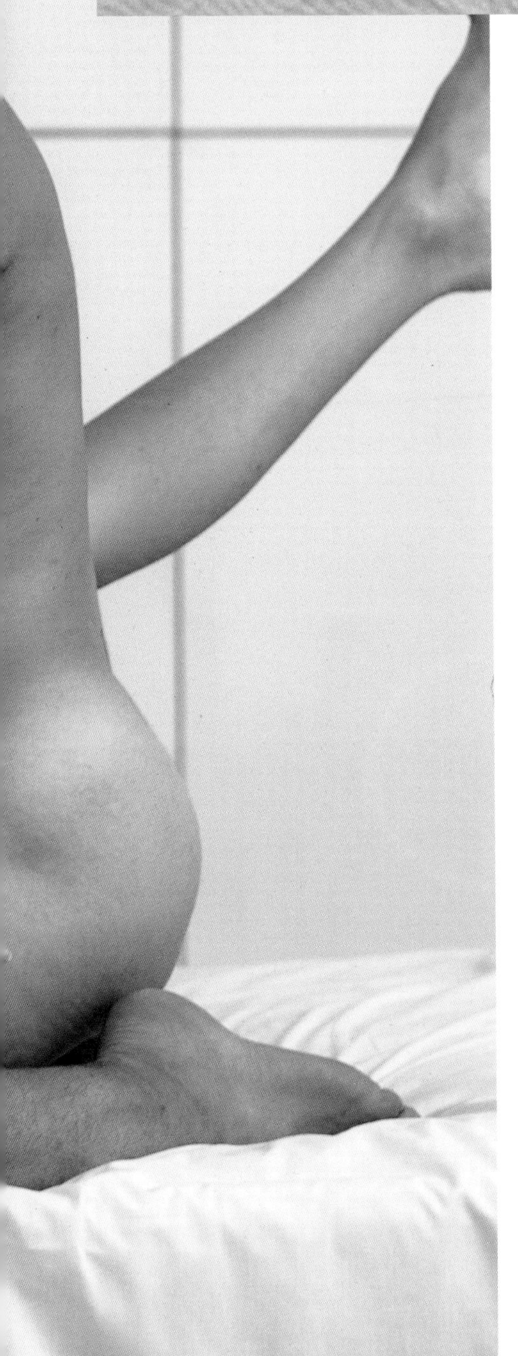

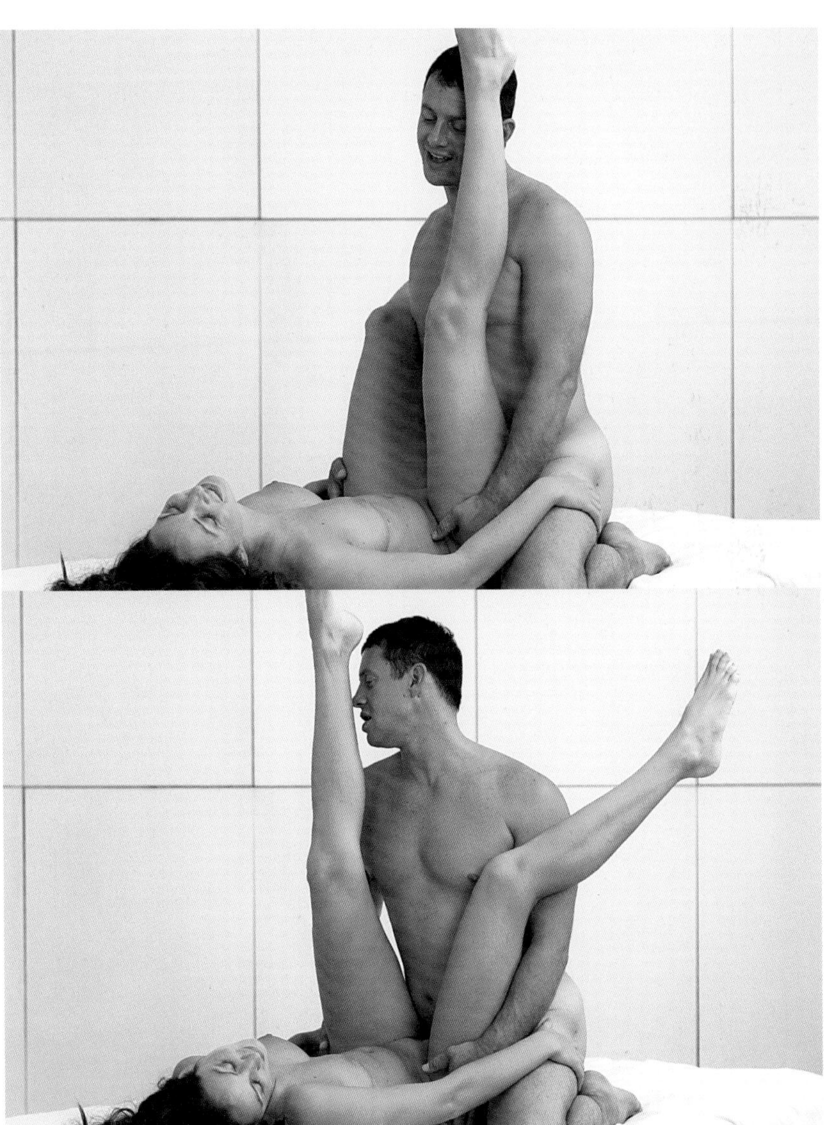

^ IF YOU BRING YOUR LEGS *almost together and then move them, you'll squeeze his penis in a completely unfamiliar way, adding new sensations to his experience of thrusting. Do tell him that you're about to perform this leg-swapping maneuver, as whacking your lover with a stray foot could ruin the moment.*

Rising

The rising positions are all about the kind of decadent, leg-up action that will create magnificent sensations. First, he needs to be on his knees, then she should lie down right in front of him and drape her ankles over his shoulders. Only adopt this stance when you are both at fever pitch, because penetration is so deep that her vagina needs to be fully expanded. Get the point of arousal just right and she'll love the experience of sudden fullness—quite apart from the palpably erotic feeling of her thighs clasping him so powerfully. He'll need to hold onto her legs to keep the action going and maintain his balance.

> YOU CAN VARY THE ANGLE *of penetration (and maybe find that G-spot of hers) by lifting her body gently. If your legs are long and you don't quite fit, use a pillow to lift her. Holding her hips is a big turn-on, as is feeling her bottom and rubbing her tummy. You can help the orgasms along by giving the occasional compliment: You might mention that her thigh pressure is intoxicating your senses and the view of her breasts unutterably gorgeous.*

This is supposed to be a passive position, but in fact your elastic vaginal muscles and gripping thigh action play a **triumphant** part. Of course, you can indulge in that "I'm so helpless, and you're such a big, strong man" **sex kitten** act if you wish, because it's so much fun. It's an especially good position when you're really ready for deep penetration. And you can just lie back now that you have his full attention focused on your **prone** form.

What works for her? ♀

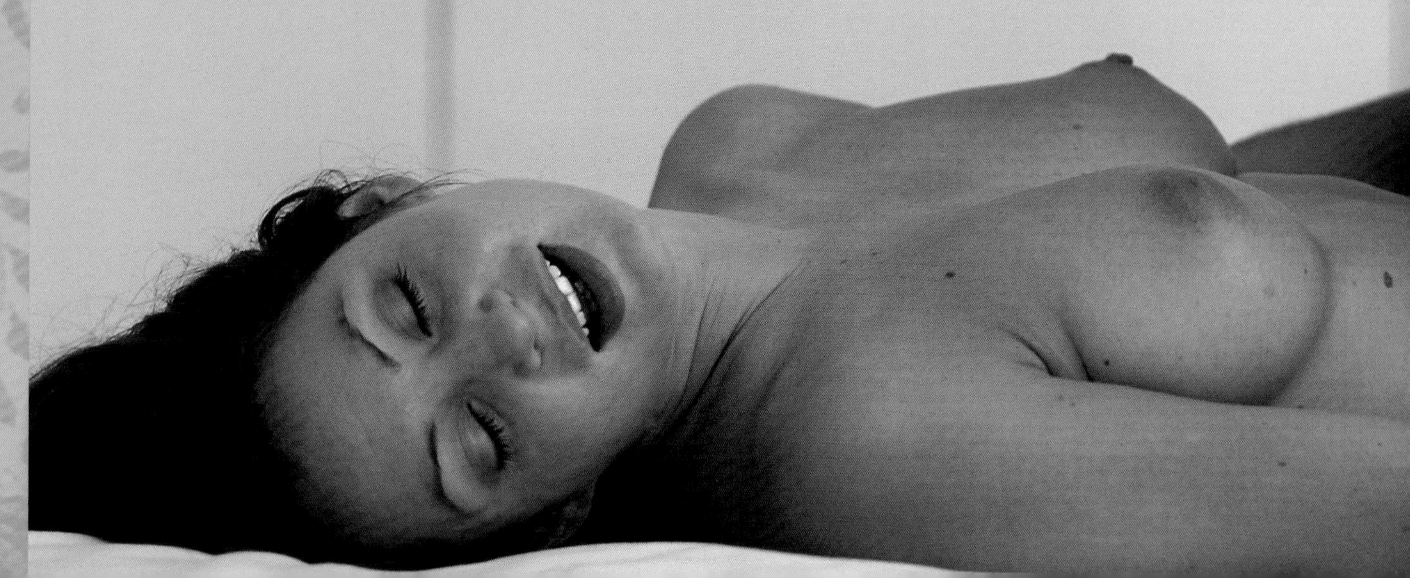

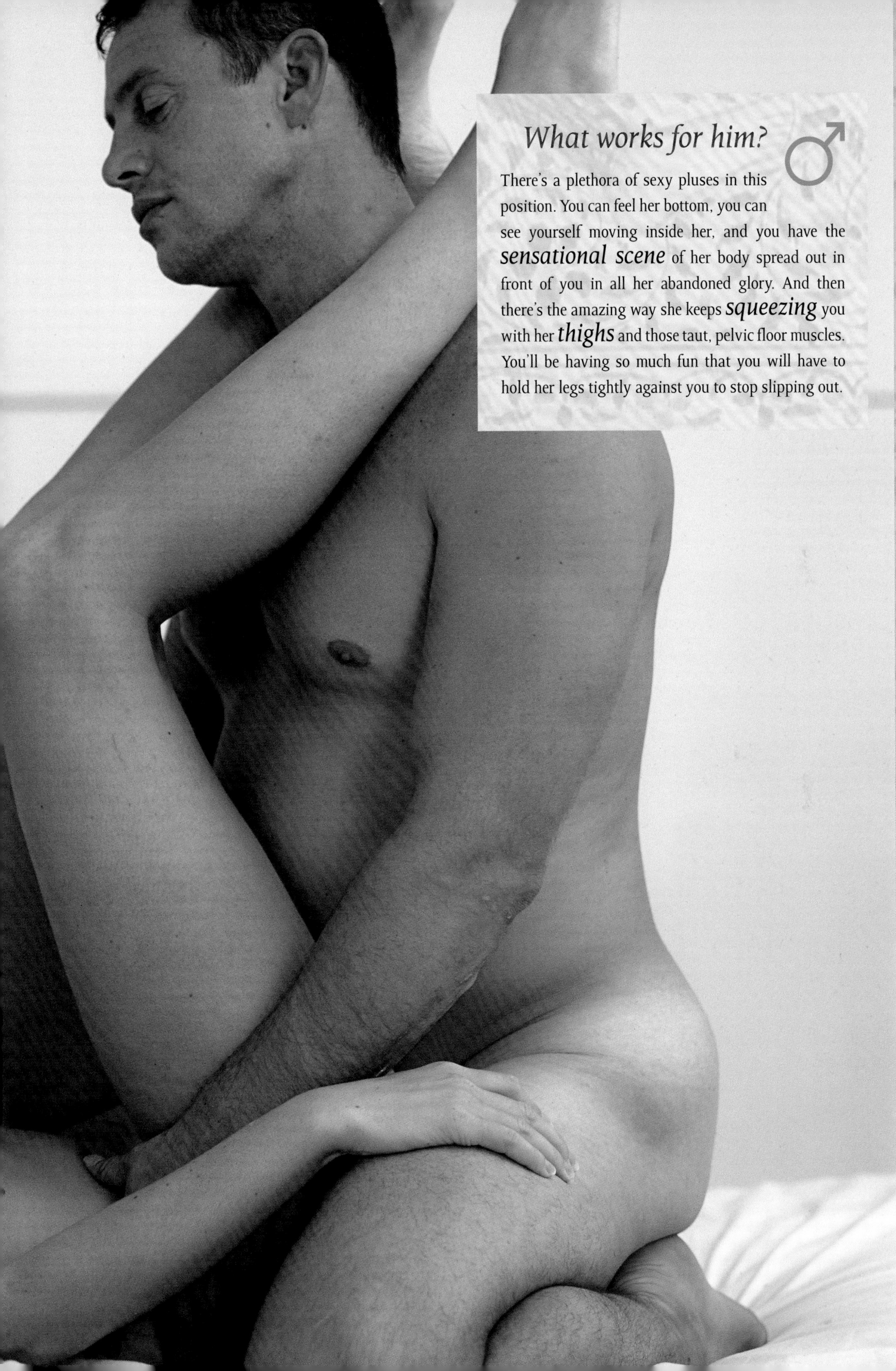

What works for him? ♂

There's a plethora of sexy pluses in this position. You can feel her bottom, you can see yourself moving inside her, and you have the ***sensational scene*** of her body spread out in front of you in all her abandoned glory. And then there's the amazing way she keeps ***squeezing*** you with her ***thighs*** and those taut, pelvic floor muscles. You'll be having so much fun that you will have to hold her legs tightly against you to stop slipping out.

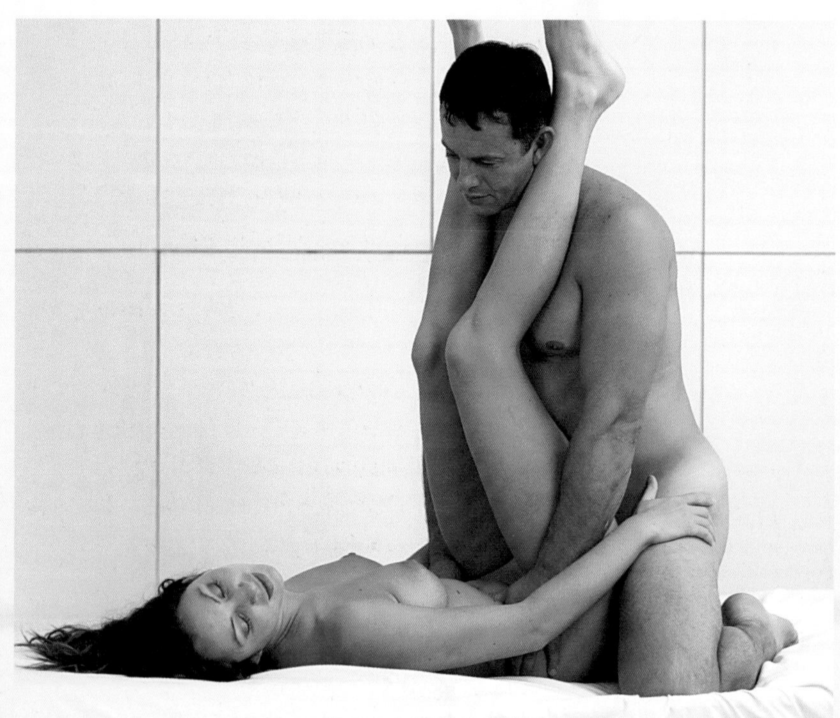

< LITTLE VARIATIONS *can make a big difference in this position, so try holding his thighs to steer his movements so that the angle is right for you. Intensify the pressure on his penis by pushing the backs of your legs against his shoulders, while squeezing his penis with your thighs. You can always treat him to a view of your hands tweaking your nipples or reaching farther south to manually enhance your pleasure.*

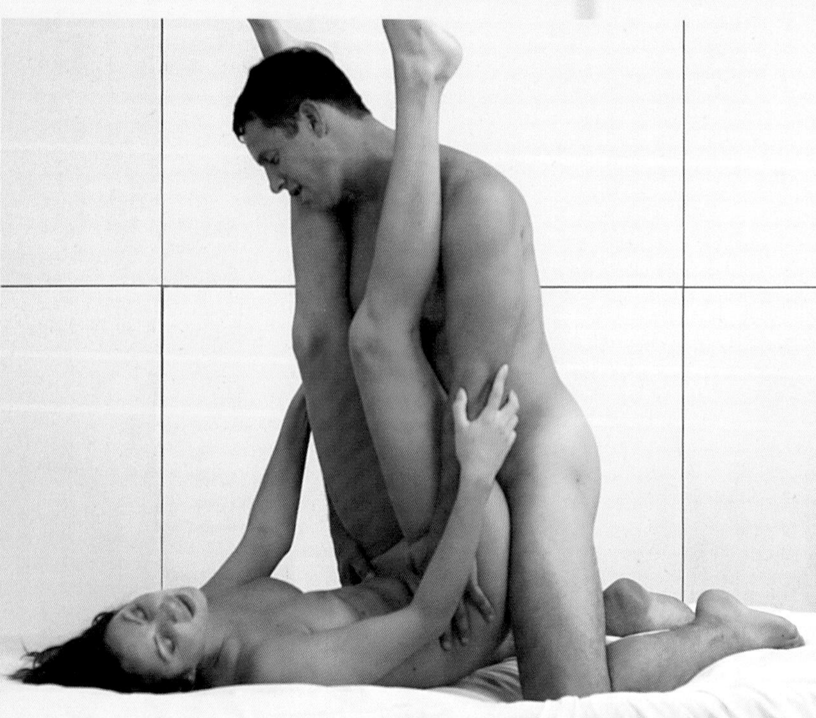

< TREAT HIM *like a climbing frame. Hold onto those manly arms and pull yourself up to get the required angle (but take care not to hurt your lower back). Make sure he's got a tight grip on your hips. There's only one word of warning here: Because he can move directly inside your vagina at this angle, he needs to make sure that he doesn't jar your cervix. Arousal is everything; when you're verging on orgasmic meltdown, let him know that it's all right to thrust wildly.*

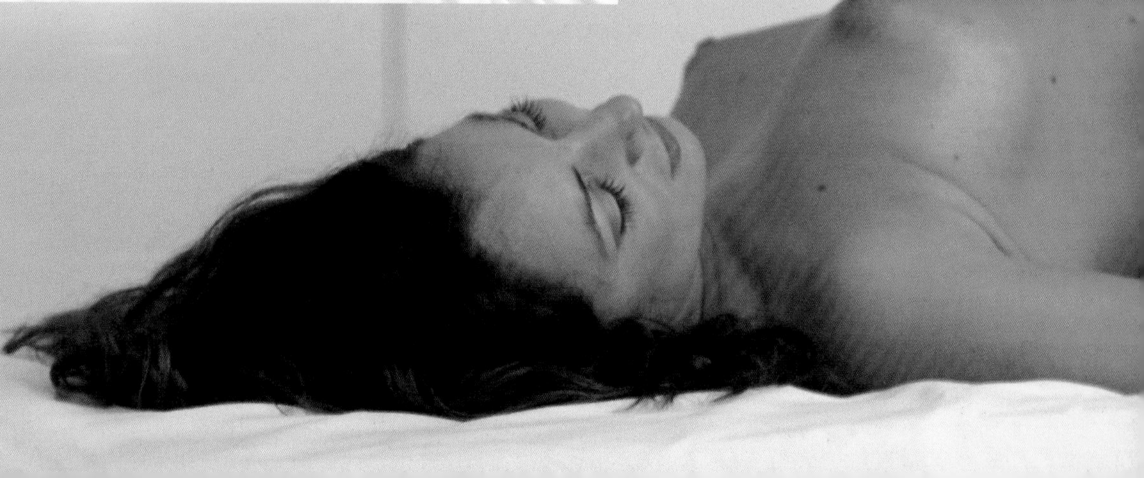

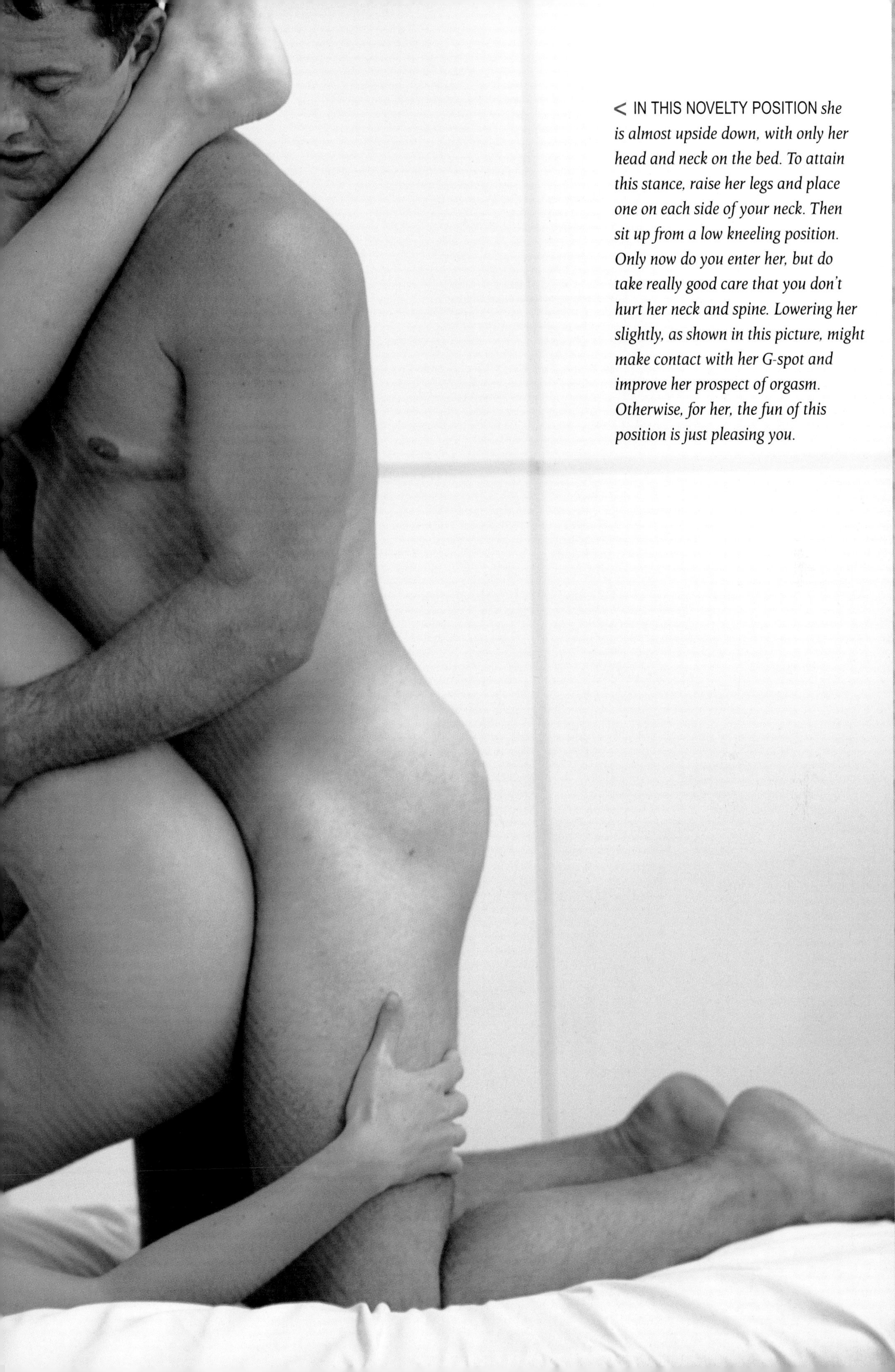

< IN THIS NOVELTY POSITION *she is almost upside down, with only her head and neck on the bed. To attain this stance, raise her legs and place one on each side of your neck. Then sit up from a low kneeling position. Only now do you enter her, but do take really good care that you don't hurt her neck and spine. Lowering her slightly, as shown in this picture, might make contact with her G-spot and improve her prospect of orgasm. Otherwise, for her, the fun of this position is just pleasing you.*

Splitting position

These legs-together positions all share an abandoned, "legs in the air" quality that makes them appealing for lovers who want to try different sensations and angles of penetration while still facing each other. For the man there is the satisfaction of manipulating the woman's body, while the woman, when completely aroused, will enjoy the depth of penetration. And the element of helpless passivity inherent in splitting positions can be passionately erotic. They follow naturally from the Open sequence, based on the Yawning and Widely Opened positions.

> THIS ANGLE *feels great for her as she drapes her legs across you while you are penetrating her vagina and touching her clitoris. You can watch her pleasure and she can watch yours (until, that is, she becomes ecstatically absorbed in her own orgasmic sensations). This is the position for her if she likes to be watched, rather than covered. Move her legs across to the other side to vary the sensations.*

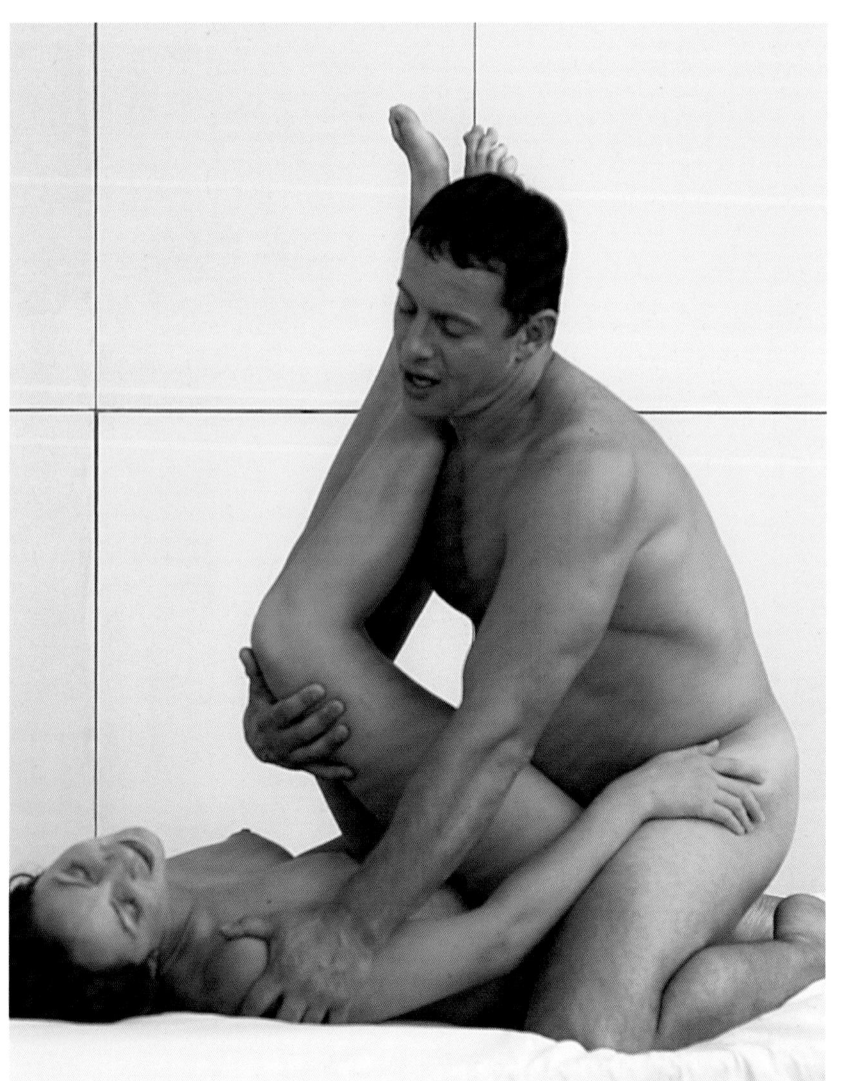

< LYING ON HER BACK, *she draws her knees up while he enters her from a kneeling position. He then lifts her legs straight up and rests them on his shoulder. Make sure you've got her into a state of complete arousal before entering, as penetration will be deep and her vagina needs to open widely to accommodate you. Keep eye contact and caress those legs. She'll love your hands roaming along her thighs, an often-neglected area that's super-sensitive.*

> HE LOVES LOOKING *at how much pleasure he's giving you, and the fact that you've given him control to move your legs around. In this position, you're clasping him not only with your vagina (it's time to make those pelvic floor muscles flutter) but also with your thighs. This maximizes the swiveling sensation around his penis, and adds to your pleasure by stimulating the front wall and sides of your vagina—yes, G-spot territory.*

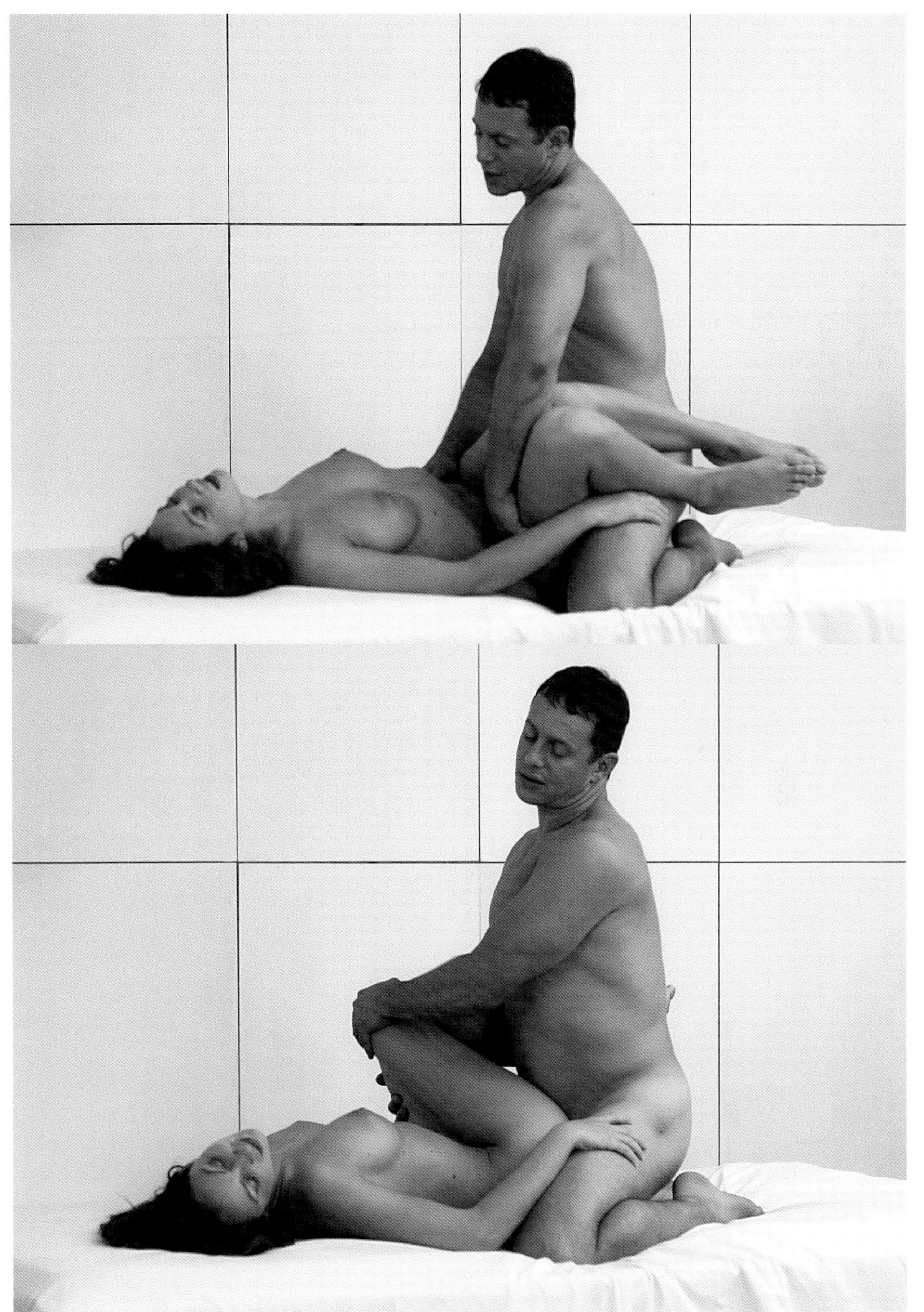

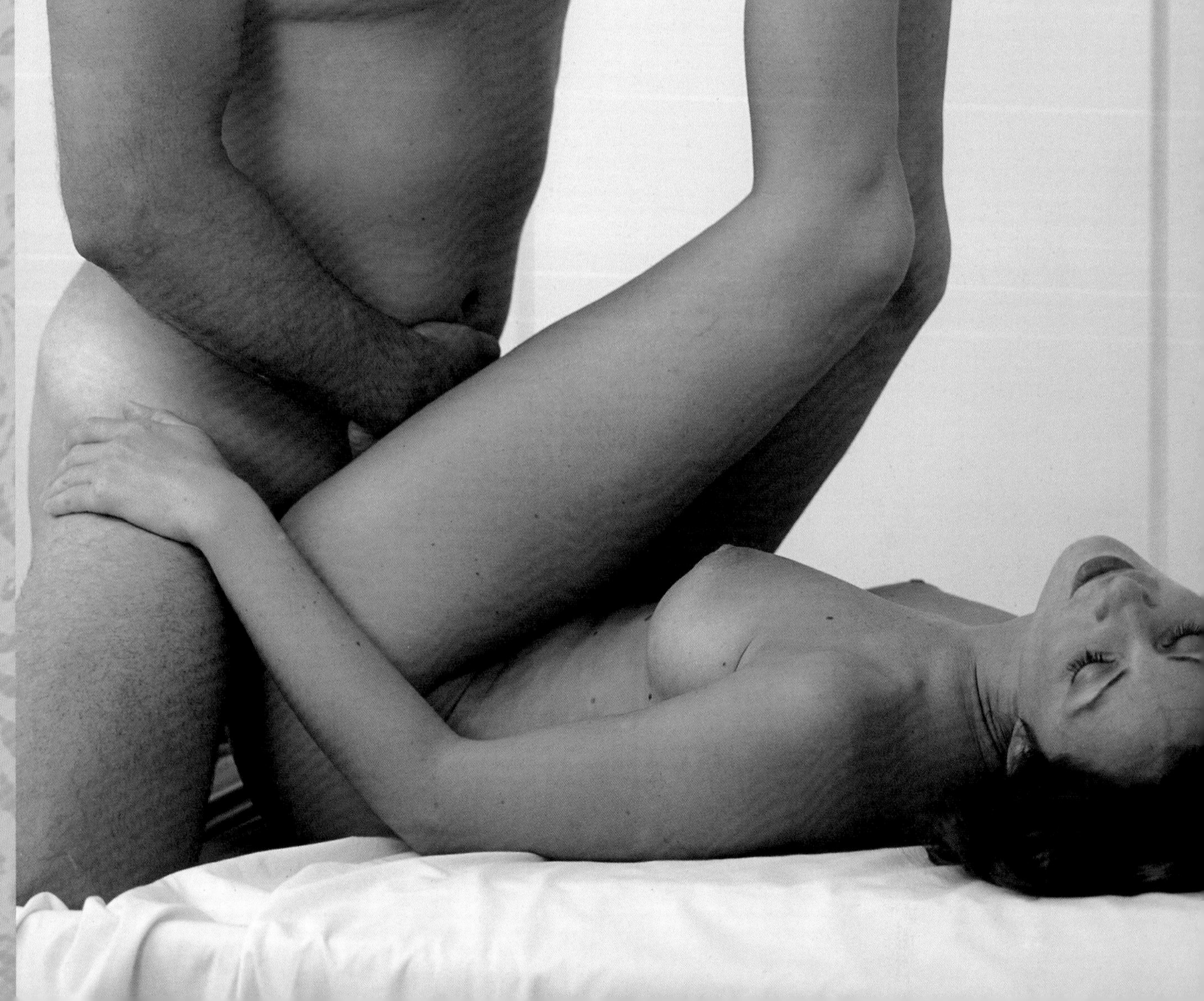

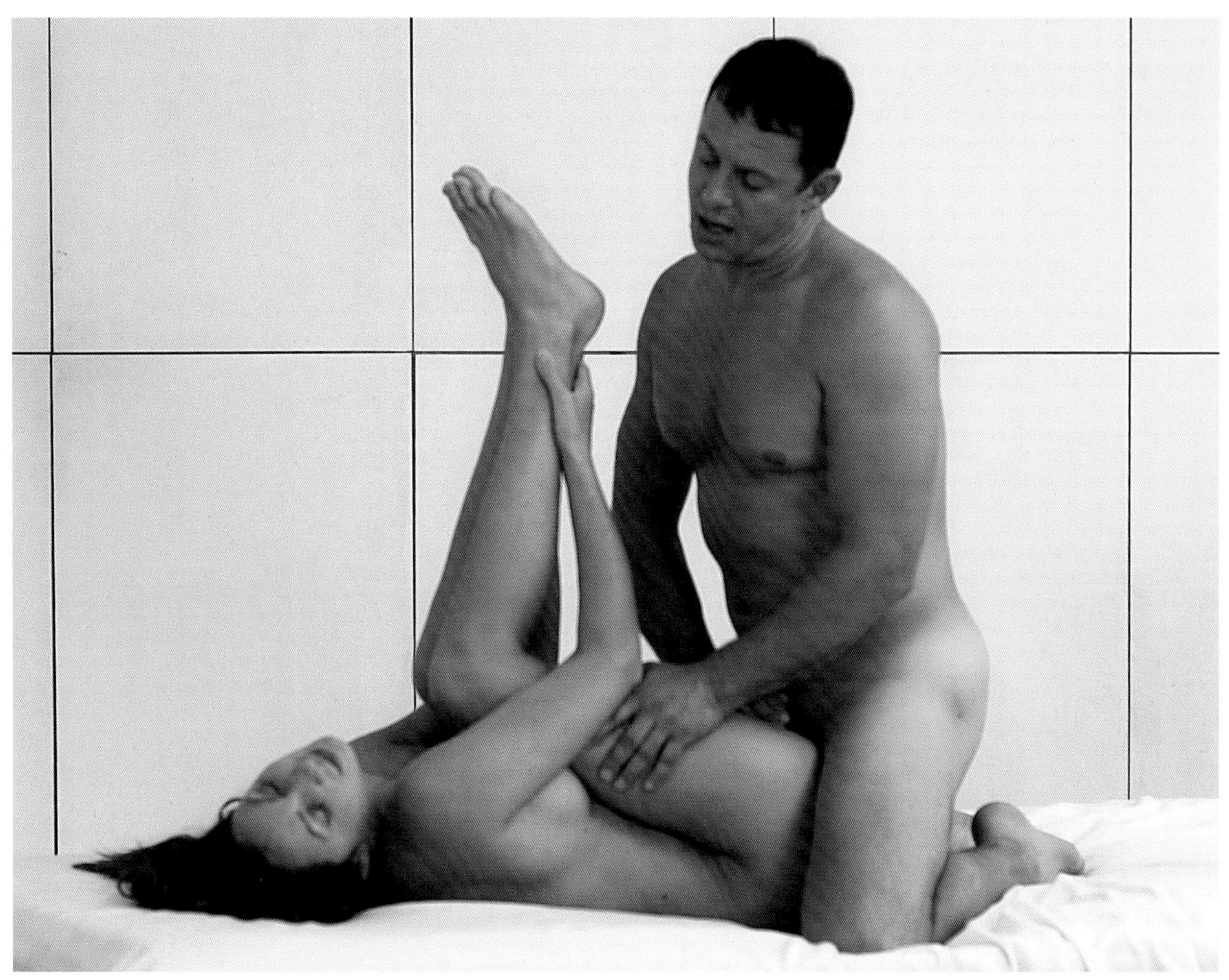

What works for him?

You can feel dominant without losing eye contact. Her legs are in easy reach for caressing, which she'll find sensual. But the biggest turn on of this position is the **swiveling sensation** around your penis, which is nothing short of mind-blowing. Older men, who may need plenty of friction to help them to orgasm, appreciate the **snug grip** of their partner's thighs and vagina and the stronger sensations this arouses.

< IN THIS VARIATION *you hold her legs away from your body, as this alters the angle of penetration yet again. She may find that it's easier to grip her thighs together and hold you ever tighter. But bear in mind that this is not the most comfortable position for her to hold for any length of time.*

^ THE KAMA SUTRA *has many references to the penis being used like a dildo, which can be enormously arousing. Tell her she is in command and must direct your member to pleasure her in any way she pleases!*

If the sight of your legs drives him wild, then this is the position to **show them off** (and they'll get the attention they deserve, especially the super-sensitive backs of your thighs). You can use his penis as a dildo and, once you've finished **amusing** yourself, enjoy the depth of penetration. Then add the fact that your thighs and vagina are causing him to experience new **levels of ecstasy** as they swirl around his penis.

What works for her?

> THIS VARIATION *has her pinned to the bed and lying on her side while you hold one of her legs across your body. You'll both enjoy the different angle of penetration. If you're engaged in role playing, the helpless abandonment that this acrobatic pose engenders can be intensely erotic for both of you. You also have a bird's-eye view of her and can experience the overtly sexual scene of your penis moving inside her. Her breasts will respond to your vigorous, rhythmical thrusting by moving in an equally rhythmical way—an incredibly erotic sight.*

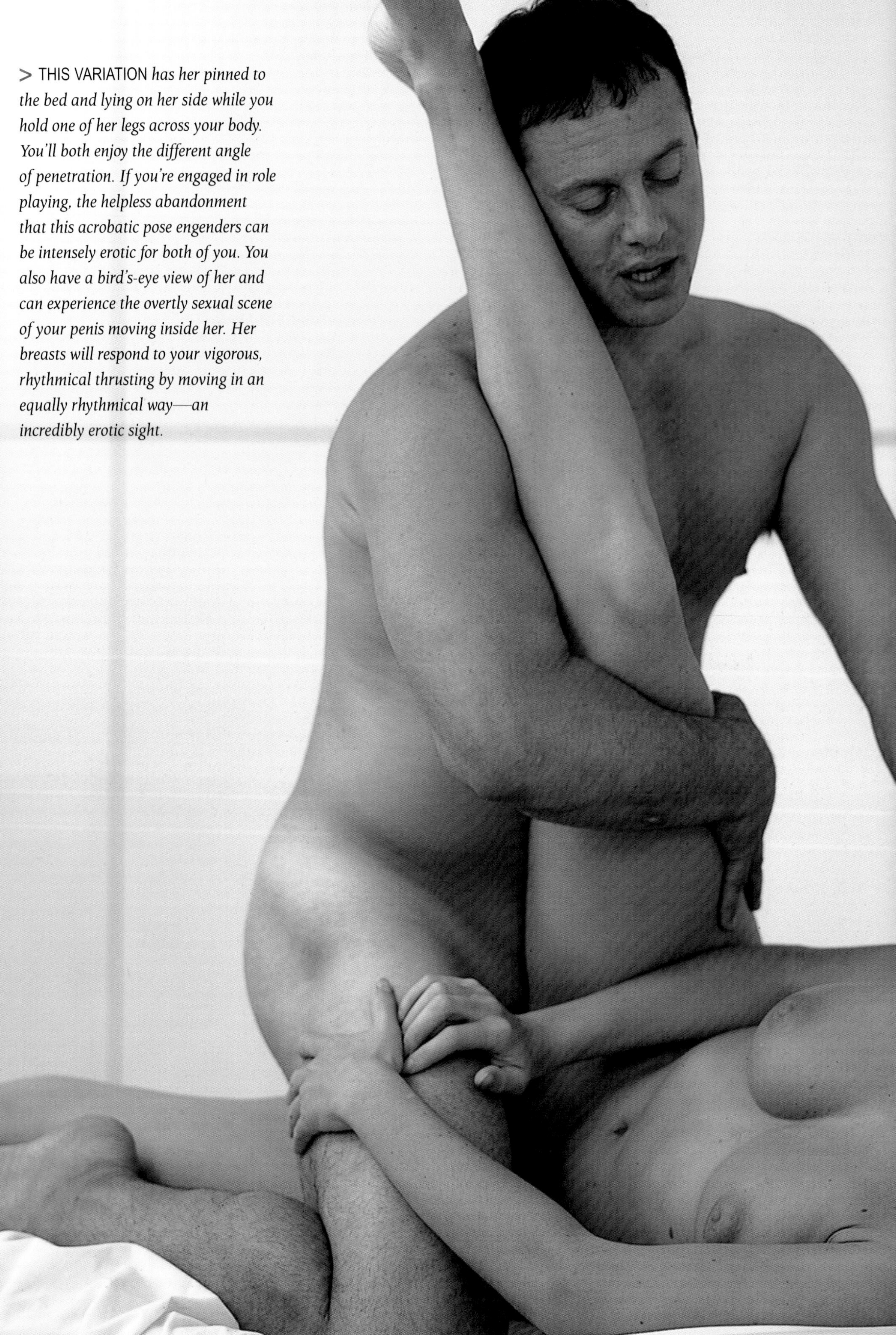

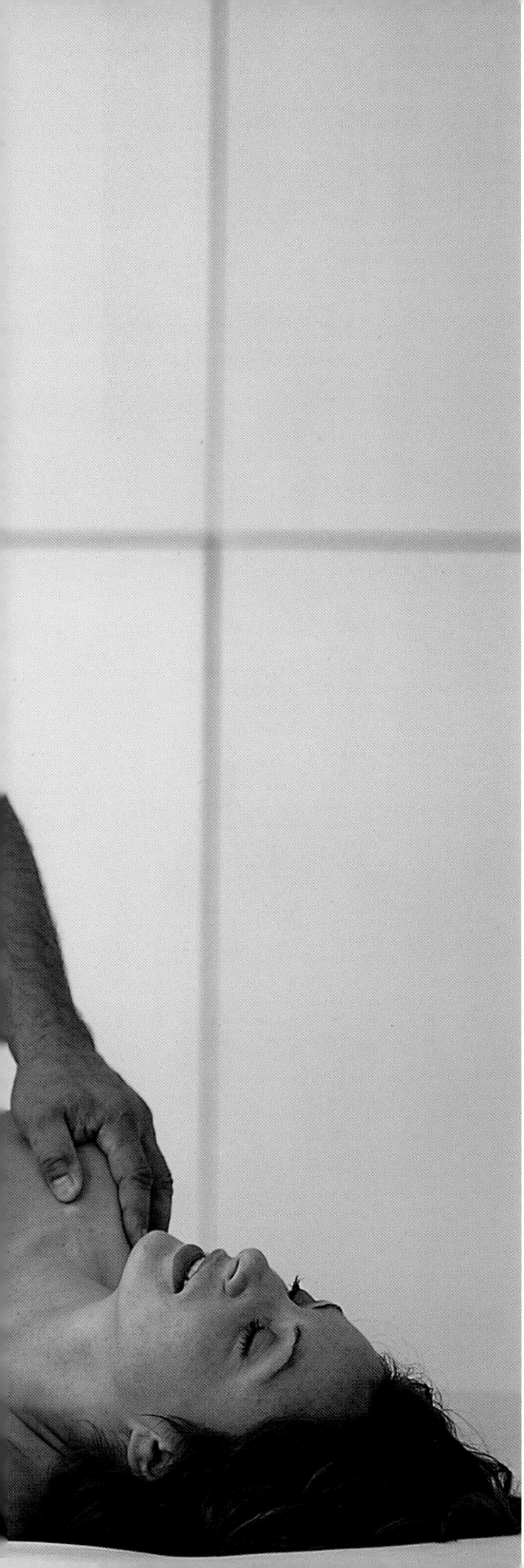

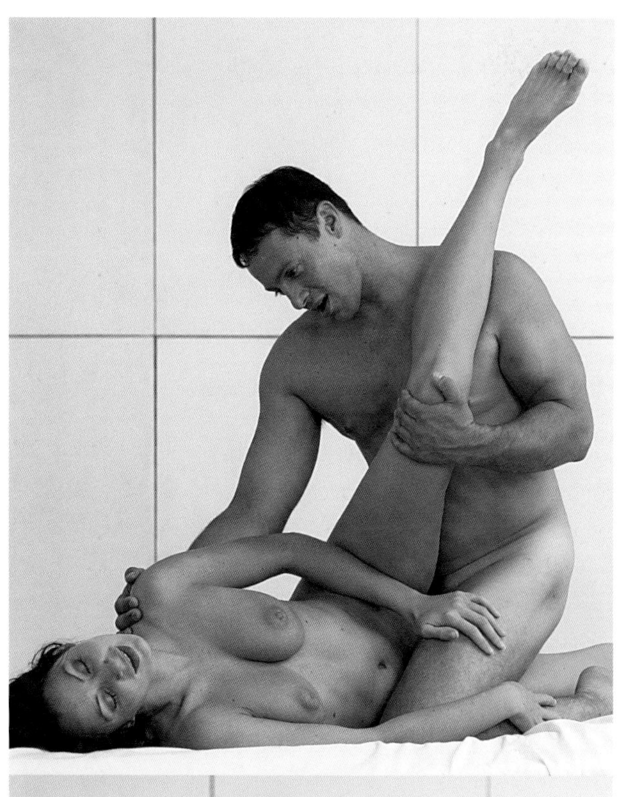

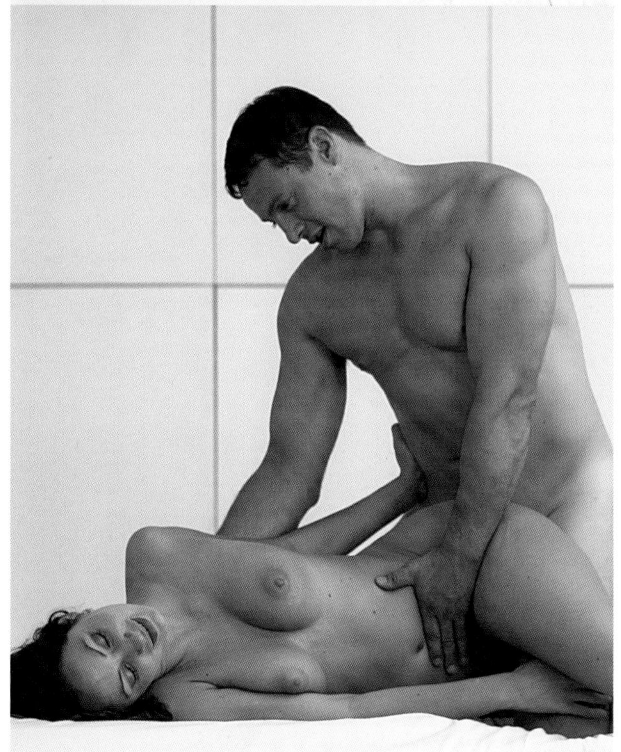

∧ THIS SPLITTING POSITION *can be part of a sequence that takes you both into the Elephant position (*see *pg. 142). This shows that you can move between positions without breaking apart (which can easily ruin the mood). Add spice by making your legs a real feature for him, and put on stockings, garters, and stiletto heels.*

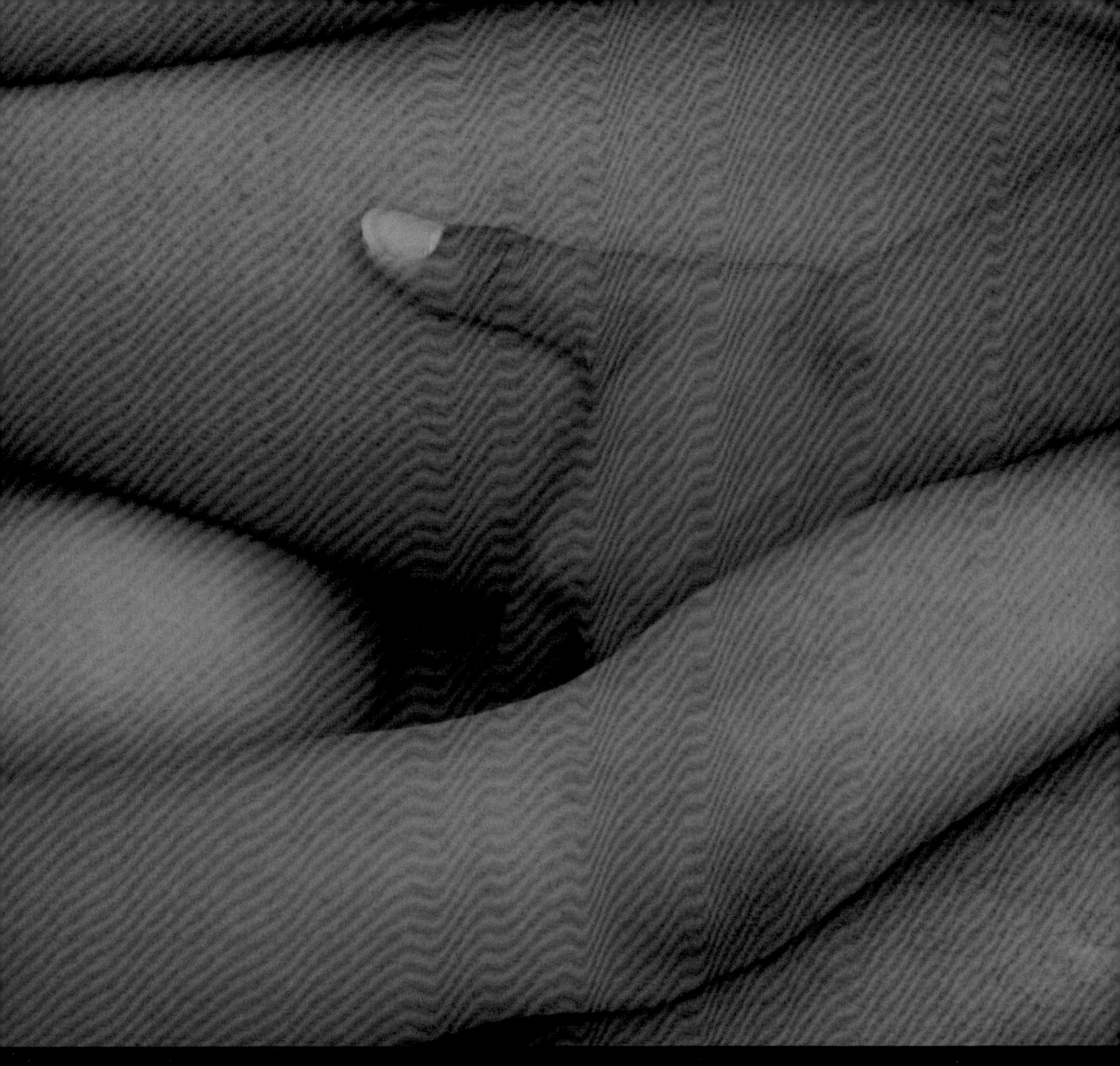

"When the legs are contracted, and thus held by the lover before his bosom, it is called the Pressed position."
KSII:VI

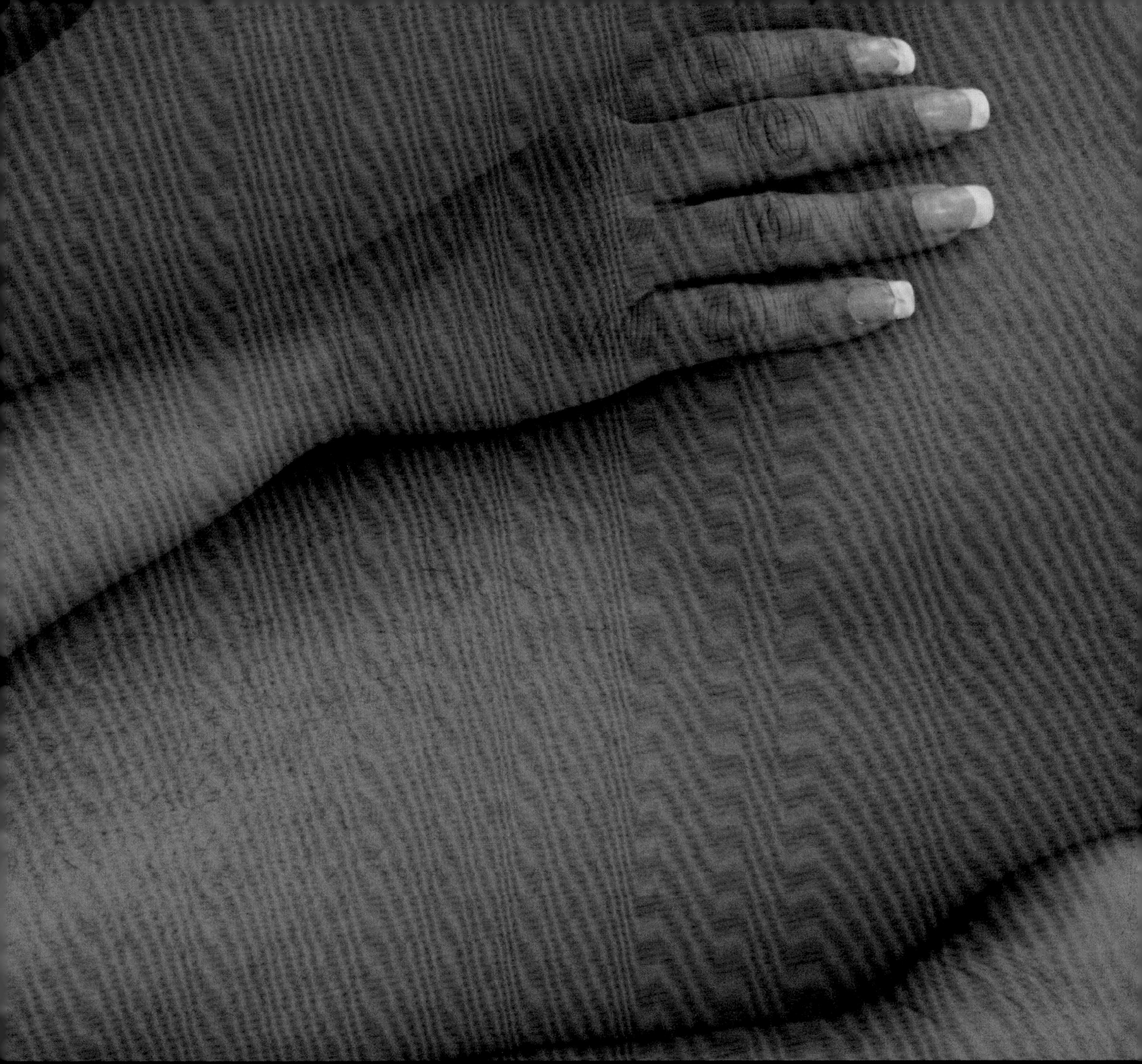

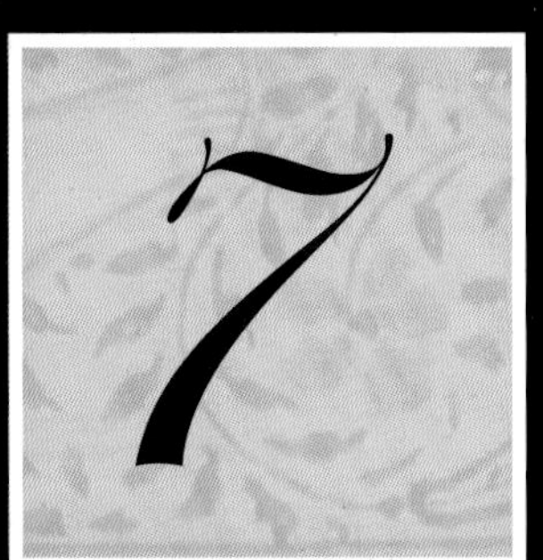

PRESSED POSITIONS

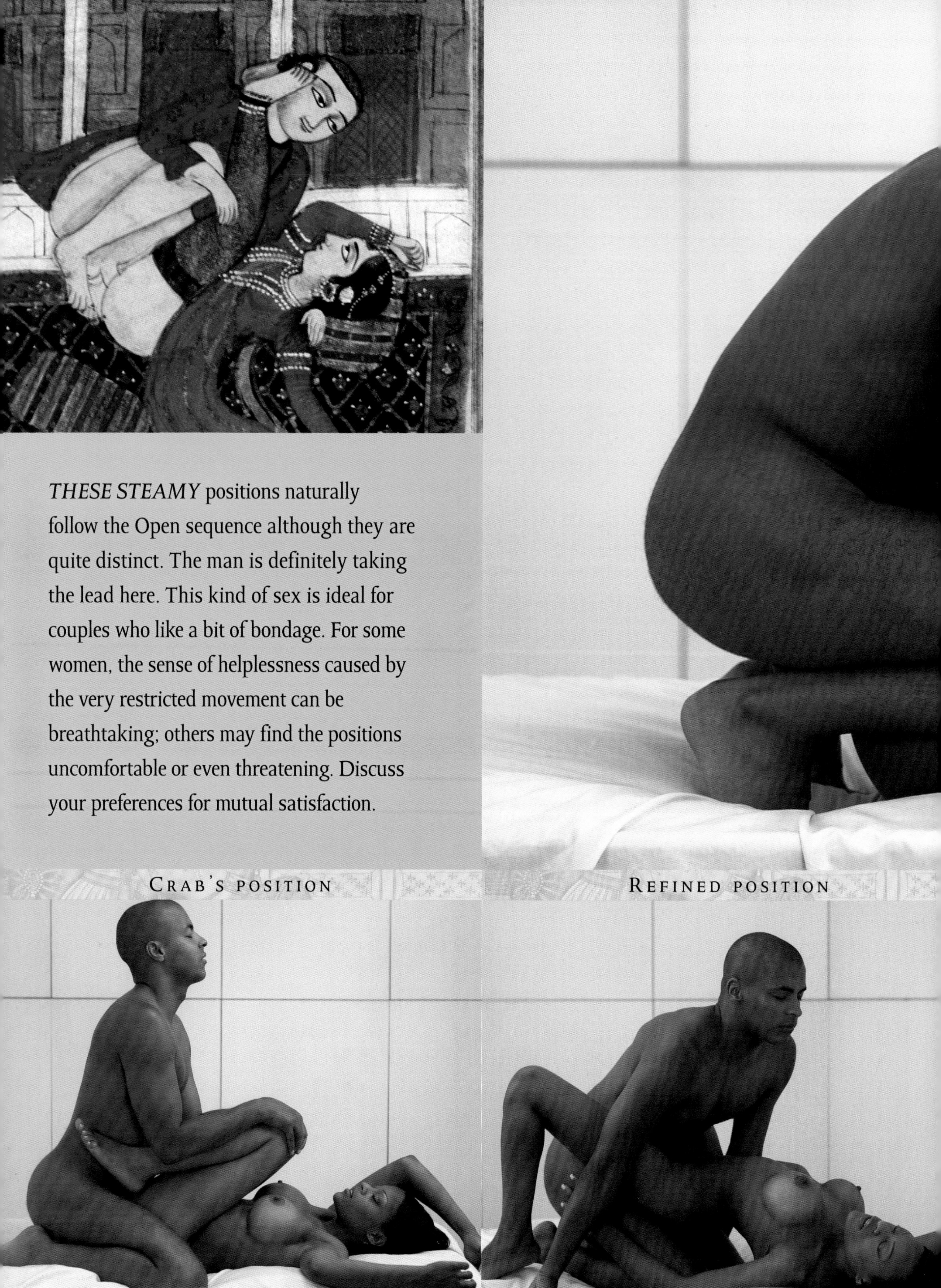

THESE STEAMY positions naturally follow the Open sequence although they are quite distinct. The man is definitely taking the lead here. This kind of sex is ideal for couples who like a bit of bondage. For some women, the sense of helplessness caused by the very restricted movement can be breathtaking; others may find the positions uncomfortable or even threatening. Discuss your preferences for mutual satisfaction.

CRAB'S POSITION

REFINED POSITION

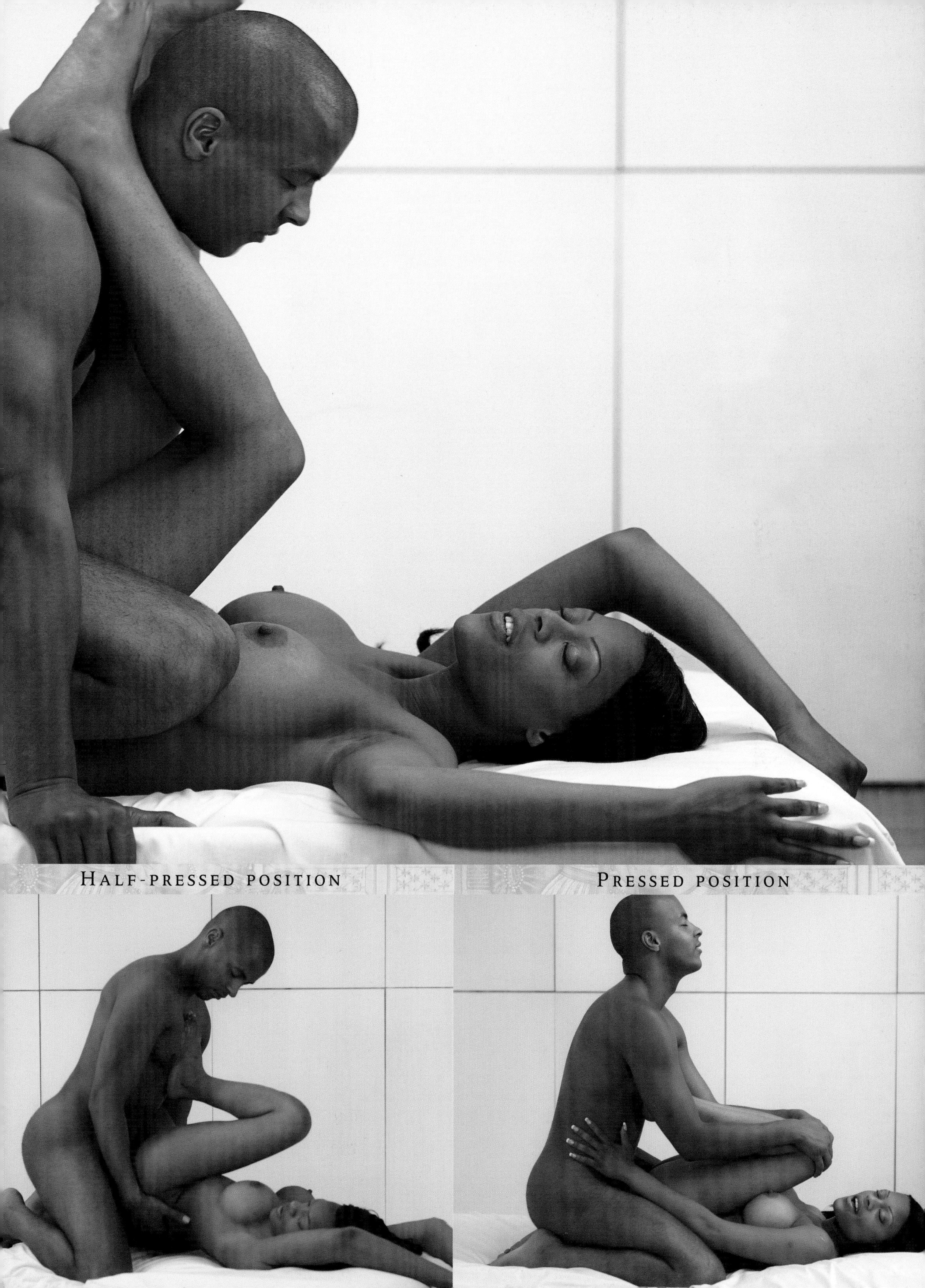

Half-pressed position

Pressed position

Crab's position

The Kama Sutra says: "When both the legs of the woman are contracted, and placed on her stomach, it is called the Crab's position." It is also known as the Intact position. Start with the open-legged position (below), a natural progression from the Yawning position, before moving on to the bent-leg position (right). Being able to look at one another maintains intimacy, but the dominance of the man's role makes these perfect for when you feel like spicing things up and getting a little bit rough . . .

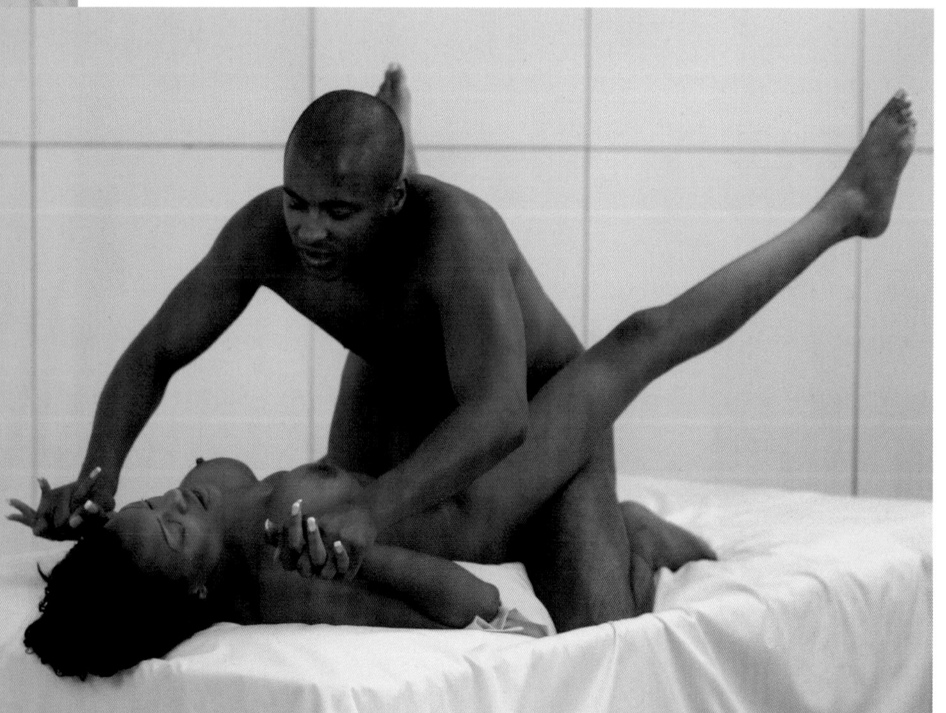

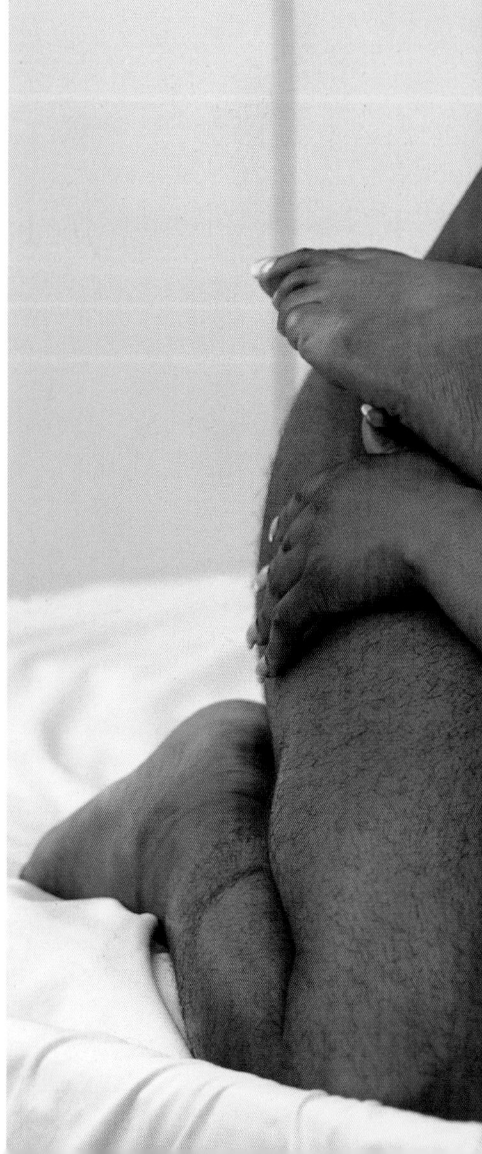

∧ FROM THE YAWNING *position, hold your lover's hands so she can't move as freely as before. This can be your signal that you want to move into more bondage play. If she is up for it, she can easily signal her willingness to comply by moving her legs close to her body to adopt the submissive Crab's position. However, be prepared for her to reject your proposition!*

> TAKE THIS ONE SLOWLY. *For some women exploring the Crab's position for the first time, the penetration may prove too deep. Hold and caress one another's legs to bring you fantastically in tune in your movements as well as to make penetration even deeper. Press your chest as close to her shins as possible. Take full advantage of the accessibility of her breasts.*

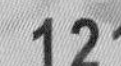

What works for him? ♂

This is a real ***ego booster*** because you are totally in control and able to dominate. It feels superb because the vaginal muscles are ***tighter*** than in other positions. Make sure your partner is comfortable and fully aroused, then benefit by watching every ***pleasurable*** change brought about—by you—in her facial expressions.

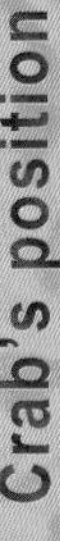

To start with, he's doing most of the work and you're getting a massive amount of the **pleasure!** As long as there is complete trust between you and your partner, this can be a truly **thrilling** experience. In this position, the **intense** erotic satisfaction gained from tensing and releasing your vaginal muscles is even stronger than usual—with your legs drawn this **close** to your body the vaginal muscles have no choice but to contract more deeply, leading to **even greater arousal**. Penetration is **deep** but, although you are underneath, the position is not out of your control.

What works for her? ♀

V MEN, USE YOUR WEIGHT *to add to the intensity of the experience—but if you're on the heavy side be very careful not to press down too hard. Use a pillow to make sure your partner's back isn't under any strain. When she is aroused, all areas around the pelvis, especially the thighs and buttocks, fill with sexual tension. The Crab's position is perfect for building this tension up to the screaming point. Tease her by holding off from penetration until she's really desperate for it. Use your penis to turn her on before entering her. Rub it against her clitoris and the insides of her thighs. If your partner still isn't aroused enough to allow penetration, make sure she stays in this position while you move downward for oral sex—the position of her legs, particularly if held firmly in place, will make the experience even more mind-blowing. When she's fully aroused, move back into position and start taking control.*

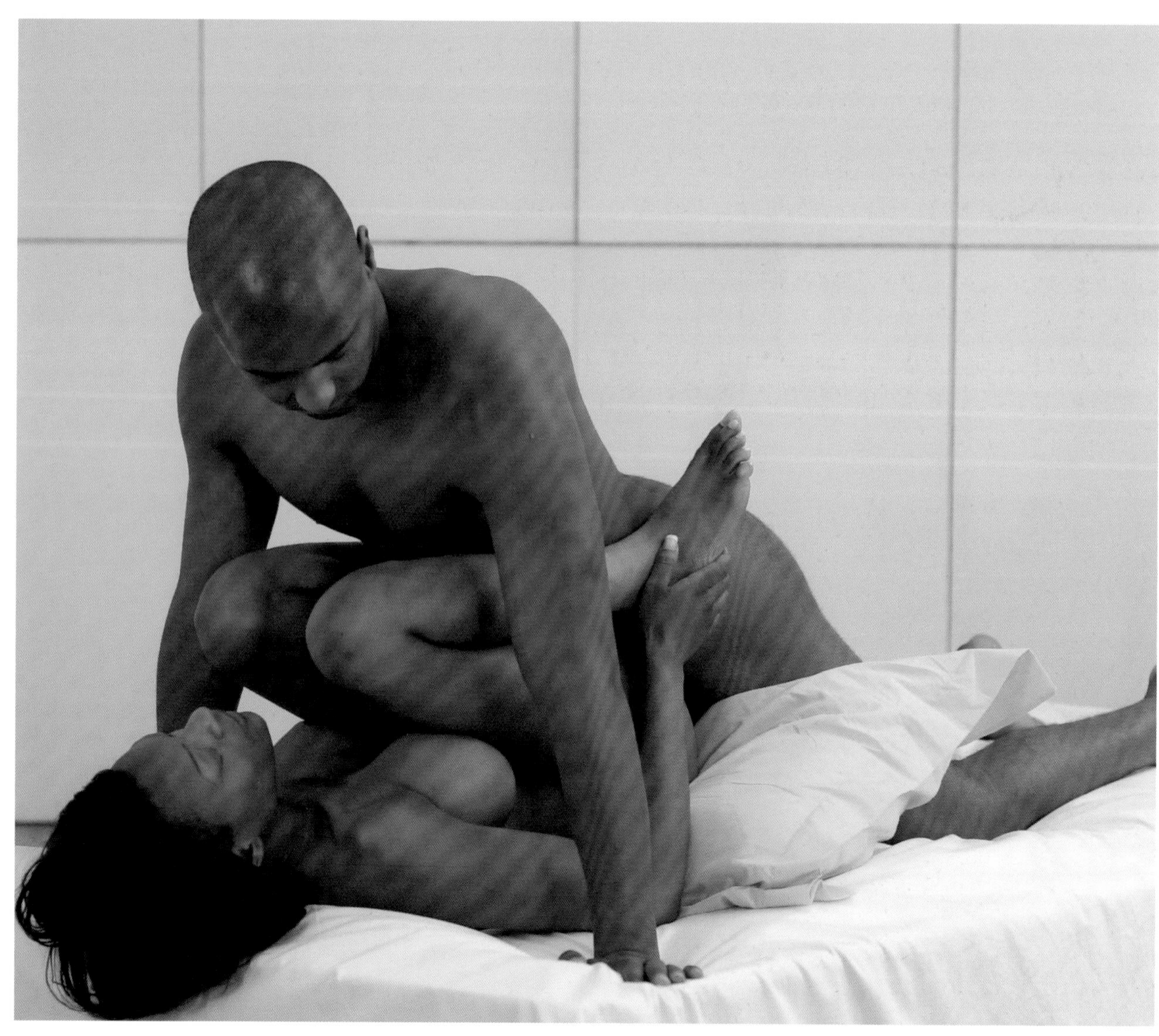

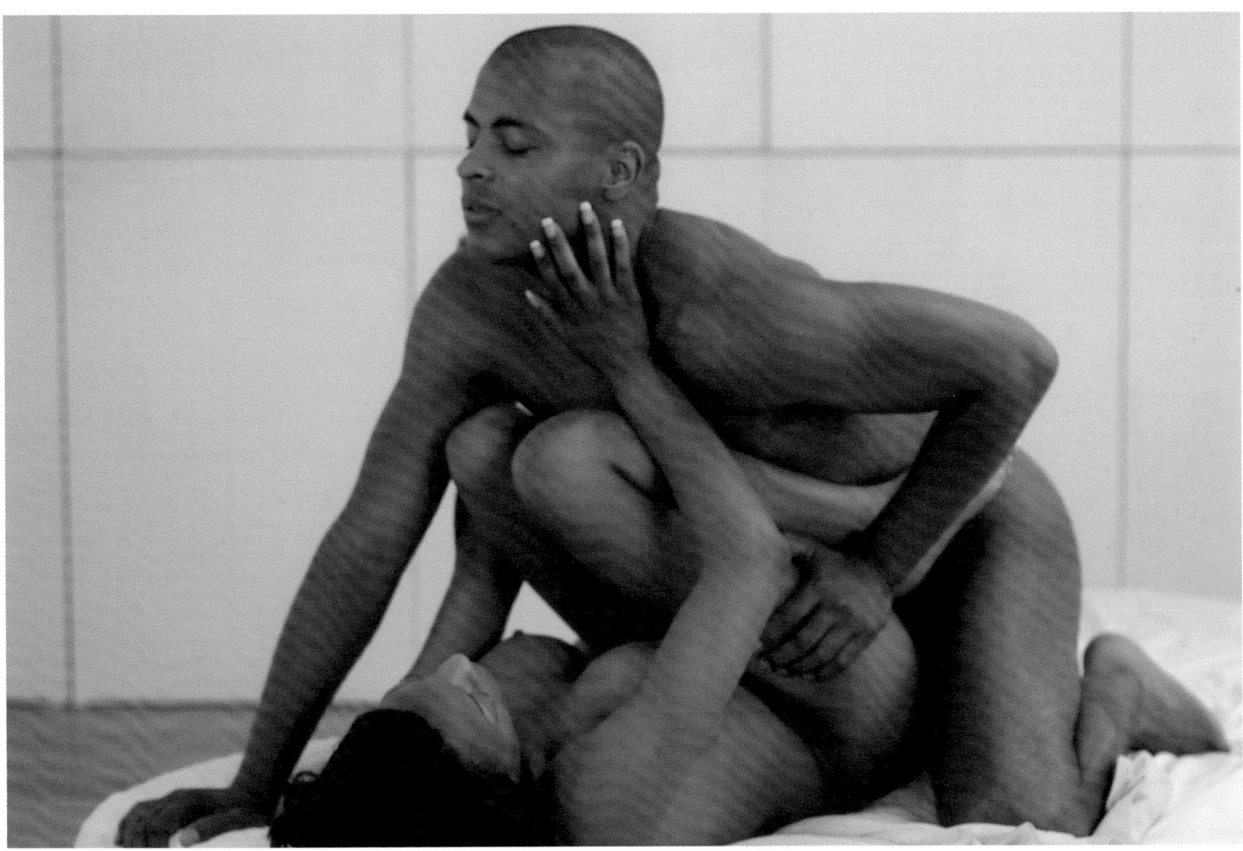

∧ DON'T LET YOUR MAN *feel he's doing all the work. Keep touching him: stroke his face, neck, ears, biceps, forearms, and anything else within range! If you're not comfortable with being submissive, tell him where to touch you and how fast or slow you want him to move.*

∨ OK, NOW YOU'VE *seriously got her attention. Do this one right and she is never going to let you go! This position requires complete trust on the part of the woman, so the reassuringly close eye and face contact are important. Whisper to her to increase the intimacy.*

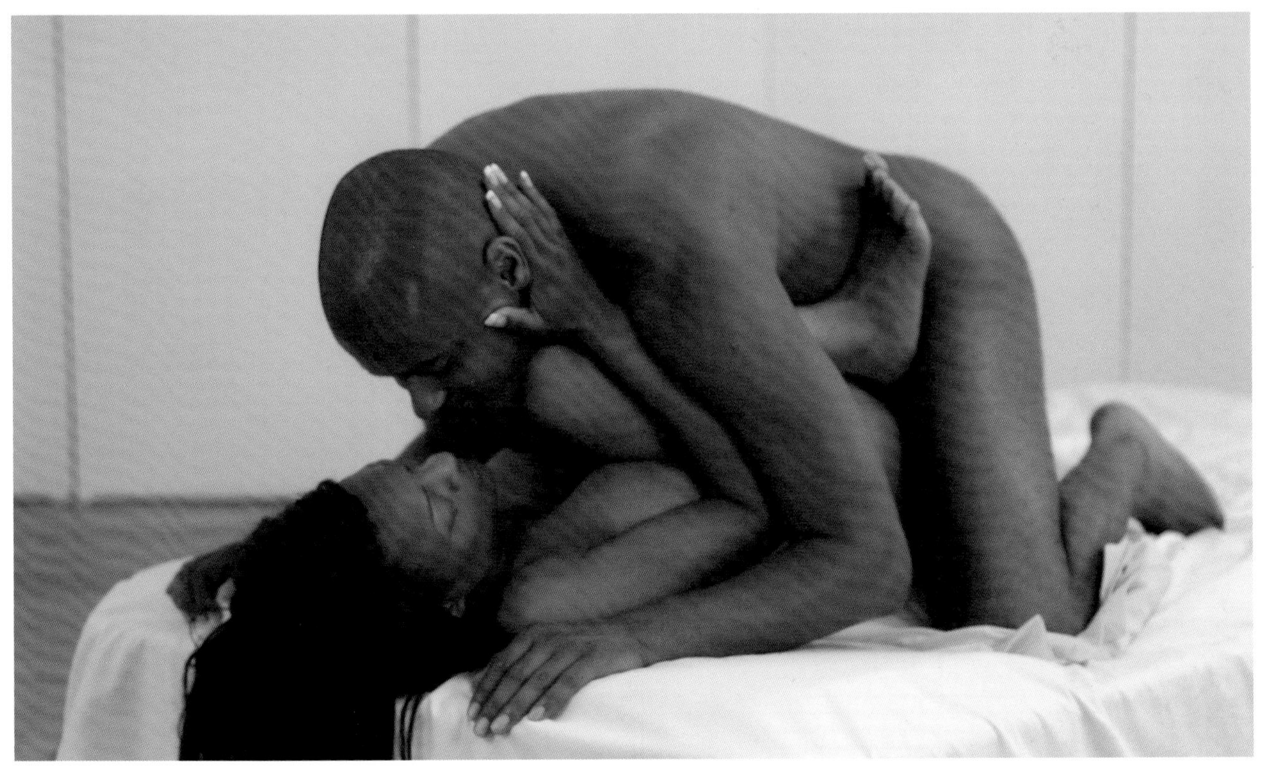

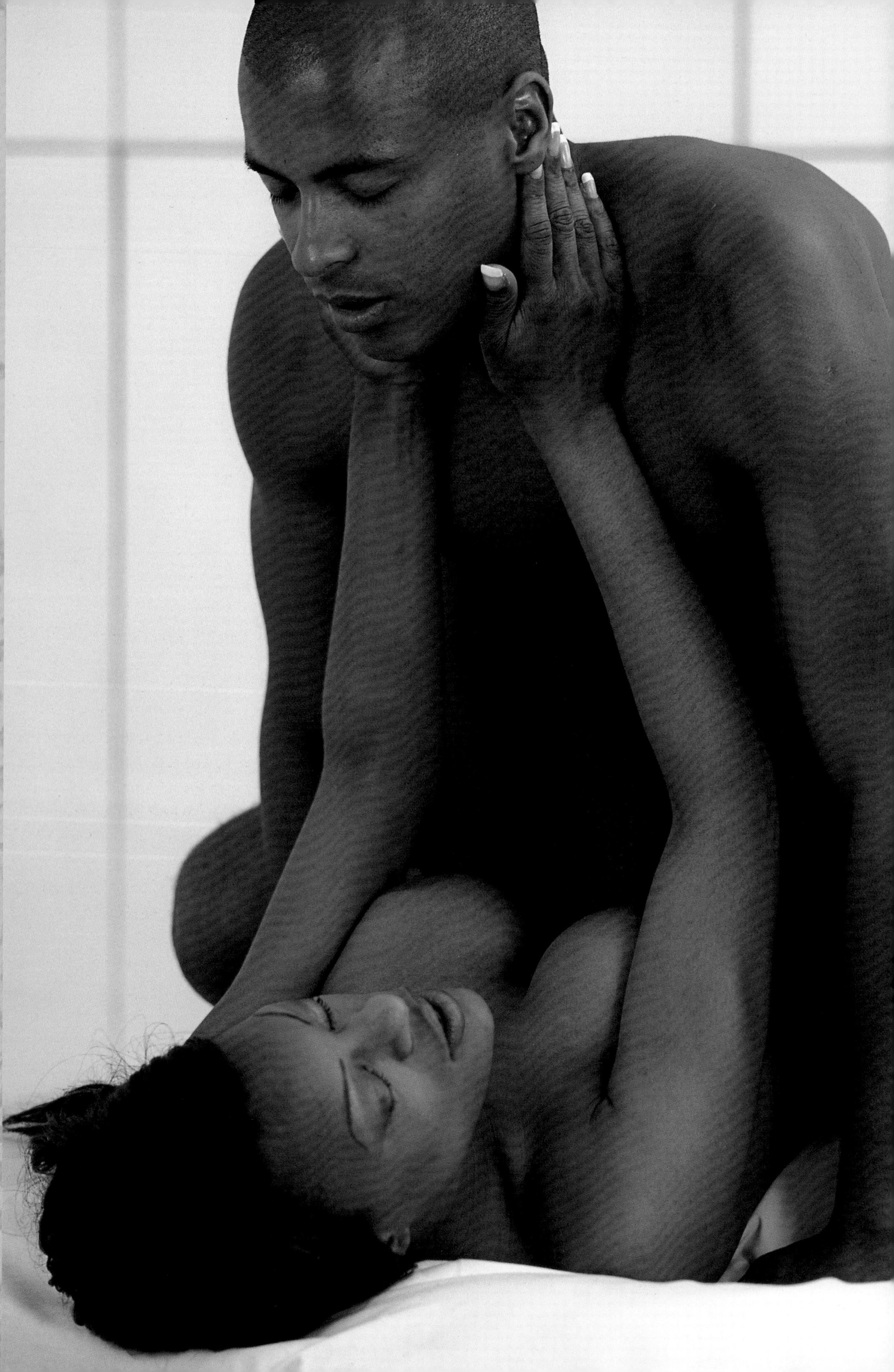

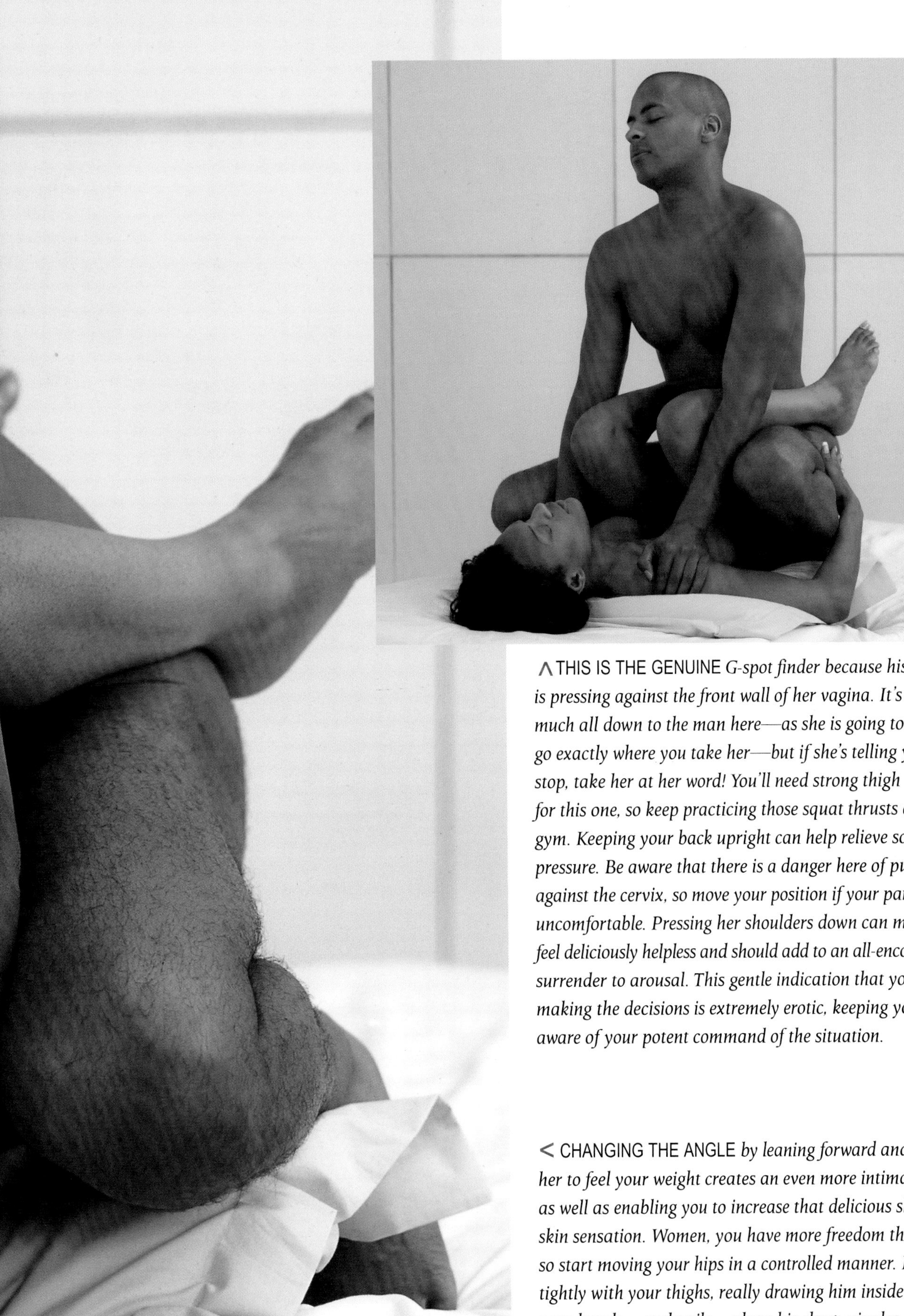

∧ THIS IS THE GENUINE *G-spot finder because his penis is pressing against the front wall of her vagina. It's pretty much all down to the man here—as she is going to have to go exactly where you take her—but if she's telling you not to stop, take her at her word! You'll need strong thigh muscles for this one, so keep practicing those squat thrusts at the gym. Keeping your back upright can help relieve some of the pressure. Be aware that there is a danger here of pushing against the cervix, so move your position if your partner feels uncomfortable. Pressing her shoulders down can make her feel deliciously helpless and should add to an all-encompassing surrender to arousal. This gentle indication that you are making the decisions is extremely erotic, keeping you well aware of your potent command of the situation.*

< CHANGING THE ANGLE *by leaning forward and allowing her to feel your weight creates an even more intimate bond, as well as enabling you to increase that delicious skin-on-skin sensation. Women, you have more freedom than before, so start moving your hips in a controlled manner. Hold him tightly with your thighs, really drawing him inside you. Run your hands—and nails—along his chest, nipples, shoulders, and neck. Tell him exactly how good this feels and be as loud as your walls allow.*

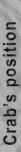

Wife of Indra

INDRANI IS THE WIFE OF INDRA, the Hindu god known as the King of the Heavens, and thus the potent deity of thunder and lightning. This complicated sexual act is named after the wife of Indra and it comes with a health warning that it is "learned only by practice." Here, the woman makes love while "placing her thighs with her legs doubled on them upon her sides." This is a position that is recommended for the deer woman because it widens her vagina in preparation for deeper penetration.

> A COURTESAN *who could "draw her legs as far back as her hair" was highly prized in Vatsyayana's day. This popular position appears frequently in Hindu paintings.*

V A WOMAN *would need to be very supple to maintain the Indrani position as described by Vatsyayana. Enjoy a simpler version by separating your thighs and drawing your knees up to your chest, thus exposing your vagina.*

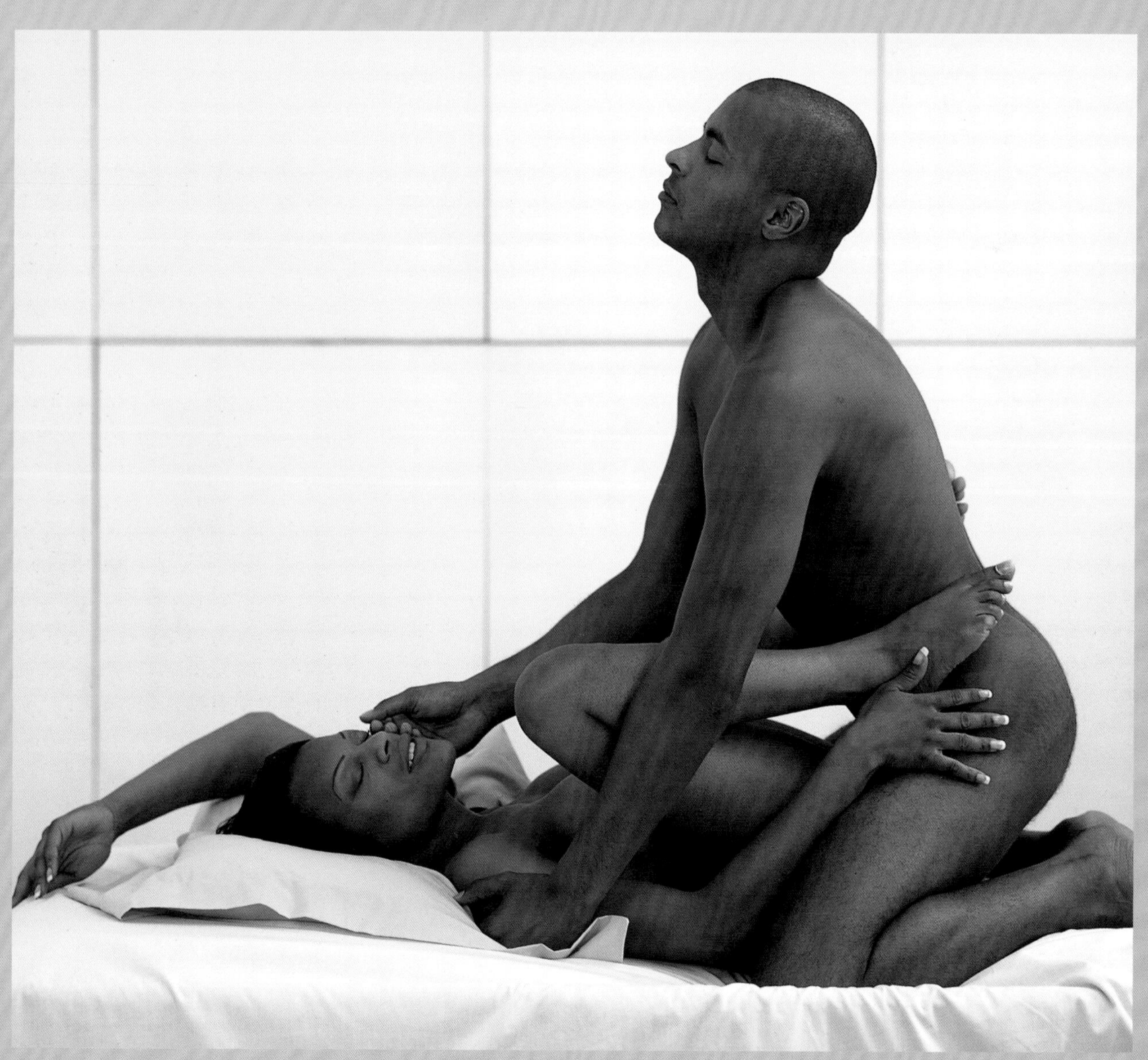

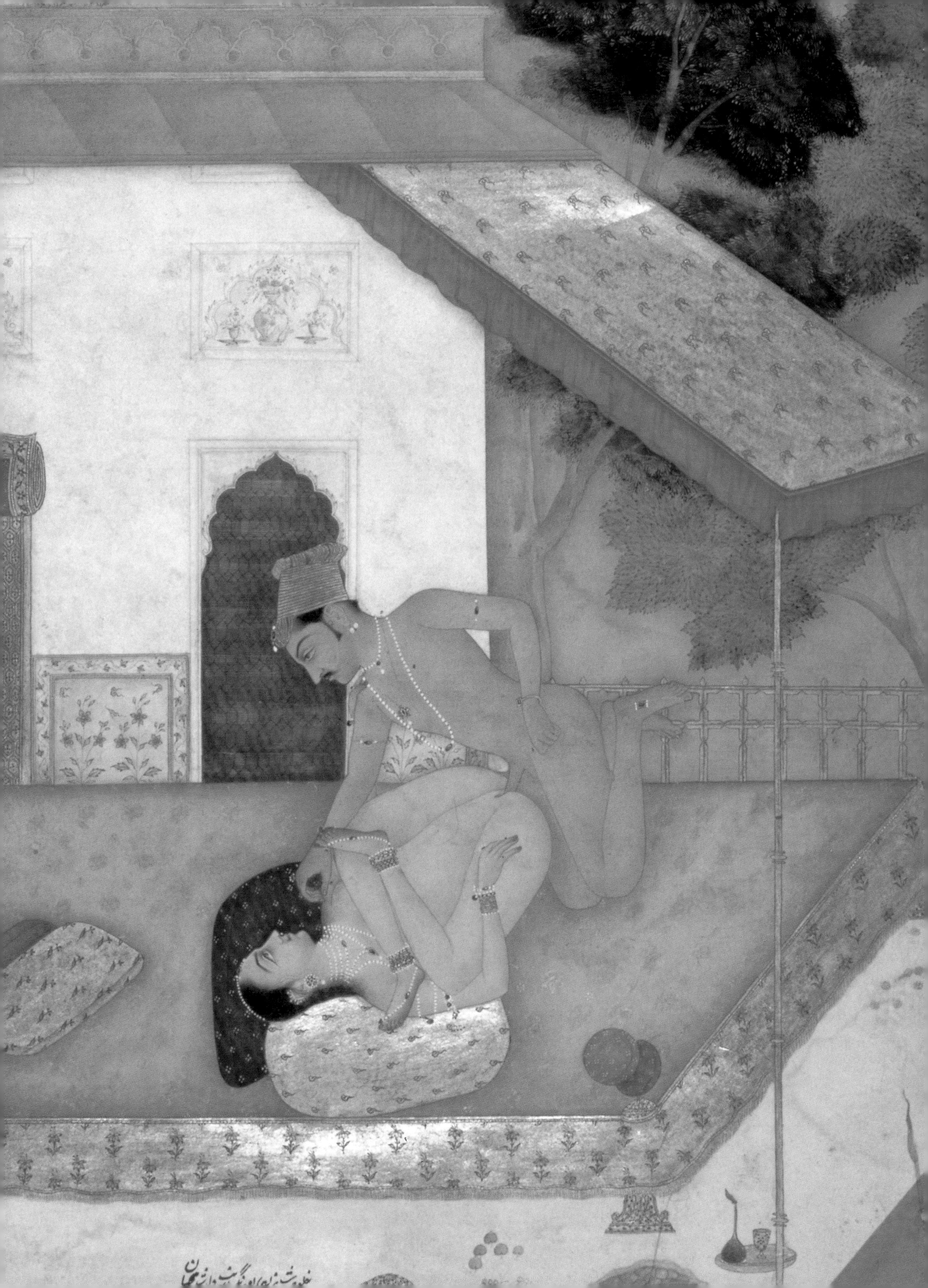

Lotus-like position

The Kama Sutra says: "When the shanks are placed one upon the other, it is called the Lotus-like position." This differs from the Crab's position because you cross your shins, as if you were sitting cross-legged in meditation. Moving into this position causes the hips to turn outwards, jutting your pelvis out at a slightly different angle. The Lotus-like position may be more comfortable for some women than the Crab's position, as it gives you more leverage to support your man's weight. It also enables you to start regaining some of the control.

> YOU NEED TO BE *extremely lithe to adopt this position. Support yourself by kneeling and place a pillow underneath her to support her weight, as this position can put strain on the neck and shoulders. Use your hands to move her buttocks until her pelvis is in the best position for both of you. Then you will have your hands free to stimulate her clitoris and anus with your fingers while your penis is inside her. This position is a natural progression from the Crab's position, which means you don't have to move away from your partner while changing from one to the other.*

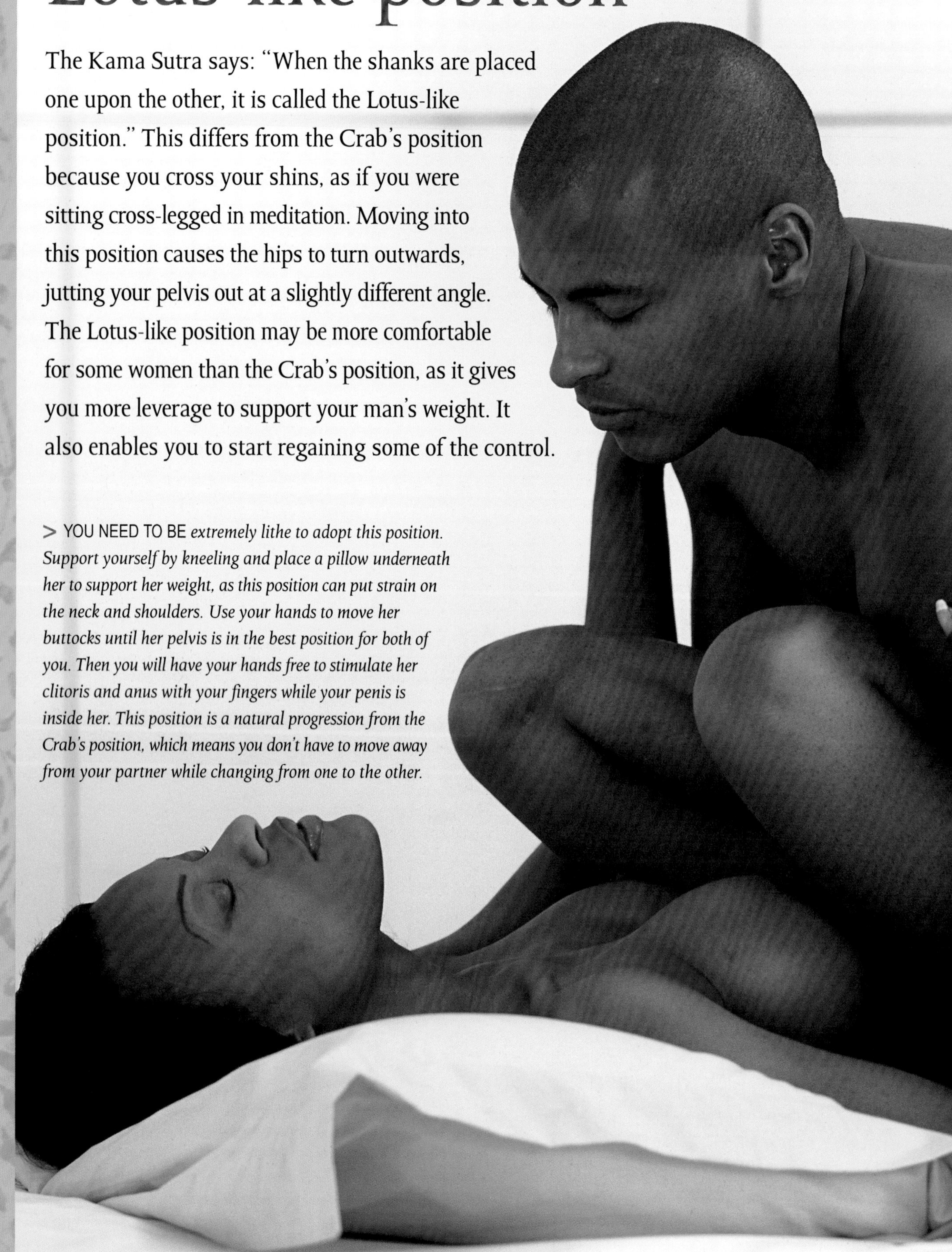

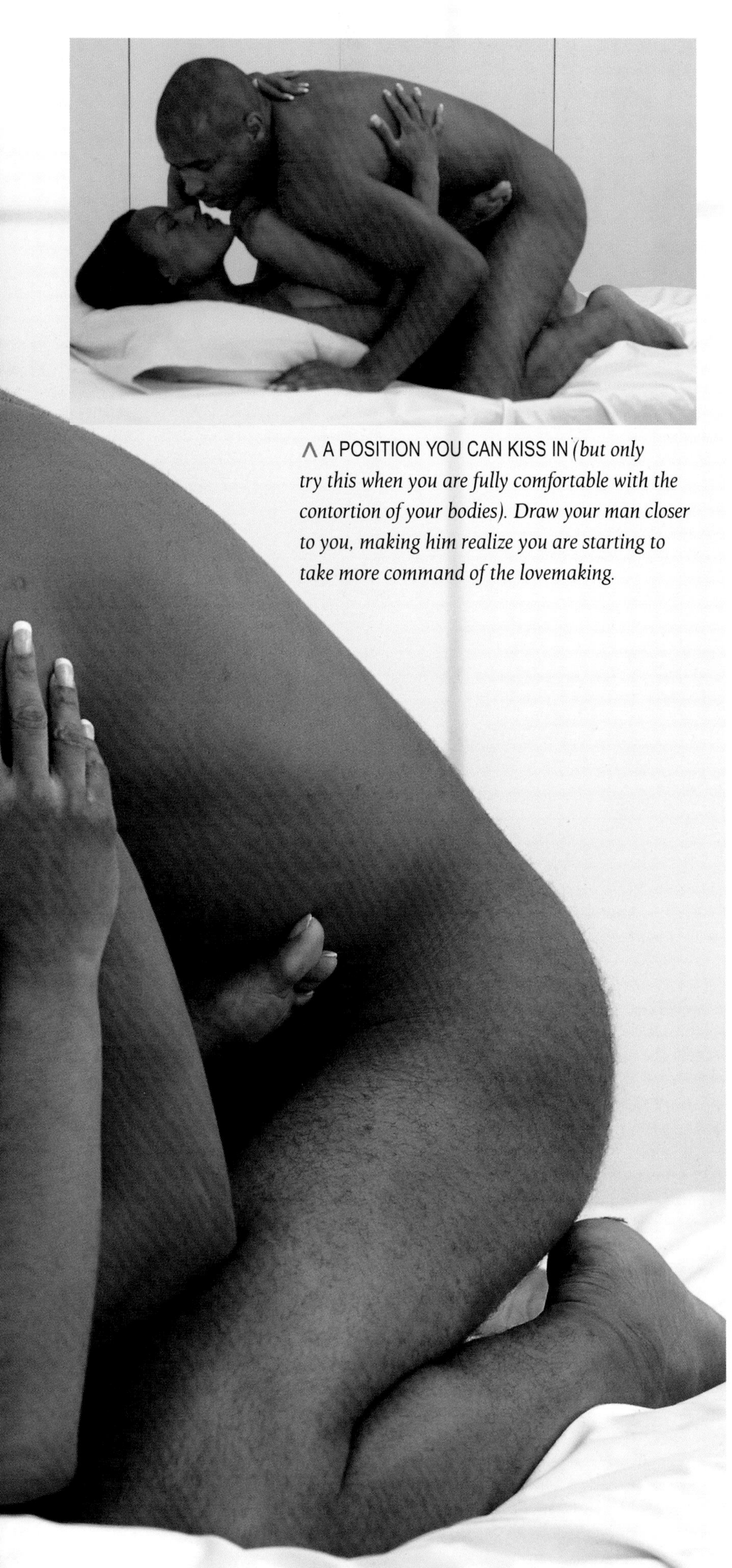

∧ A POSITION YOU CAN KISS IN *(but only try this when you are fully comfortable with the contortion of your bodies). Draw your man closer to you, making him realize you are starting to take more command of the lovemaking.*

The Lotus position

The true lotus position, as practised in yoga and meditation, is even more difficult to perform than the Lotus-like sexual position. Many people find it impossible to contort their legs and ankles into the correct places to sit in the lotus position—and even if you do manage it, you will need time and practice to become relaxed and meditative.

Another equally difficult kind of position, as espoused in the Kama Sutra, is the Packed position. This is described as, "when the thighs are raised and placed one upon the other." This is probably only possible for contortionists!

All of these positions are difficult to perform unless you are naturally very supple. Don't try to force your partner's legs into the correct position—remember, practice makes perfect.

Refined position

The pressed positions require a lot of stamina, as well as strong leg muscles. The Refined position offers time out from more demanding positions, while maintaining the excitement. In this position the woman continues to gain more control. This can be a welcome progression after being so submissive in the earlier pressed positions. Freedom for the woman to move her legs and to change the angle of her pelvis means penetration can be deeper, more varied, and perhaps more mutually satisfying.

V WHILE HE SUPPORTS *your weight by placing his hands on your buttocks (any excuse!), your fingers are free to explore . . . With your legs around his waist, you can change the angle and length of penetration. Tilt your pelvis up and down and tense your thighs to bring you even closer to his genitals. Squeeze your vaginal muscles to grip his penis more tightly. The opportunity for self-stimulation of the breasts means both lovers are kept happy.*

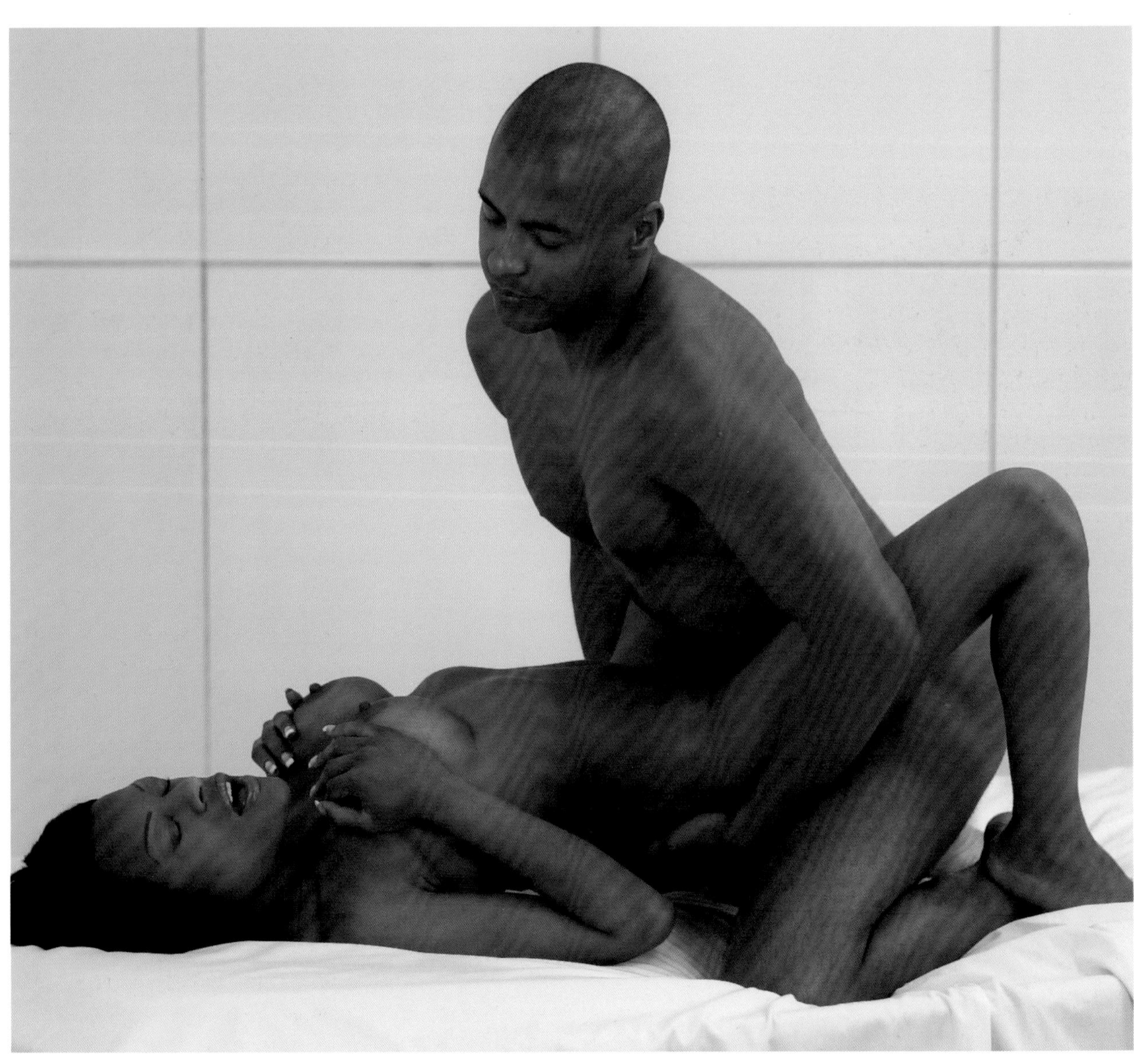

> IN THIS POSITION *you can stroke her breasts, buttocks, neck, face and thighs, while she is writhing around in front of you. As your lover sensuously arches her spine, her lungs, abdomen and diaphragm will expand, enabling her to breathe more deeply. An increase in oxygen will greatly increase her sexual excitement, so this position should intensely heighten her orgasm. Arching the back also helps open the vagina, which makes deep penetration more easily achievable for women who may find other deep-penetration positions uncomfortable.*

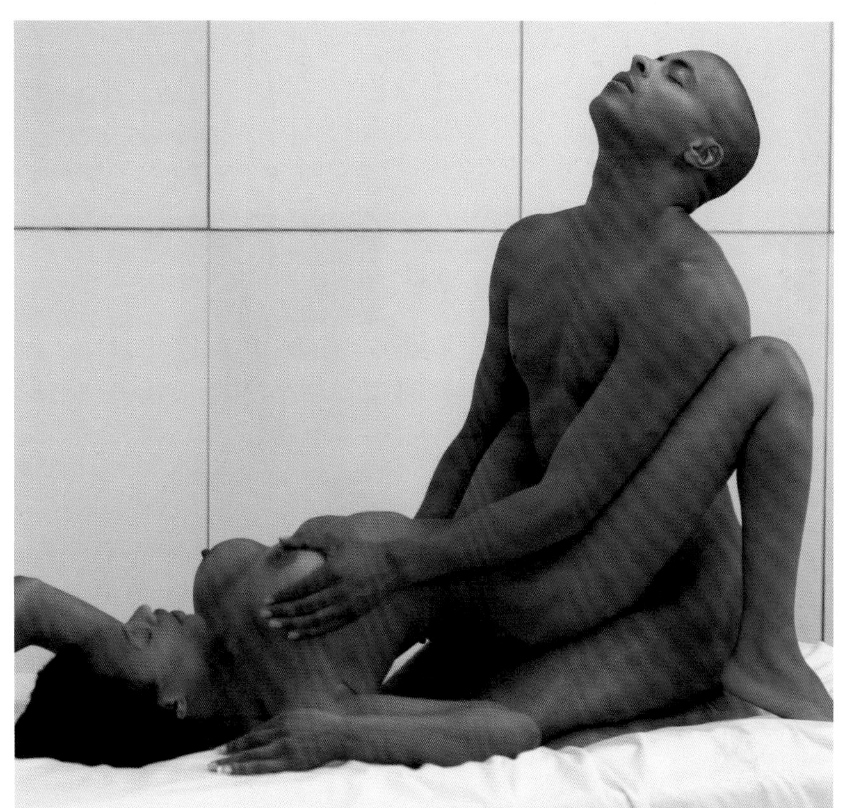

What works for him? ♂

You're able to observe every fluttering change in **her body** and face. You're in control of when penetration takes place. Plus you get to **fondle** her buttocks. What more could you want?

You can **stimulate** your clitoris while he is inside you—the best of both worlds! You'll also enjoy the knowledge that your partner is achingly **absorbed** in what he can see and hear.

What works for her? ♀

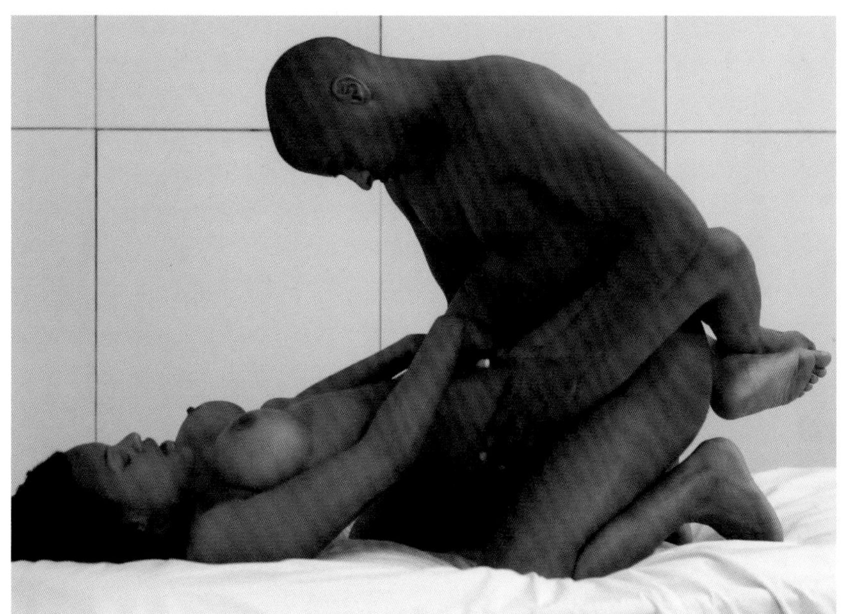

< CHANGING THE ANGLE *in this way allows for every man's fantasy—the ability to watch his lover bringing herself to orgasm while he is inside her. Lock your ankles behind his back and push yourself against him as an aid to clitoral stimulation. While your lover is pleasuring herself, caress her thighs, buttocks, and arms, making her orgasm even more intense. Knowing that you are mesmerized by the movements of her fingers will increase her pleasure even more. This is one moment in lovemaking when you are absolutely forgiven for not making eye contact with each other!*

Half-pressed position

According to the Kama Sutra, "When [from the Pressed position] only one of the legs is stretched out, it is called the Half-pressed position." This is good for women who want to exercise more control and avoid deep penetration. You can vary the sensation by alternating the legs, as though you are bicycling with your man between your thighs. You can also bend one leg over your lover's shoulder and stretch out the other leg, then alternate that position. This is known as the Splitting of a Bamboo (*see* pg.104).

> THIS PAINTING *clearly depicts the Half-pressed position, although here the woman is half upright while the man supports her weight with a hand behind her back. The lovers are gazing passionately into each other's eyes.*

V THIS POSITION *can be changed. Try it with your foot nudging against your lover's belly, with your foot pressing against his chest, or with your foot resting against his shoulder.*

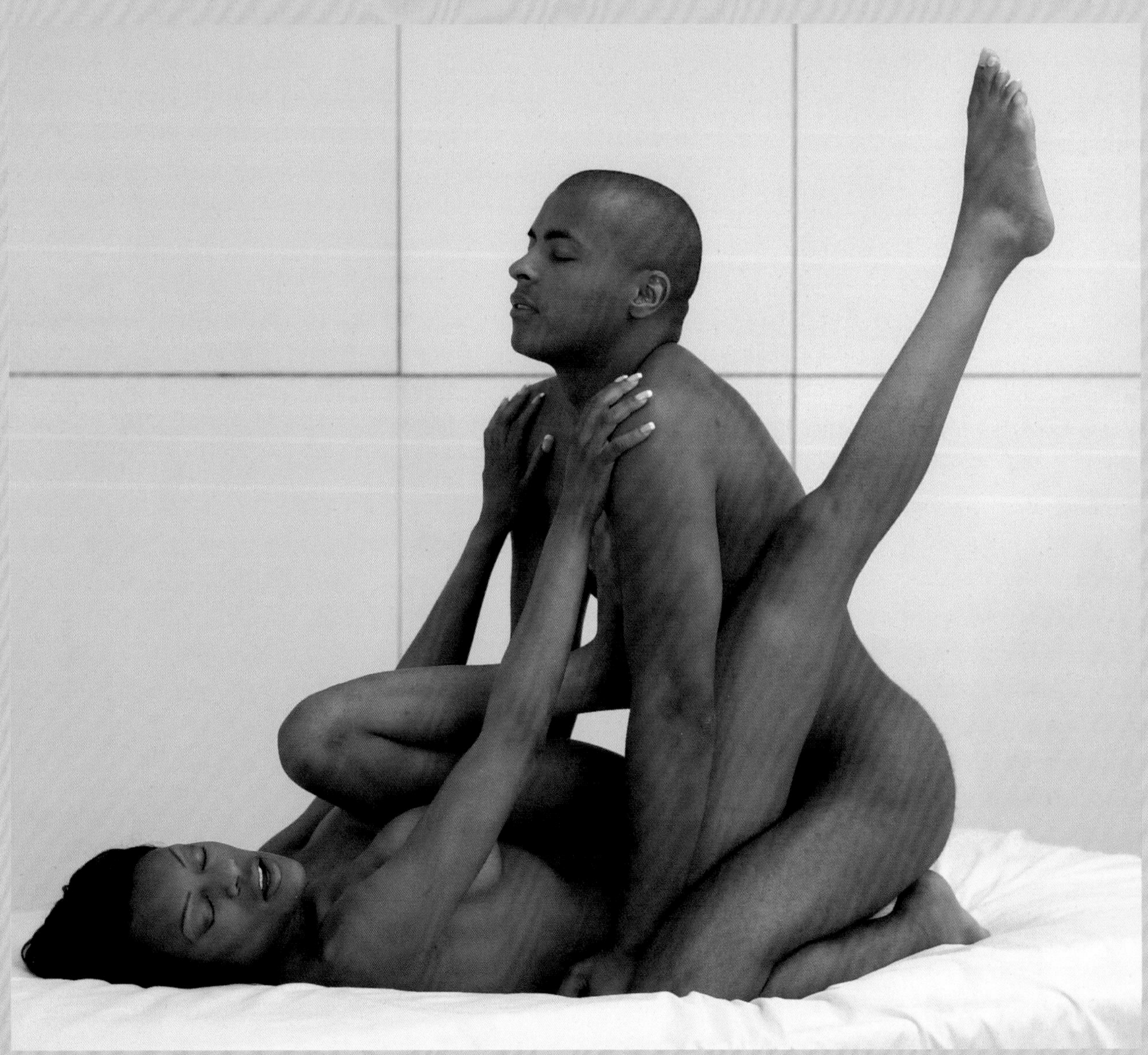

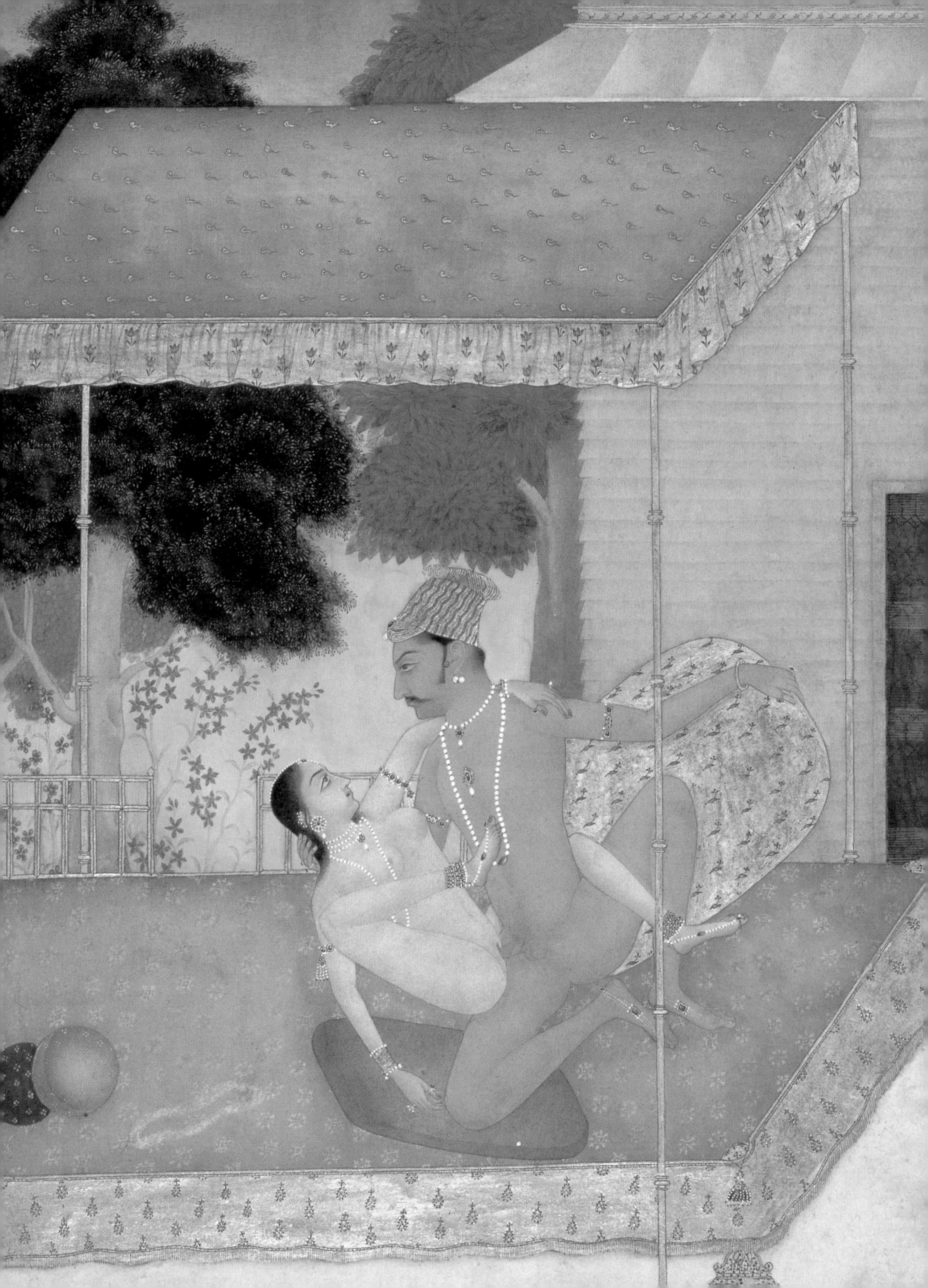

Pressed position

This is especially good for couples who like deep penetration. You are able to maneuver your lover into exactly the right position, while she maintains firm contact with your body with her hands and feet. To protect her back, support her spine against your thighs or with a pillow. This is the ideal position for men who get especially turned on by the sight of their woman's buttocks (and is there any man out there who doesn't?). To increase her arousal, caress the areas around her inner thighs, perineum, and anus.

> BEFORE ENTERING *your lover, tantalize her by rubbing your penis against her buttocks, clitoris, and the outside of her vagina. Stroke from her knees to the tips of her toes, then run your hands all the way back and along the outside of her thighs to her buttocks. Add a bit more spice to this position, when you're in the throes of lovemaking, by gently raising her buttocks, so her back rounds.*

Foot fetish

Kissing, licking, nibbling, and biting her feet can turn a woman to jelly. Maintain sexy eye contact all the while. Holding her ankles gently is an erotic indication that you are in control of her body and about to take full responsibility for her pleasure.

Ladies, all you have to do is make sure your feet are kept in perfectly kissable condition!

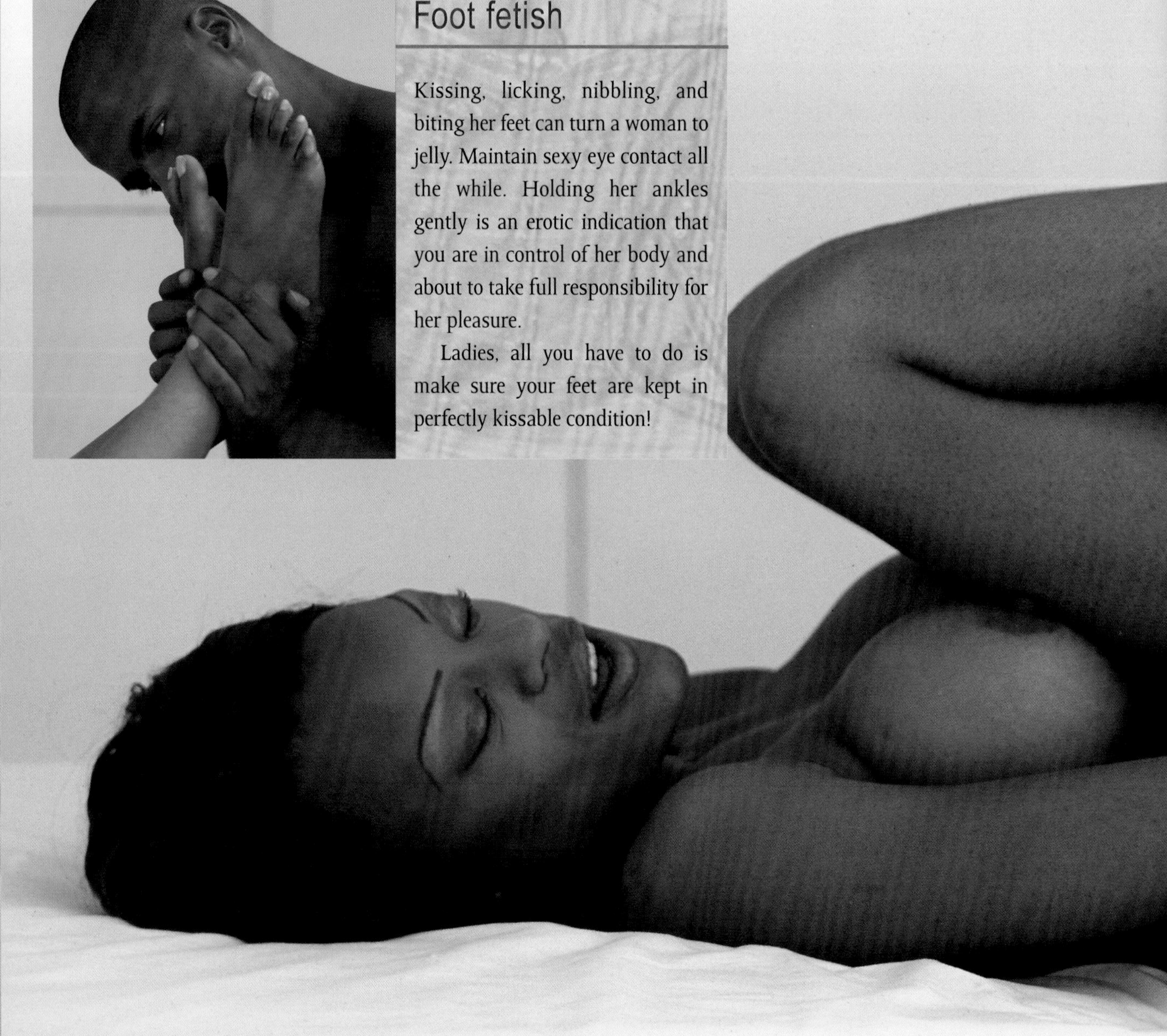

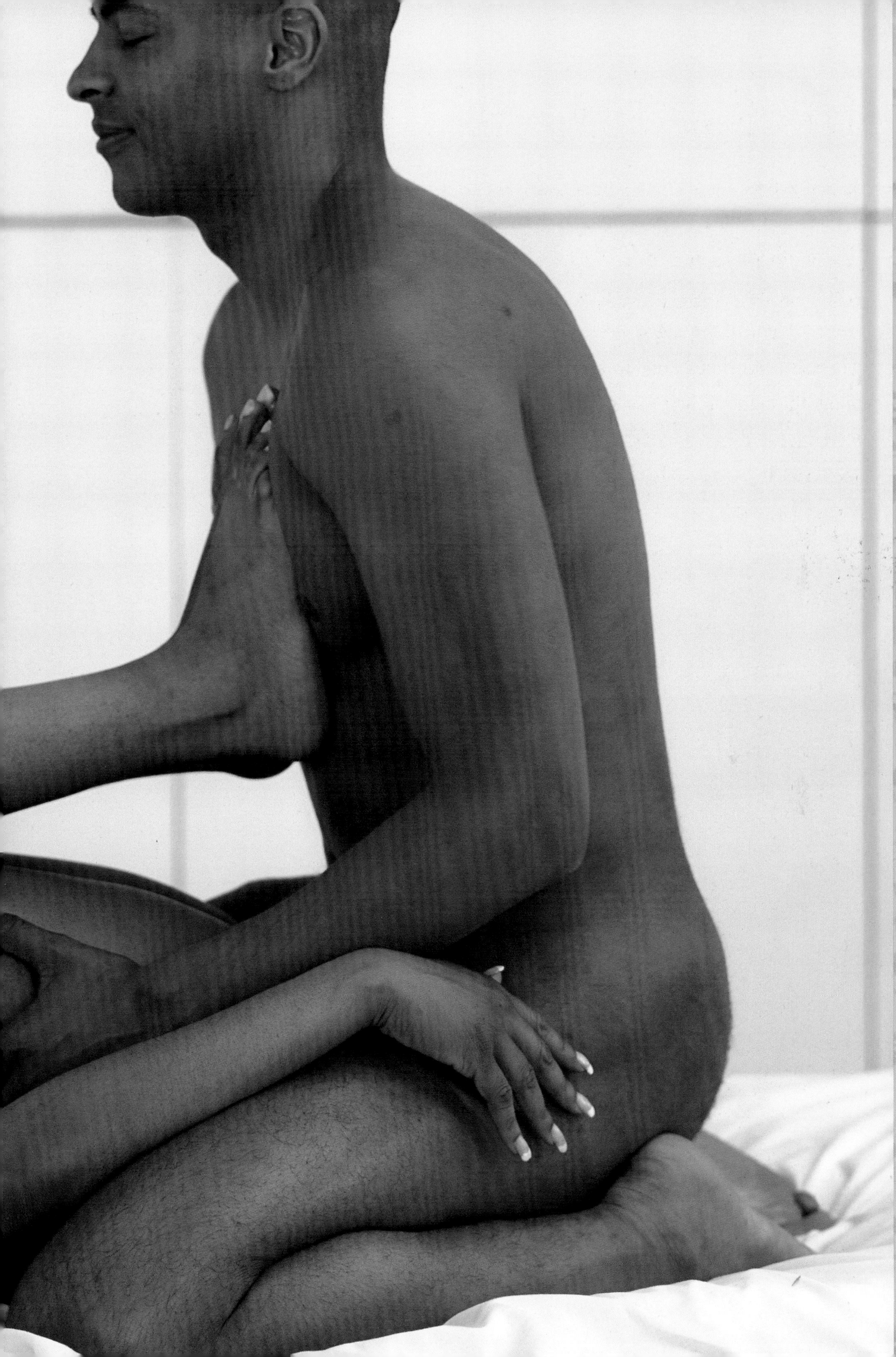

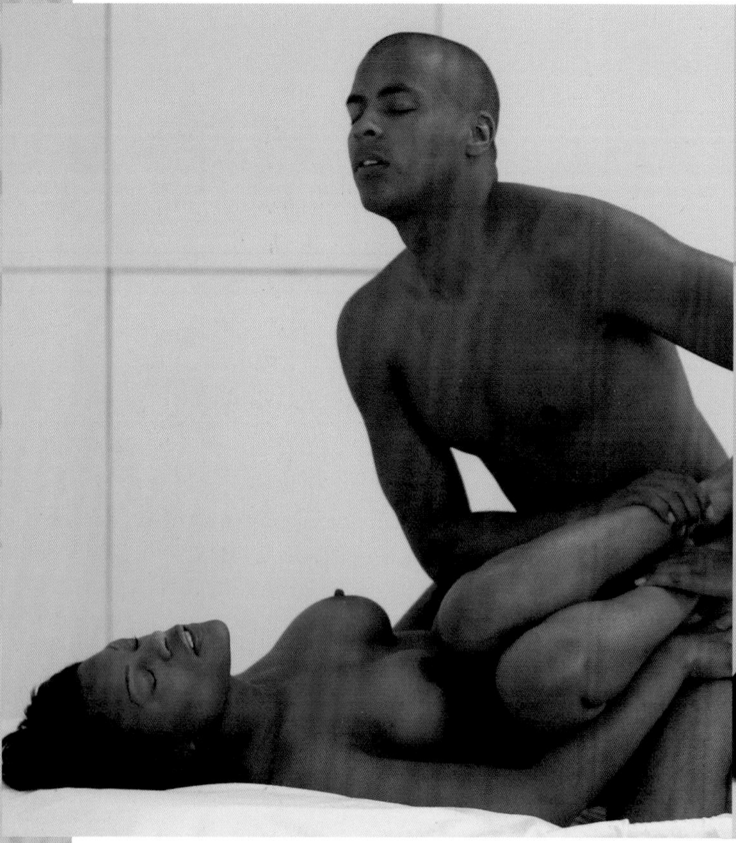

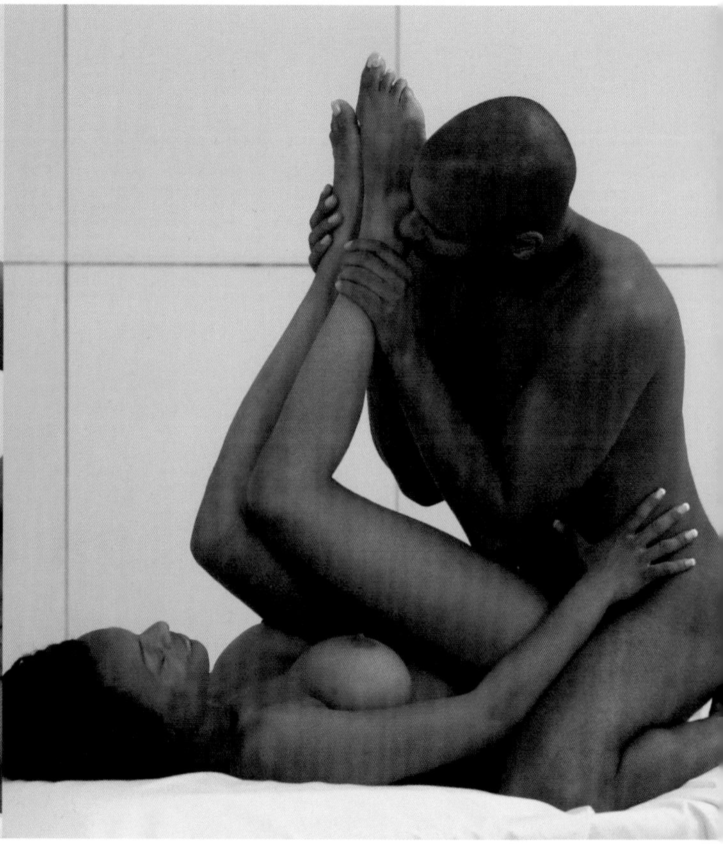

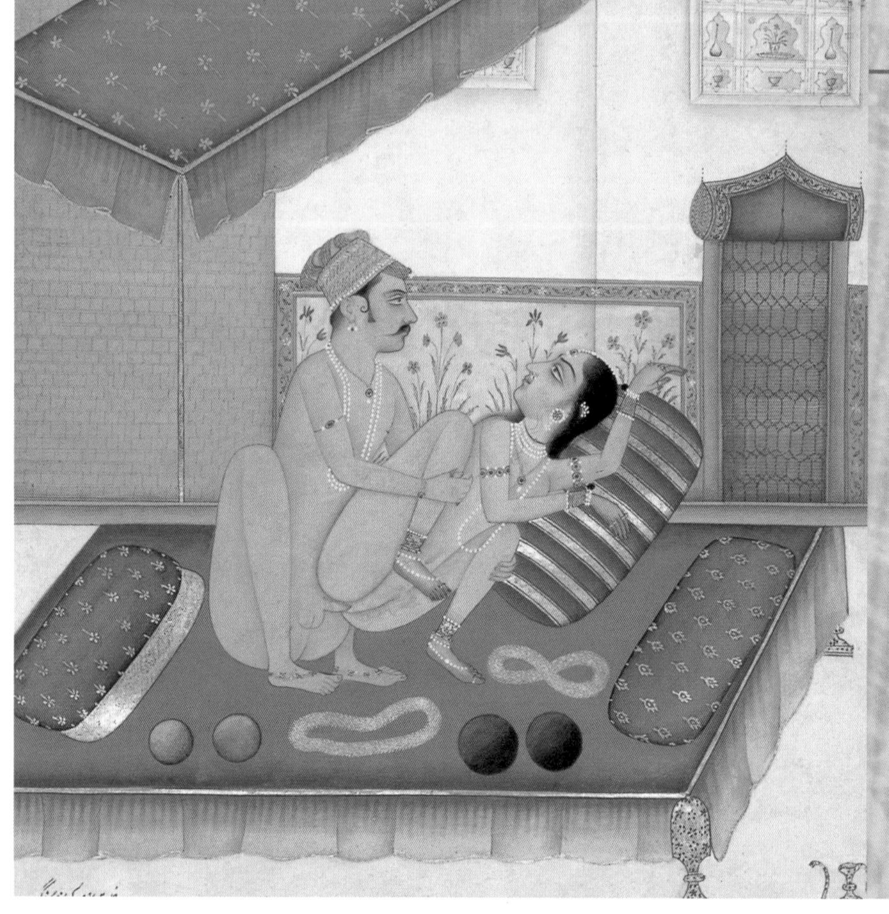

Side rear entry

A variation on the more usual "doggy style" of rear entry. In this position the woman reclines with her back to her lover, partially resting on her side and supporting herself with her elbow. A pillow or cushion also helps in supporting her body. This position allows the man to sit instead of kneeling up, making the experience more relaxing for both partners. Rather than the woman holding herself relatively still while the man performs most of the pelvic thrusting, in this version of rear entry the man remains more static and it is his partner who moves her pelvis backward and forward to bring him to orgasm.

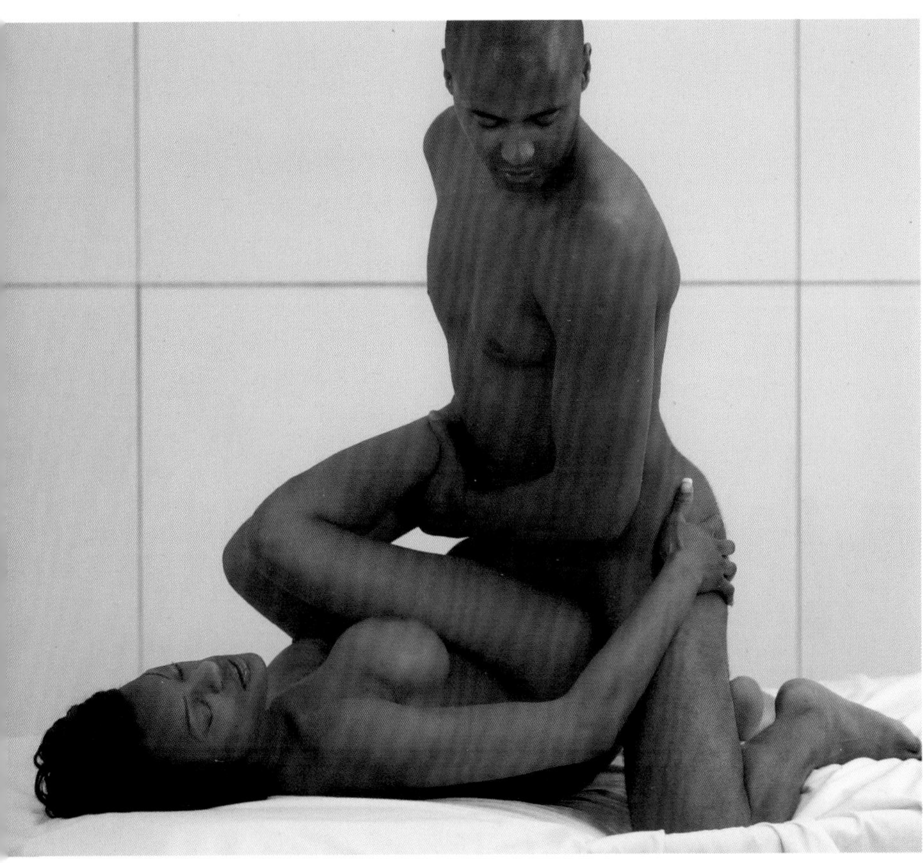

< AN EXCITING *variation on the Pressed position. Hold your lover's ankles and slowly move her legs from the side to the center of your body, then down to the other side. Clasp her ankles and press her feet against your waist before starting again in the opposite direction. Vary the moves by elongating or slowly bending her legs so that her vaginal muscles contract around your penis. Reflexologists believe that pressing gently against her Achilles' tendon at the heel should stimulate her pelvic region even more. The action can become increasingly vigorous as your arousal heightens. If she likes you to play a little rough this will drive her crazy. The side position presents a highly erotic view of your partner's breasts and the sensuous twisting motion can bring you both to a wonderful orgasm.*

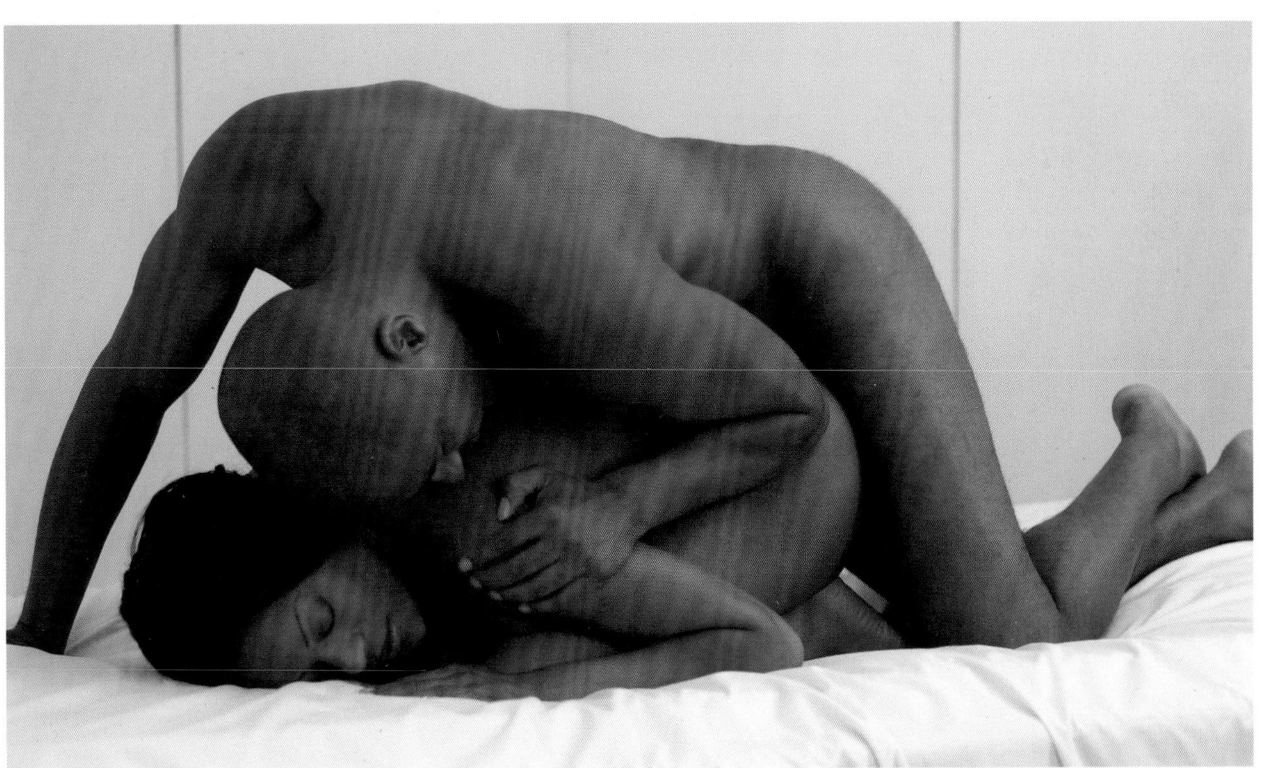

∧ TO TAKE THE DOMINANT ACTION ONE STAGE FURTHER, *turn your lover all the way over onto her knees and explore the supremely erotic rear-entry positions (see Chapter 8). However, this position can also be surprisingly tender. Check that she is not feeling too vulnerable. Kiss your lover gently on her face, neck, and shoulders and enjoy the nerve-tingling sensations as your chest brushes against her exposed back.*

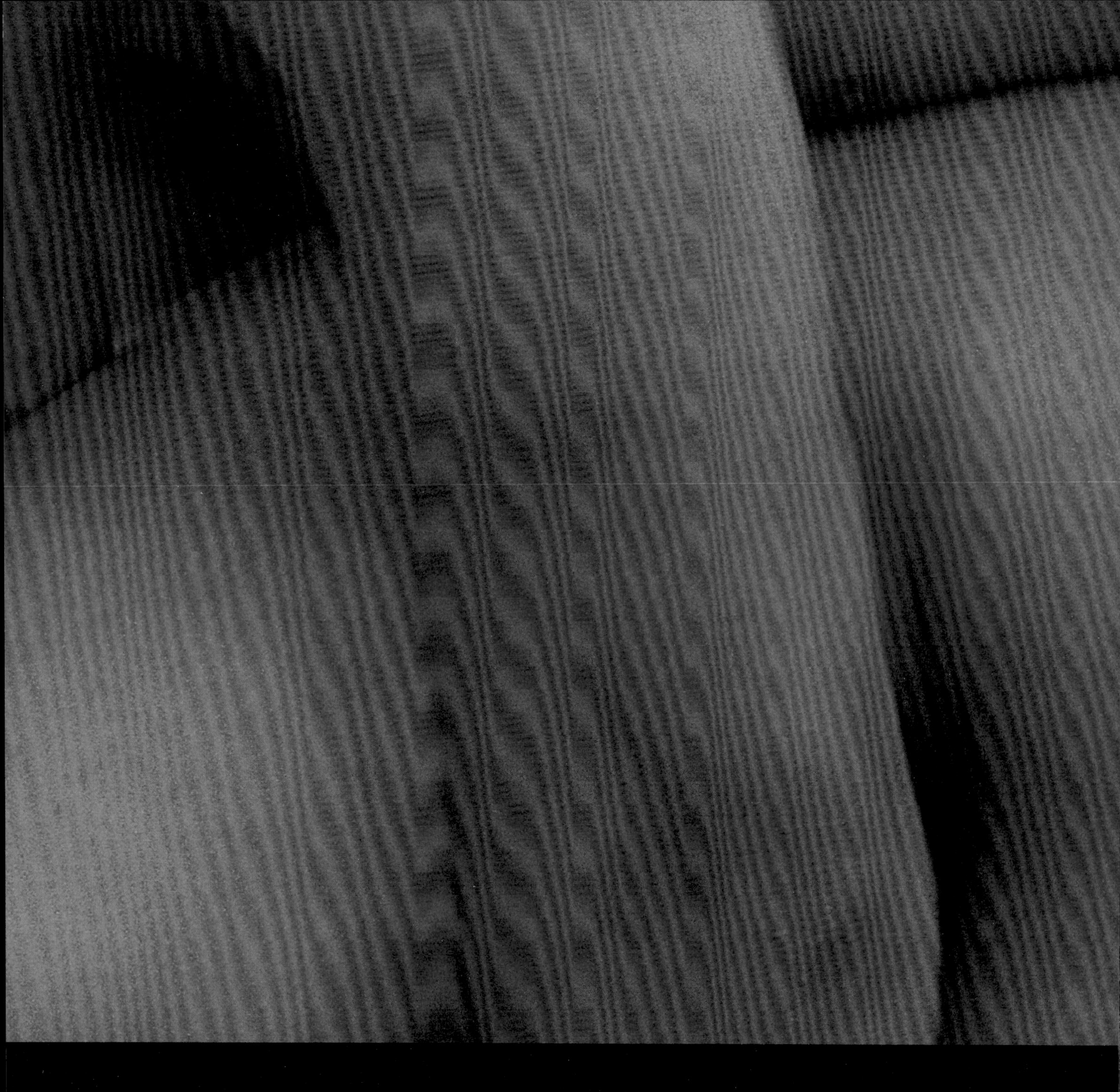

"An ingenious person should multiply the kinds of congress after the fashion of the different kinds of beasts and of birds."

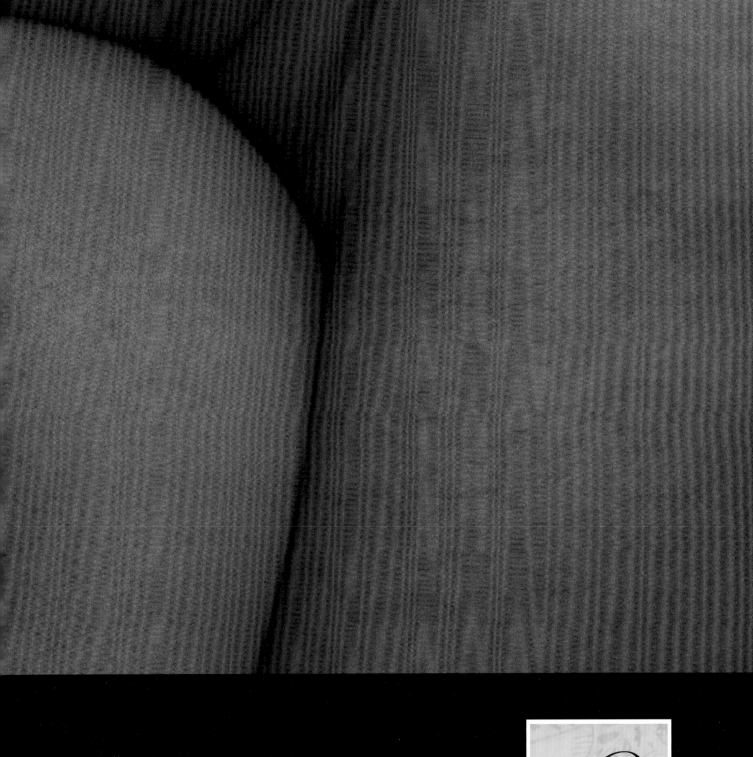

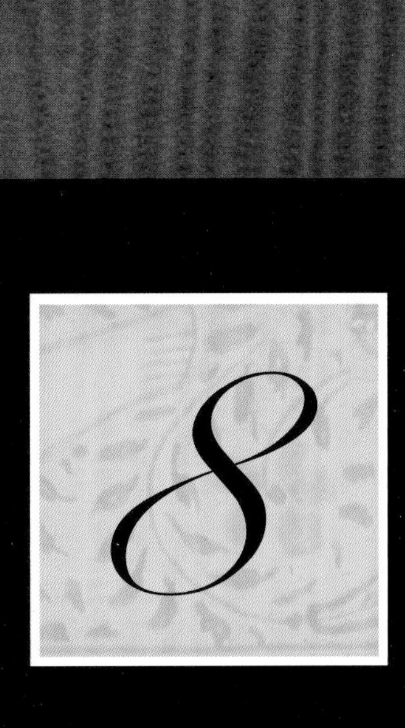

ANIMAL POSITIONS

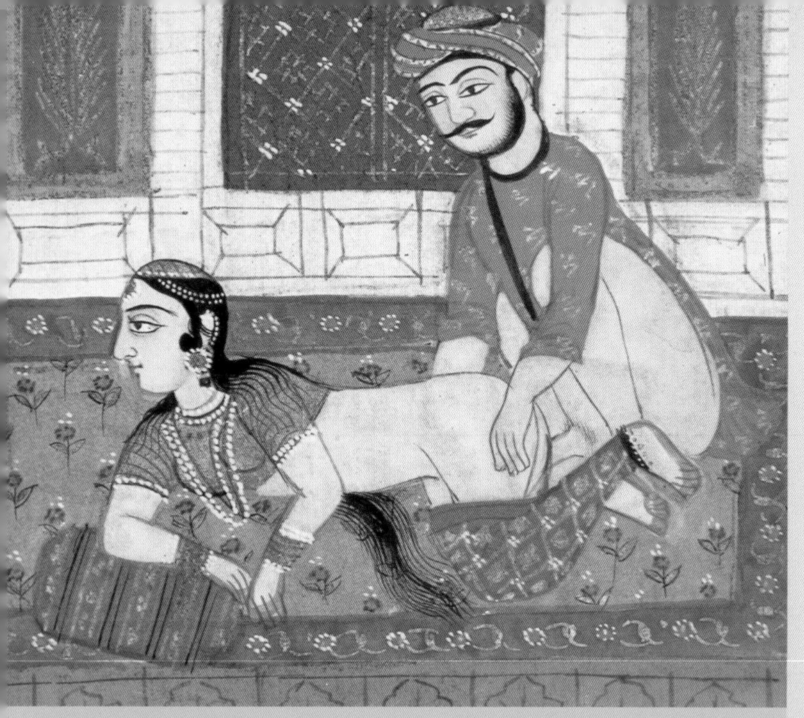

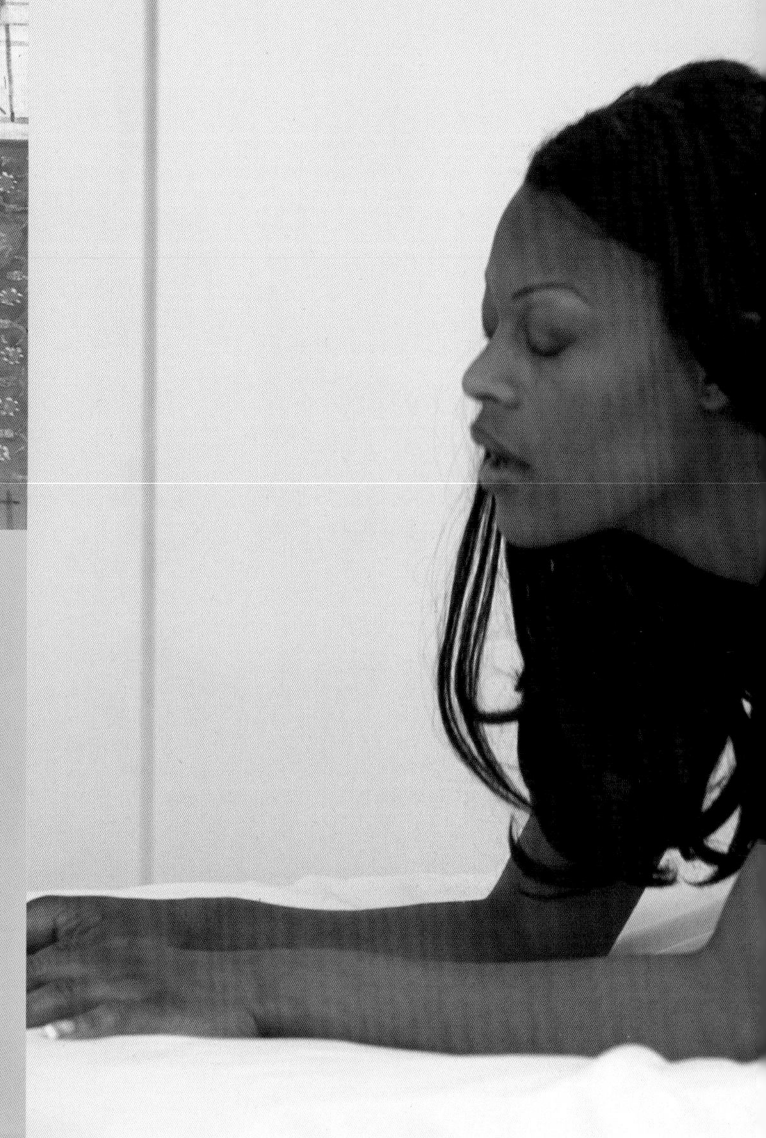

VATSYAYANA BELIEVED that animals could teach us a thing or two about sexual technique. These rear-entry positions are a steamy form of role-play—adding spice by adopting the characteristics of certain animals. Animal positions allow primitive feelings to surface, which is part of their special eroticism. Lovers can leave their civilized selves behind and revel in unadulterated carnal delight.

ELEPHANT POSITION

DOG POSITION

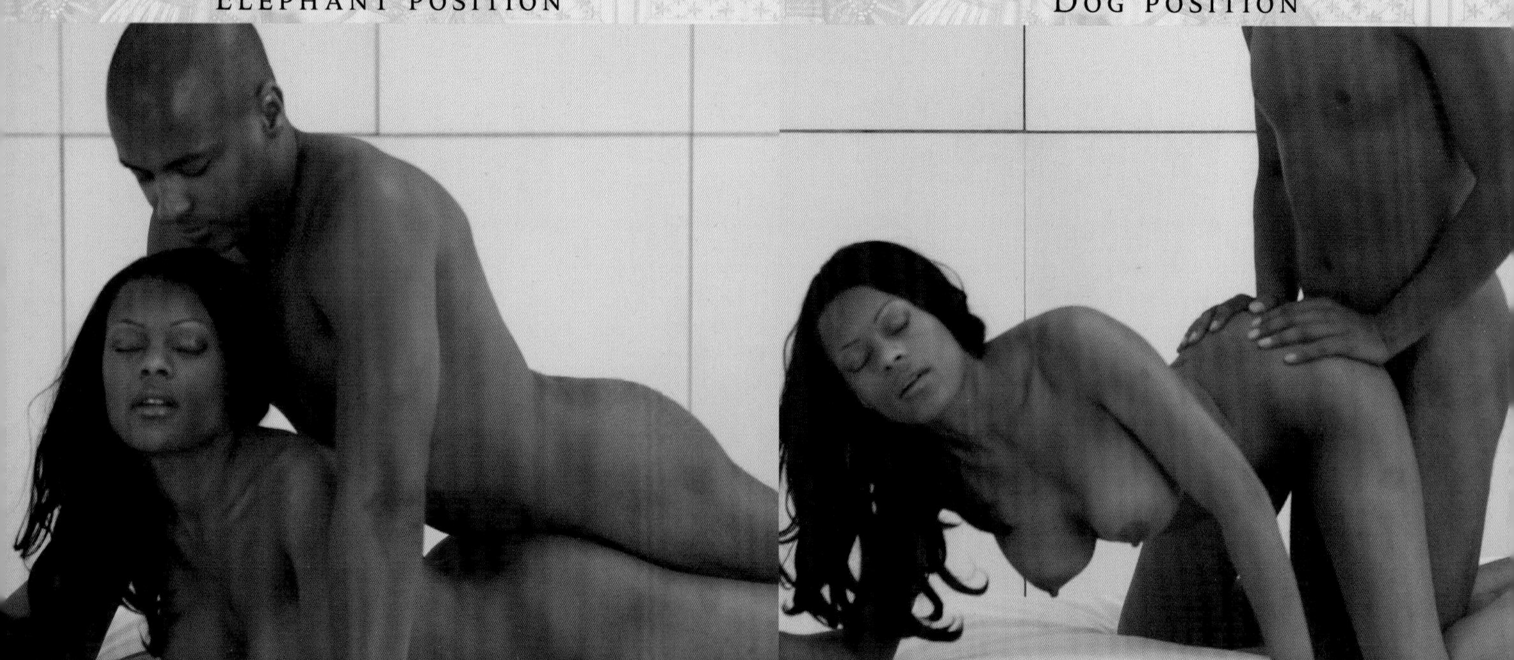

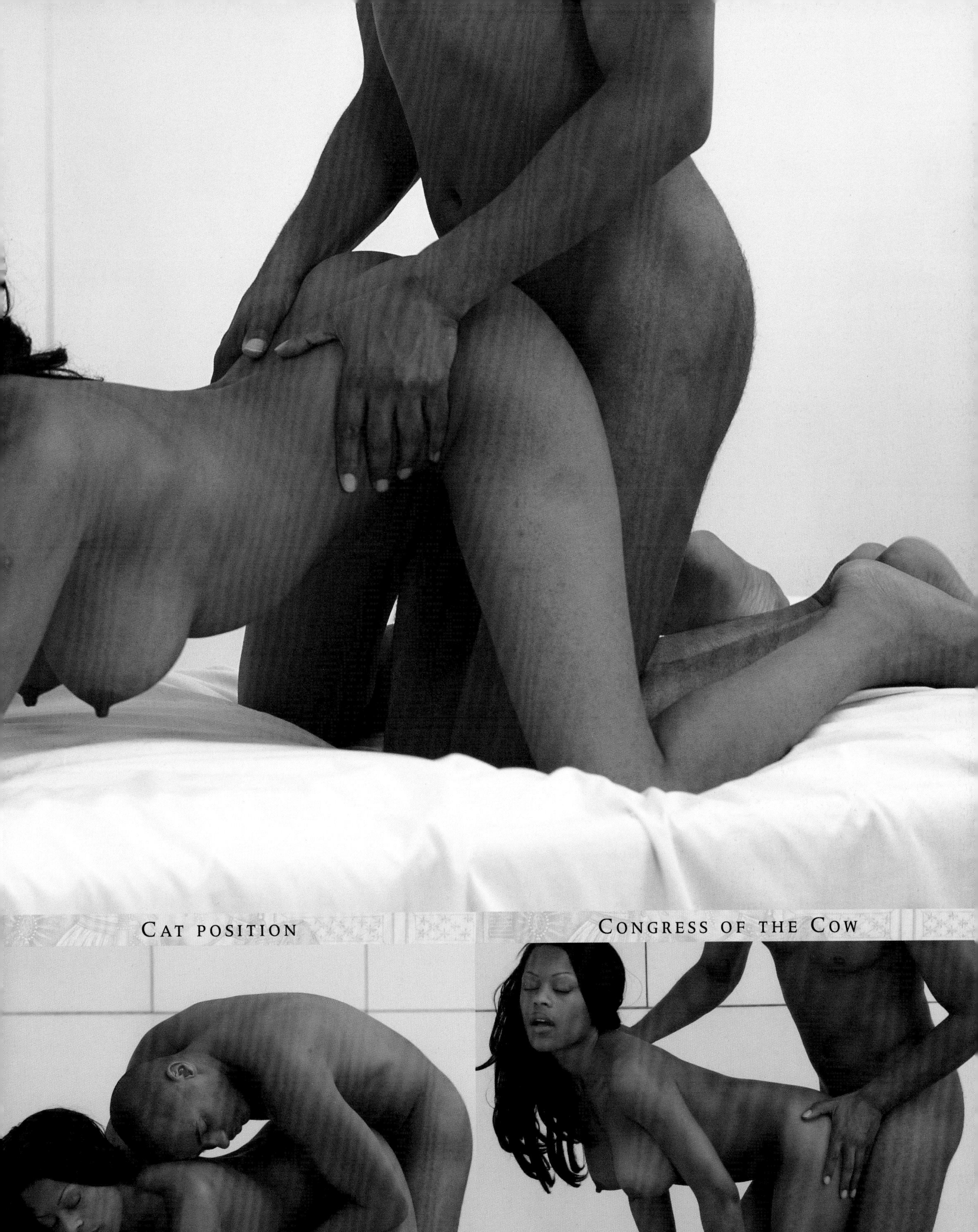

Cat position

Congress of the Cow

Elephant position

The Elephant position is described in the Ananga Ranga: "The wife lies down in such a position that her face, breasts, stomach, and thighs all touch the bed or carpet, and the husband, extending himself upon her, and bending like an elephant, with the small of the back much drawn in, works underneath her, and effects insertion." It has everything—G-spot activation angles, deep penetration, and head-to-toe body contact. Relinquishing kissing and eye contact frees up other senses and introduces a pure animalistic dynamic.

V THIS POSITION *creates a gentle, erotic power play. You offer him your whole body to cover; he feels delight that you are giving him "control." He needs to support his weight, caressing not crushing you. He gets to feel your buttocks and body against him, and can still kiss and nibble your neck and shoulders. Once he is inside, you can create stronger sensations by pressing your thighs together, so who has control now?*

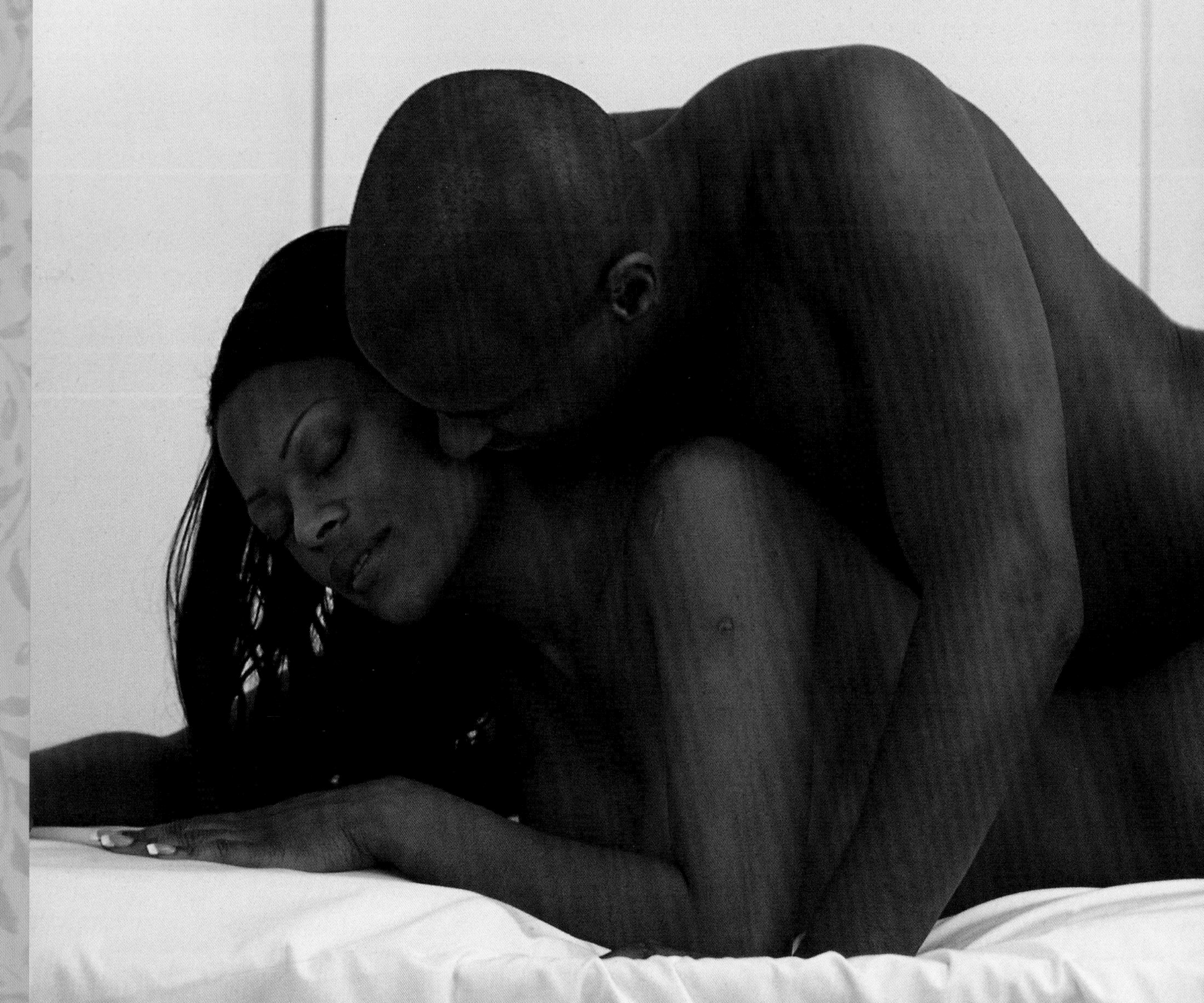

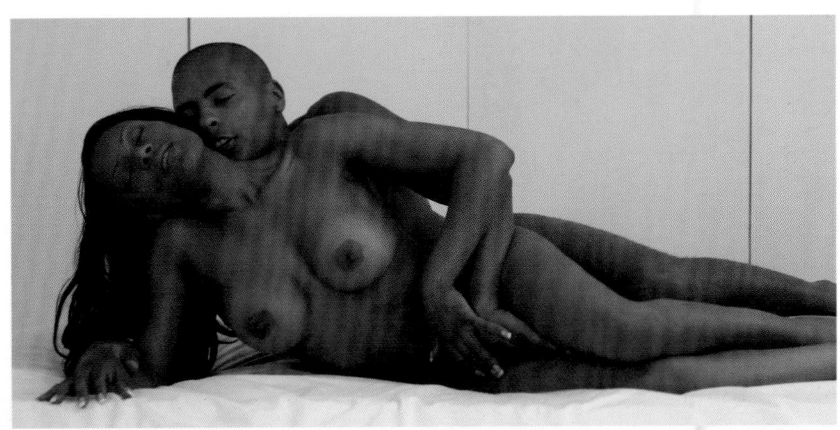

< THIS POSITION *is an excellent way to initiate the Elephant position. Snuggle like spoons, making it easy for him to caress your breasts and stomach and stimulate your clitoris (and you can help too). Turn up the bestial buzz by going into the full lying flat position or tone it down by moving sideways. It's easy to move in and out of this position, as the mood takes you.*

> THE ELEPHANT POSITION *can turn into a banquet of orgasmic sensations. It's perfect for women who love to be caressed everywhere while enjoying deep penetration. Experiment to get exactly the right angle—add a well-placed pillow. Raise and lower your feet to contract your vagina around his penis. He can also use his toes to get better leverage as he thrusts.*

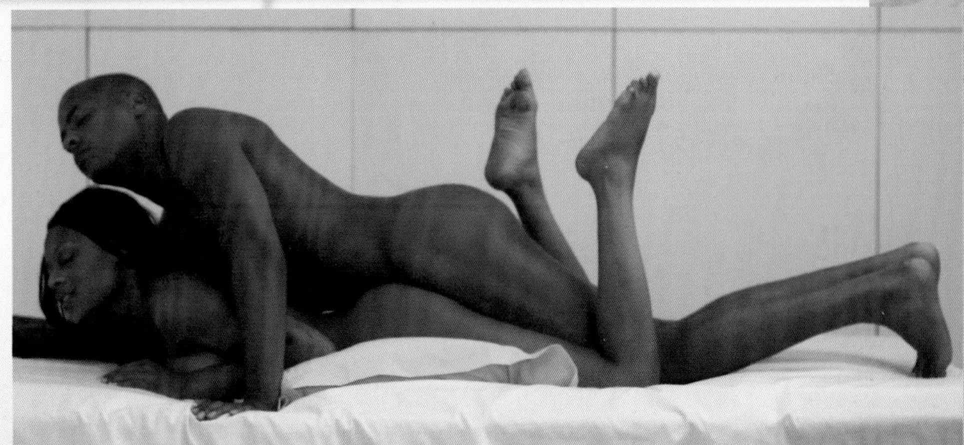

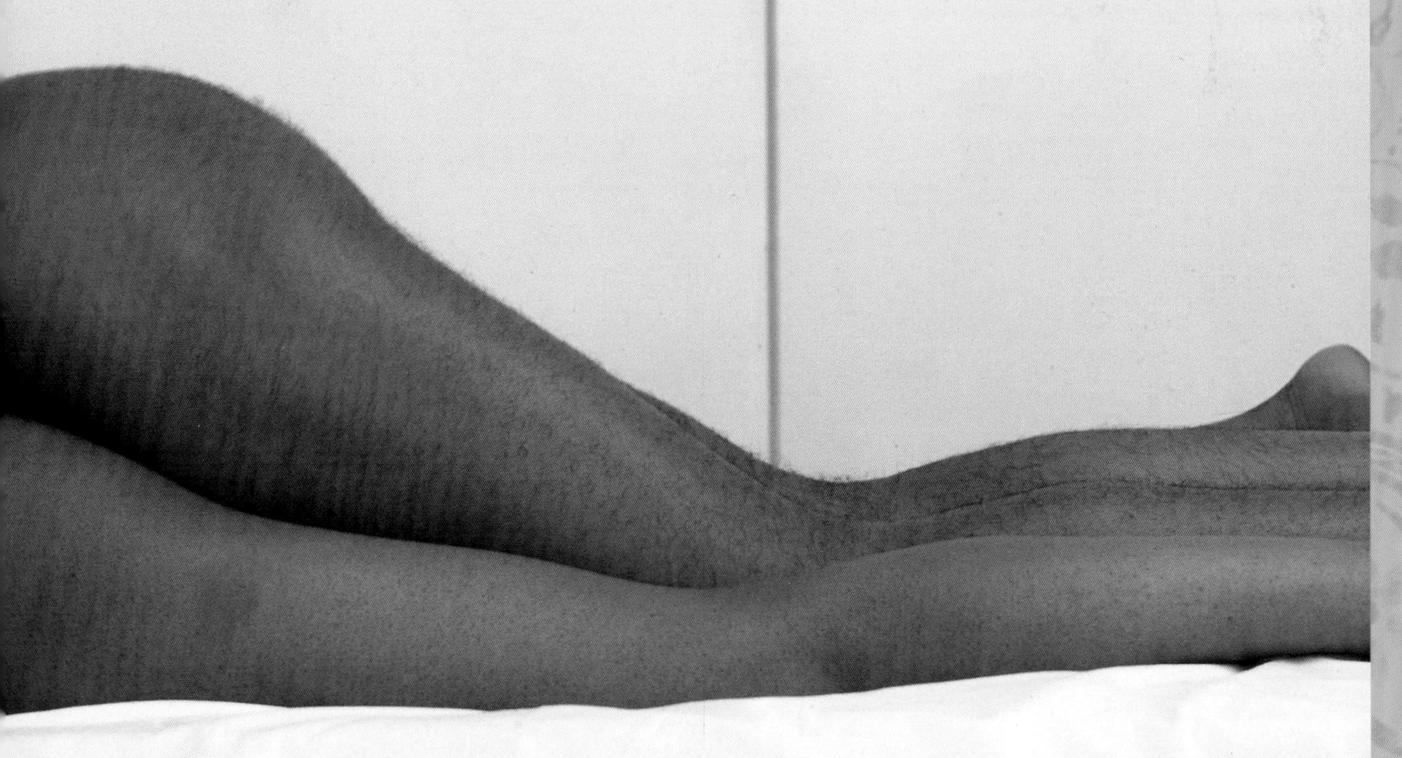

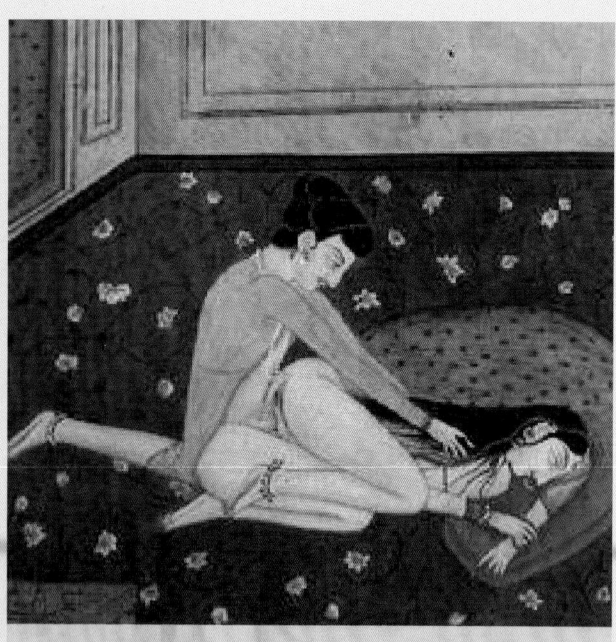

Stretching

Invest in some huge cushions to try this variation on the Dog position. It's like an inverted version of the Splitting of a Bamboo position (when she pretends to be a windmill, and moves her legs athletically around). You'll find that if you stretch and move your legs, you can squeeze his penis in some pretty interesting ways. Another plus is that you can also vary the angle and depth of penetration.

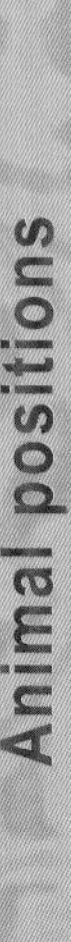

Dog position

This position is unashamedly erotic. Emulating animals allows us to abandon ourselves to pure carnal pleasure. Throw out modern attitudes to this position and their attendant inhibitions. It's not the most intimate position, and there is an inescapable element of passivity in all rear-entry positions for her. But if you are both clear about your boundaries, congress in this position can be explosively sensual. After all, trust is the foundation of headboard-rattling sex, not who's behind, above, or below.

V FACE IT, *looking at your butt turns him on. Some women don't like displaying their derrière, but bending over makes buttocks look pert and breasts swing enticingly. There is also the delicious sensation of his pounding against your sensitive perineum and anus. And you can push back against him to set the rhythm.*

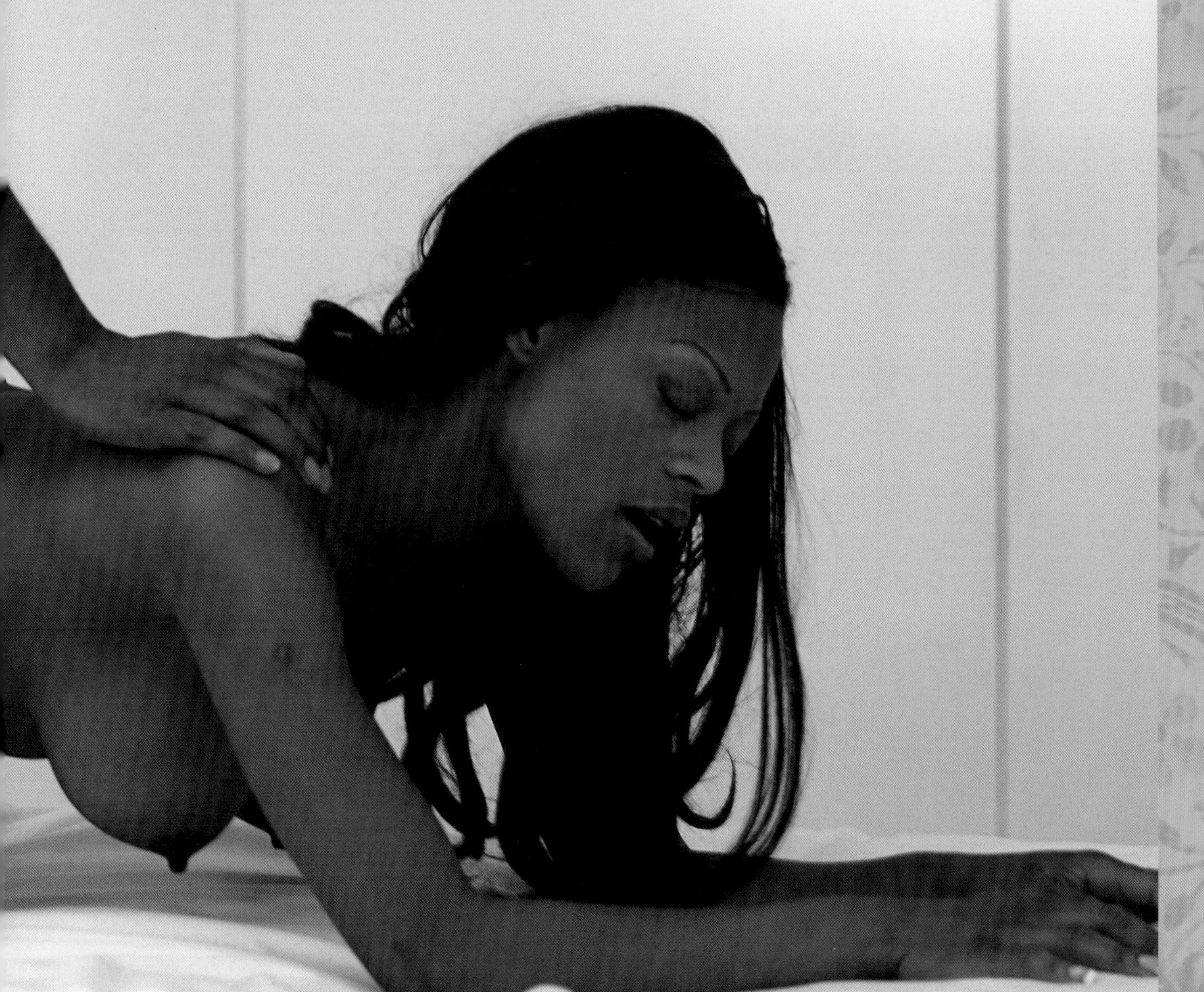

Cat position

Who wouldn't want to be a cat? Cats unequivocally say "yes please" to pleasure, milking that feline grace and cuteness for all it's worth. Look and learn. You might be a powerful puma exuding danger and prowess or a seductive, diamond-collared Persian. It doesn't matter. To get full appreciation of the Cat position, crank up your sensuality levels and prepare to stroke, nuzzle, bite, scratch, and purr. Also, and this is important, bask in the attention you're getting as your god-given right on this planet.

> THERE'S SOMETHING DEEPLY *sexy about this position. You can arch your back and rub up against him while he strokes you. Luxuriate in feline-inspired sensuousness. If you're really in character, copy mating cats by softly biting the back of her neck (but only if you know that she'll meow with gratification). Mother cats do this to kittens to make them relax when they lift them, and it's the same principle here.*

You can leave your *everyday self* behind and enter the *jungle*. Without eye contact, "wild life" takes on a completely new meaning. By closing your eyes you can focus purely on your own pleasure for a while, enjoying every delicious sensation. Let those *fantasies* out and revel in *role play*. Physically, rear entry positions are great as they allow him to penetrate deeply, stimulating the front wall of the vagina (which has trillions of nerve endings), just right for activating a *G-spot* orgasm. Get the angle right and it may be a while before you can be persuaded to face him.

What works for her? ♀

What works for him? ♂

A) You feel like the king of the jungle. B) You get to see and feel all of her from *behind* and touch her at the front, plus you'll get fantastic friction on the coronal ring of your penis. Now you need to ask your partner to *play*. You'd feel vulnerable turning your back, so make sure she's happy. Make her laugh at your animal antics, explain that you're an *alpha lion* and she's an utterly *gorgeous lioness*. Nobody wants to be described as a dog, but comparing her to a cat will flatter and appeal to her, so that getting into "character" heightens the *excitement*.

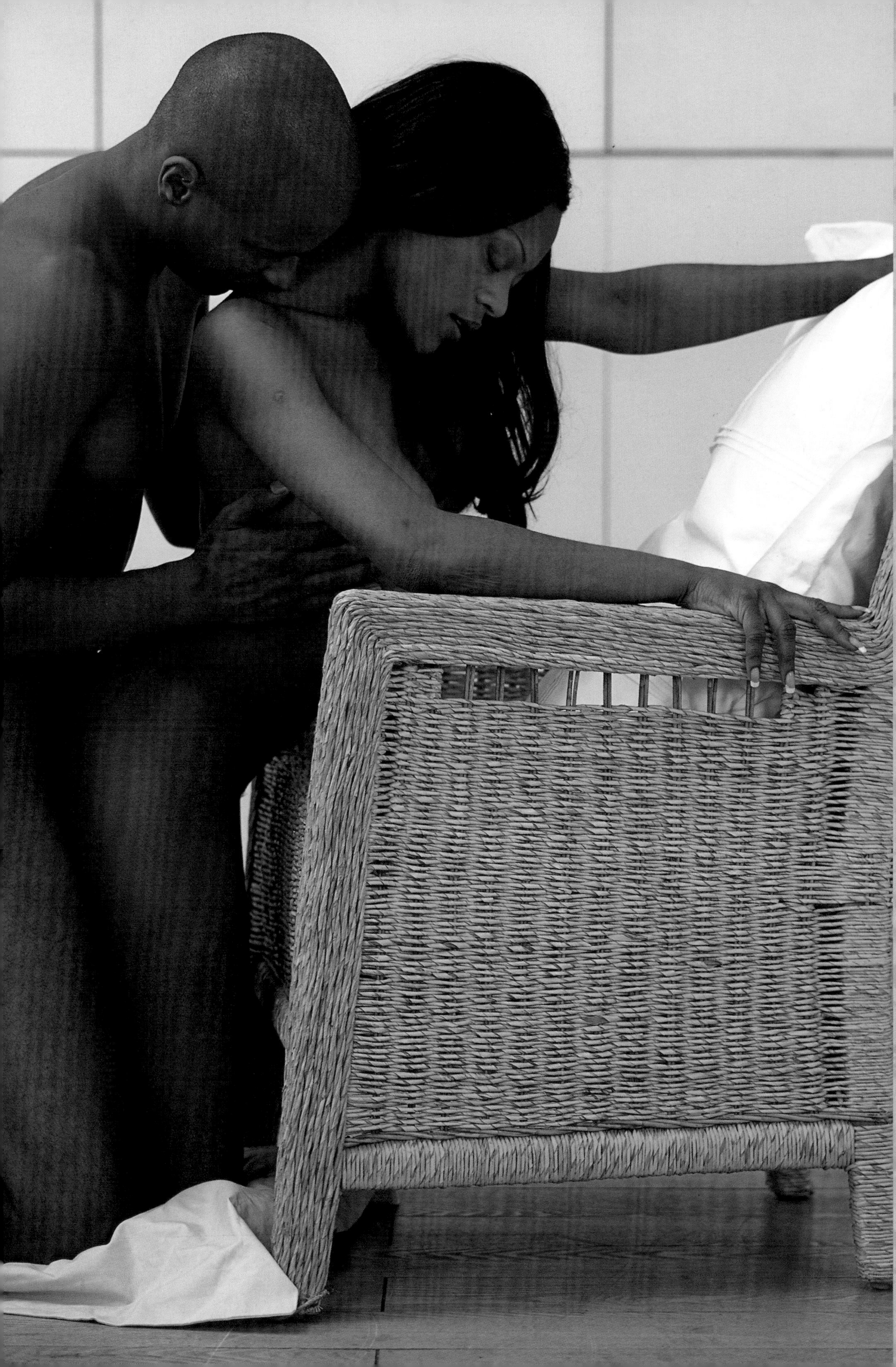

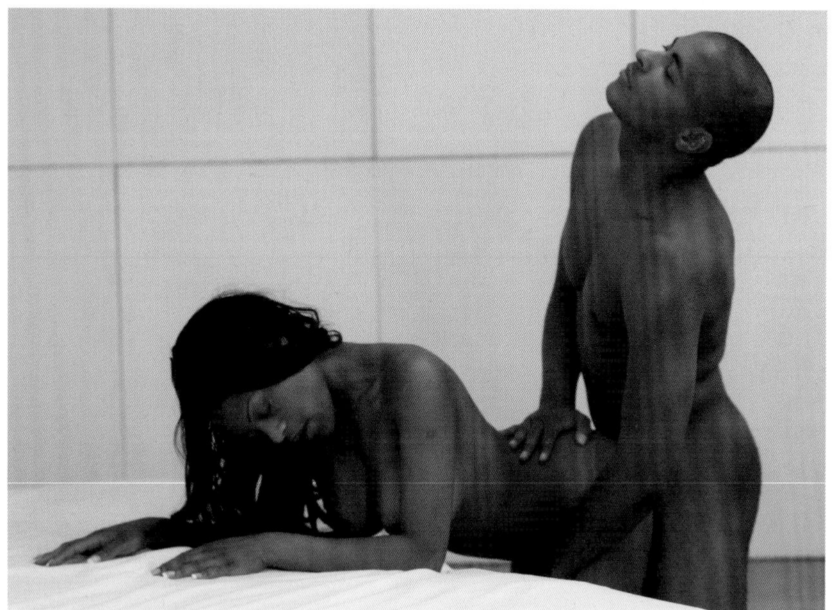

< GIVE HER MORE *to meow about. Reach around to touch her clitoris. There are between 6,000 and 8,000 nerve endings right there. Rub too hard and you'll dull rather than excite. The trick is to keep your stimulation light and indirect (the clitoris isn't a "push and play" device). Heighten the sensuality by rubbing her back and massaging the top of her bottom.*

> SHE MAY ARCH HER BACK, *offering you her gorgeous breasts for your lustful attention. Avoid going straight for the nipple. Yes, it is tempting, but if you really want to turn the heat up, make circular movements using your fingertips, especially under the breast moving up first to the cleavage.*

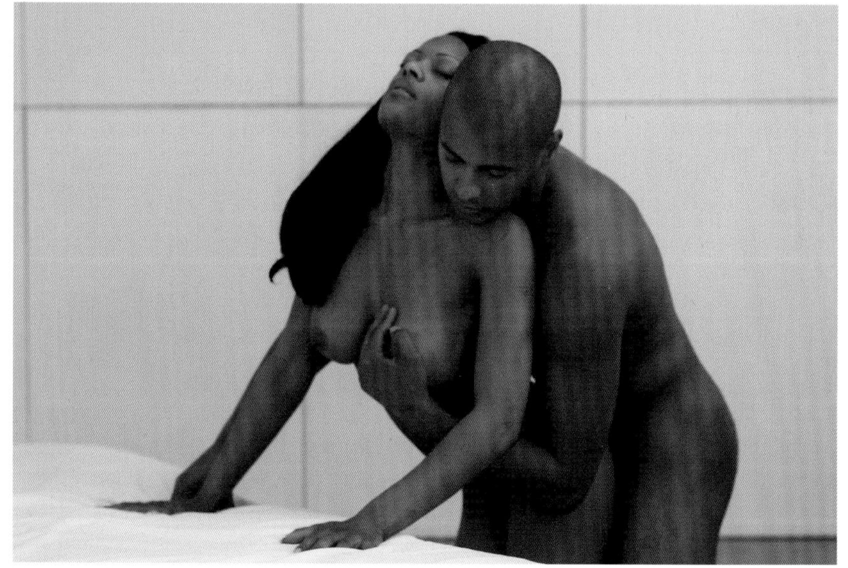

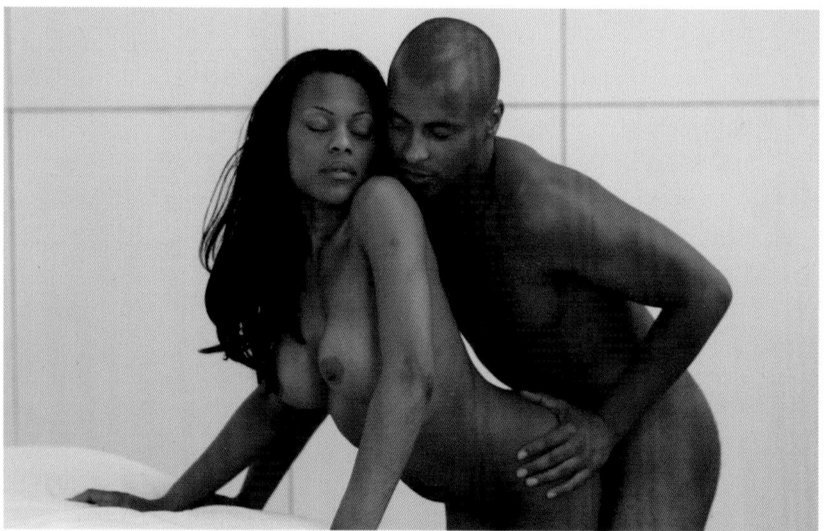

< PUSH AND STEER *against one another to get exactly the right angle. Put more erogenous zones on the map by caressing her upper thighs and tummy. Is she purring yet?*

> THIS ILLUSTRATION *demonstrates that, even though rear-entry positions are detached, you can achieve a certain amount of intimacy. The occasional loving glance can help to reassure your lover. Compensate her with kisses and whispered compliments.*

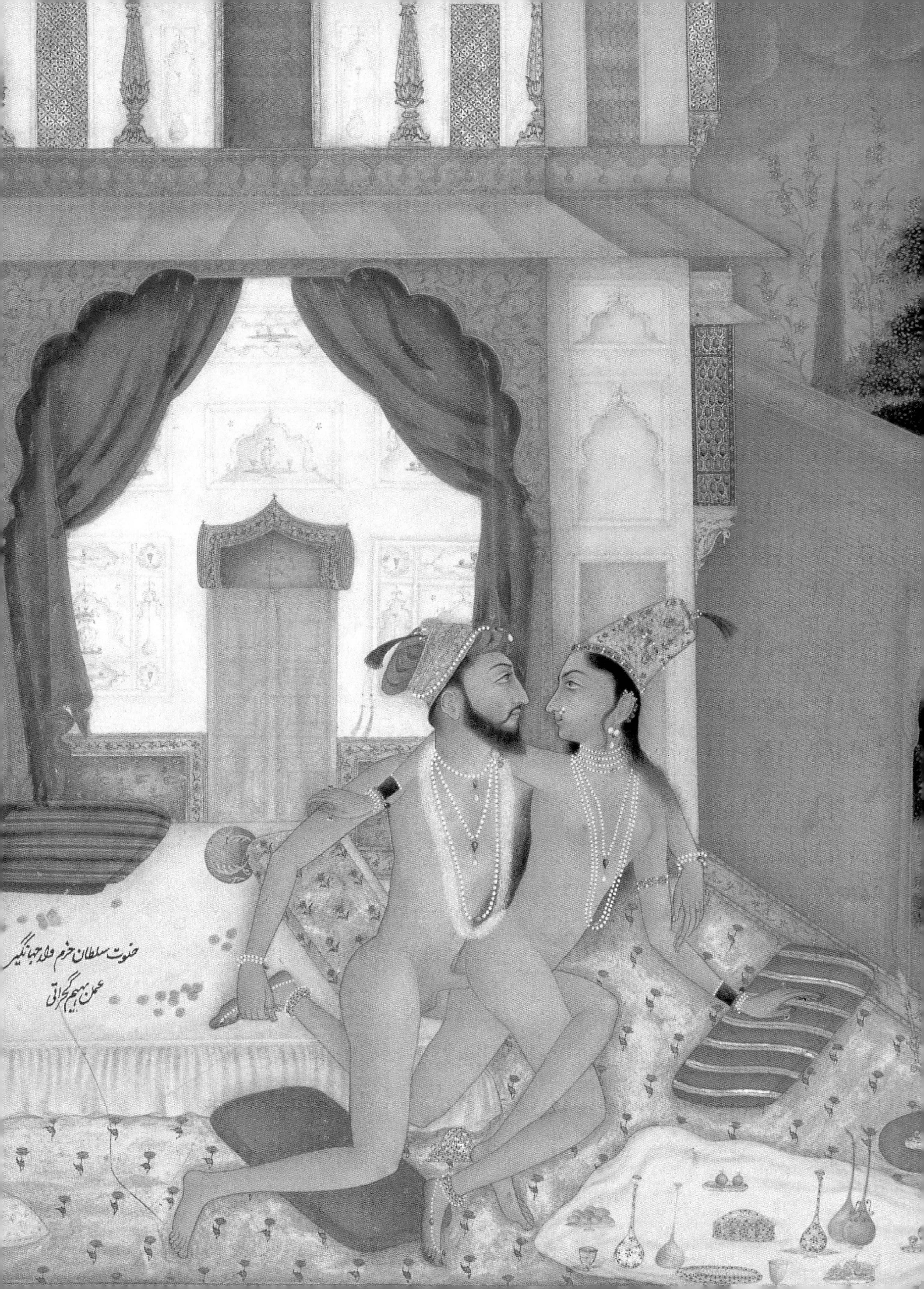
خلوت سلطان خرم ولد جهانگیر
عمل بهیم گجراتی

Congress of the Cow

The Ananga Ranga says: "The wife places herself upon all fours, supported on her hands and feet (not her knees), and the husband, approaching from behind, falls upon her waist, and enjoys her as if he were a bull." It is very demanding for her. You'll probably need to experiment quite a bit to make it workable. Focus on her, as she can feel that you're emotionally disengaged, but if you've enticed her into a frenzy beforehand she'll be having such a good time herself that she won't notice you may be fantasizing madly.

> TAKE CARE *with this challenging position. It's difficult for her to keep her legs straight and hands flat on the floor. Also, she'll get a rush of blood to the head and her breathing may become constricted. This alters her perception. If she climaxes, she might experience a sensational orgasm, if not, she could end up with a headache.*

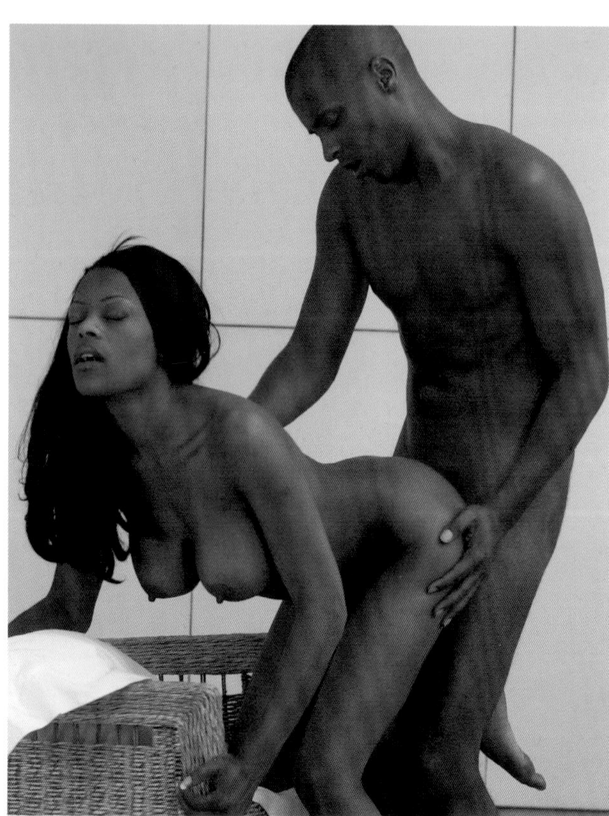

< HANGING ONTO THE FURNITURE *is a great way to enjoy this position. She can rest part of her weight and anchor herself without the problems of letting her head hang down. This also gives her the ability to control the depth and rhythm of your thrusts. Meanwhile, you can enjoy watching yourself moving inside her, holding her hips and caressing her.*

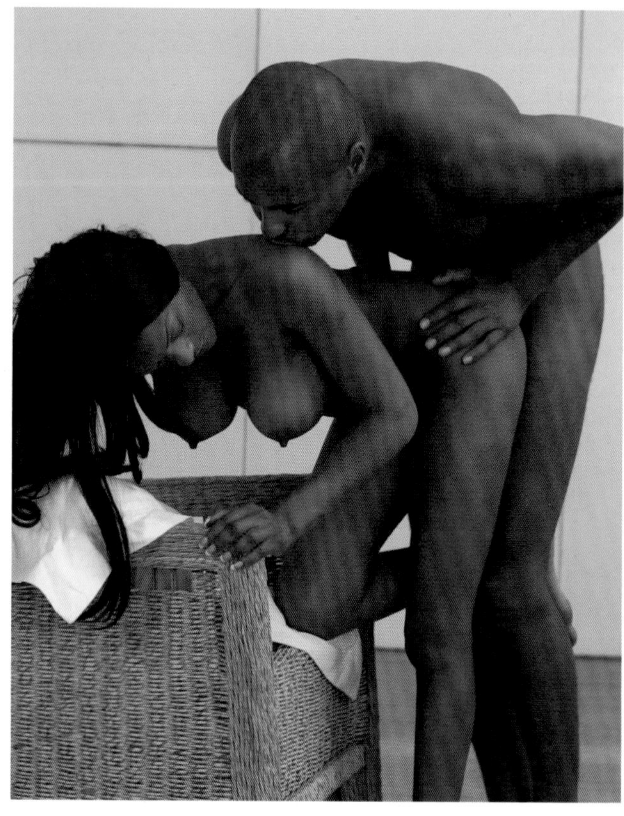

> NUZZLING, KISSING, AND CARESSING *are all part of showing her that you're connecting with her, in the moment. Let her move against you to find out what she really wants. She can change the pace and alter the sensation by changing the tilt of her hips and moving her thighs closer together. Kiss her shoulders and neck tenderly and remind her how incredibly gorgeous and sexy she is.*

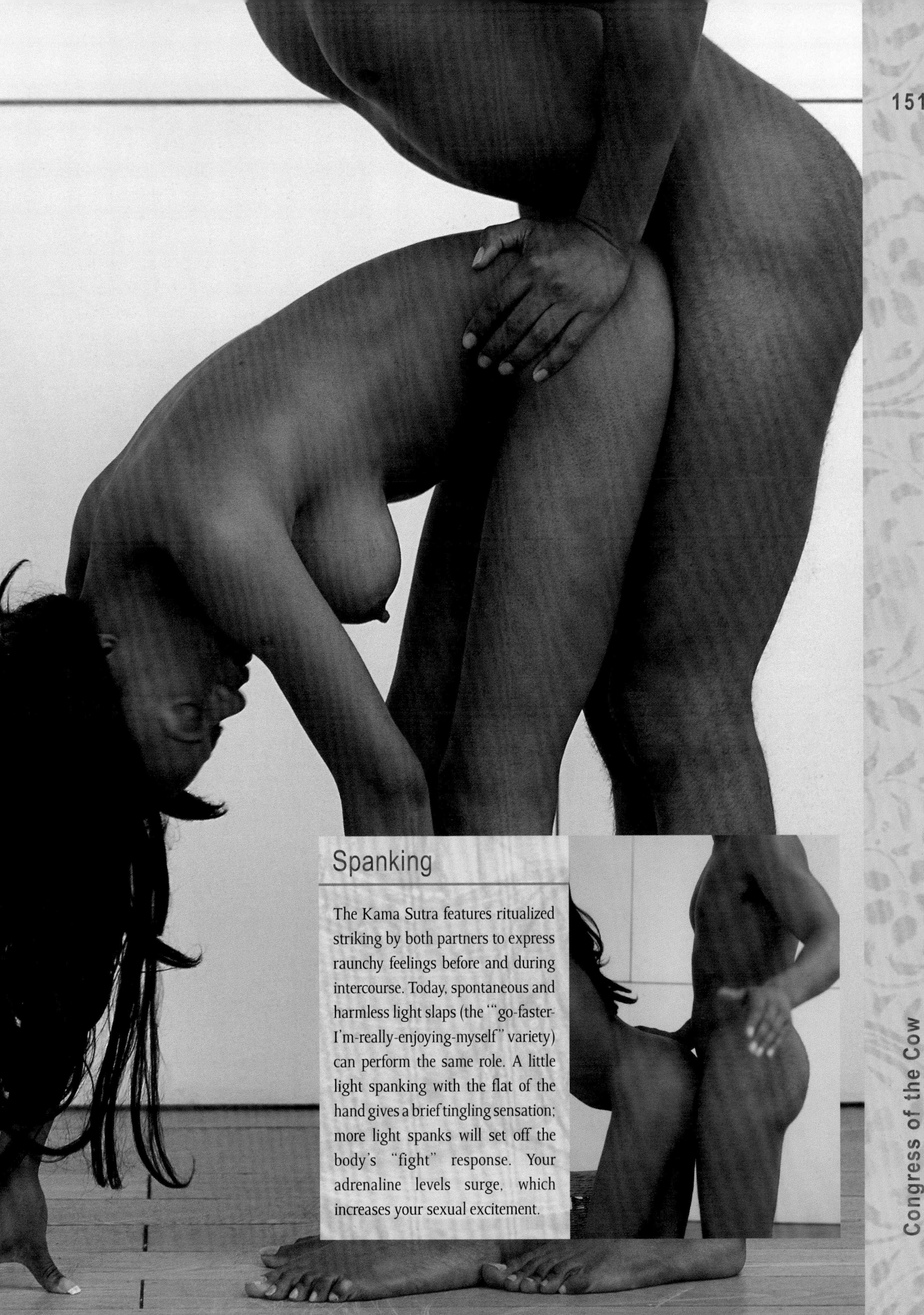

Spanking

The Kama Sutra features ritualized striking by both partners to express raunchy feelings before and during intercourse. Today, spontaneous and harmless light slaps (the '"go-faster-I'm-really-enjoying-myself" variety) can perform the same role. A little light spanking with the flat of the hand gives a brief tingling sensation; more light spanks will set off the body's "fight" response. Your adrenaline levels surge, which increases your sexual excitement.

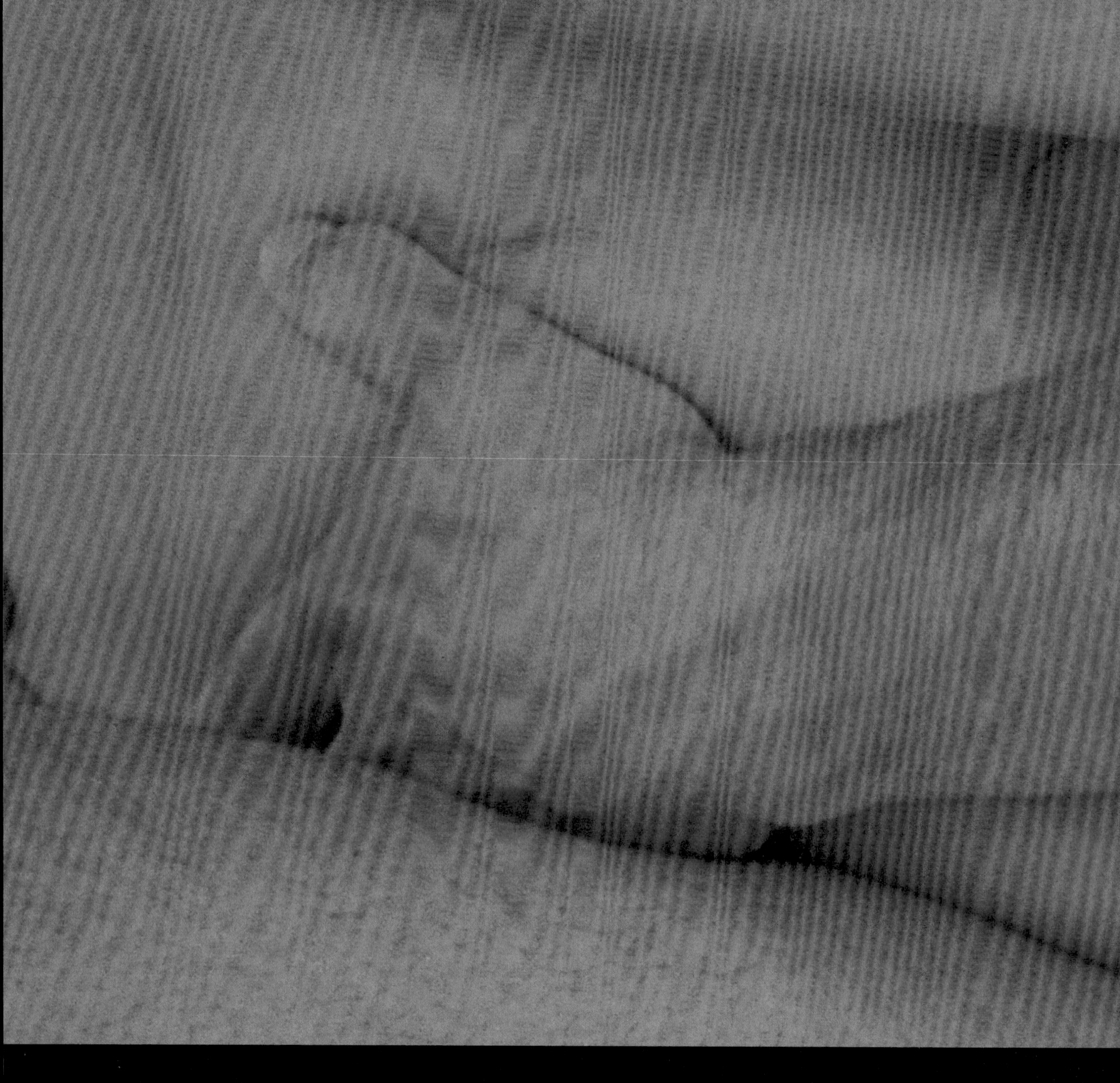

"Though a woman is reserved, and keeps her feelings concealed, yet when she gets on top of a man, she then shows all her love and desire."
KSII:VIII

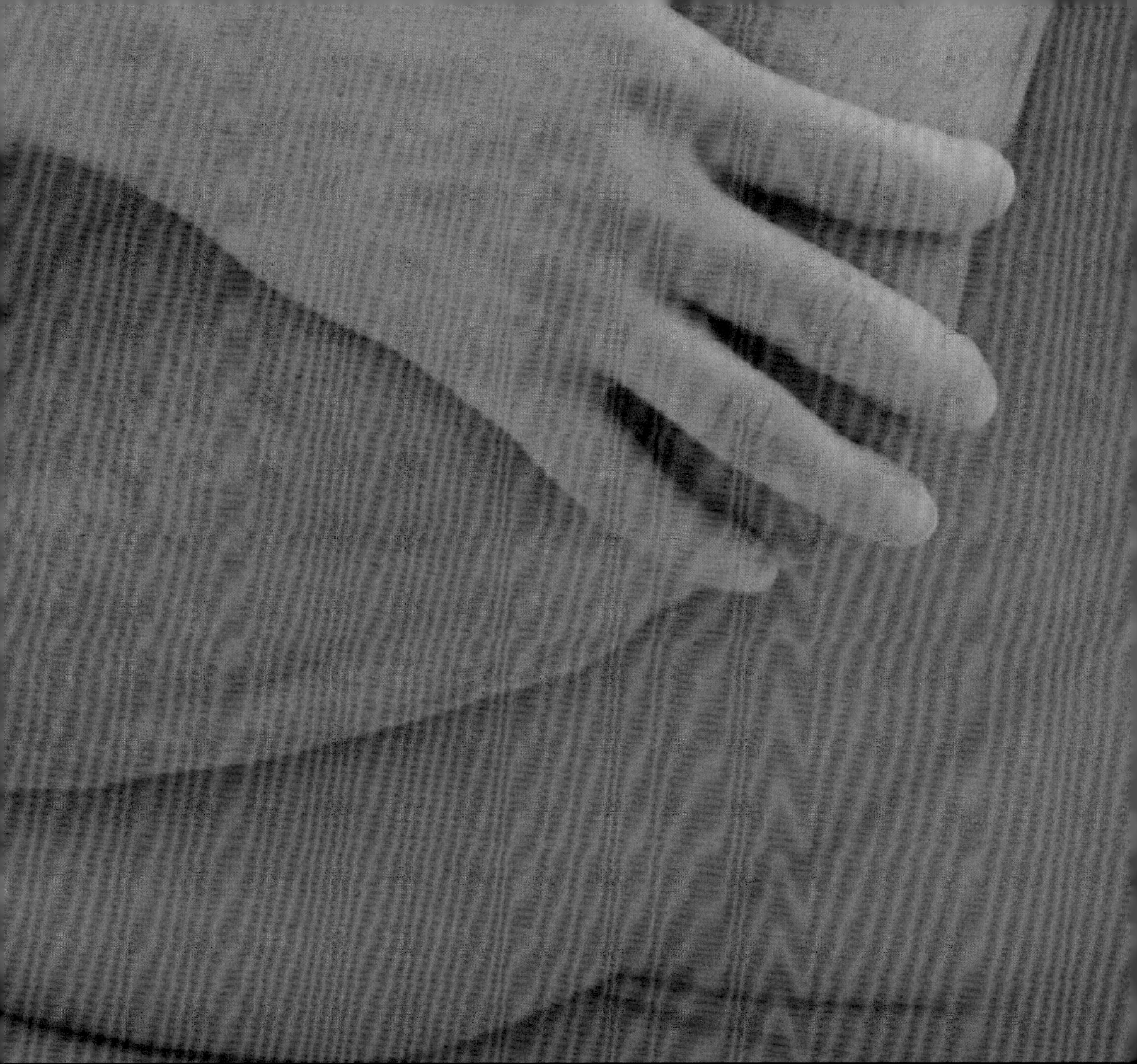

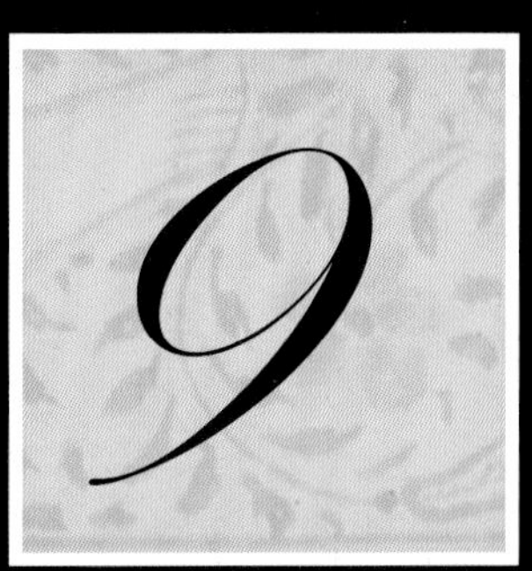

TOP POSITIONS

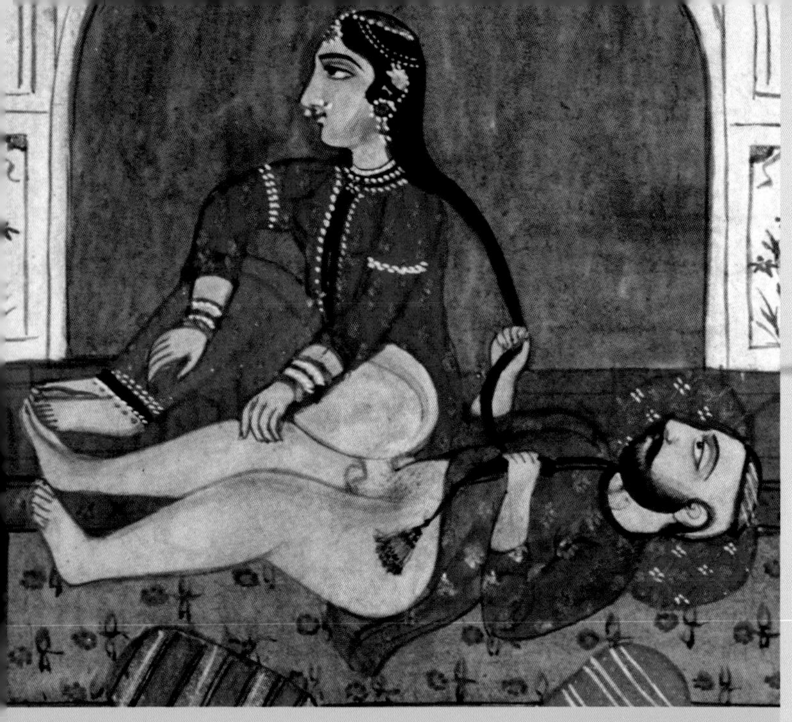

THE WOMAN-ON-TOP positions are united by two themes: the importance of satisfying female desire, and the eroticism of role reversal. The Kama Sutra took women's pleasure seriously, noting that a man could learn what his partner liked by allowing her to play his part: "A man should gather from the actions of the woman of what disposition she is, and in what way she likes to be enjoyed."

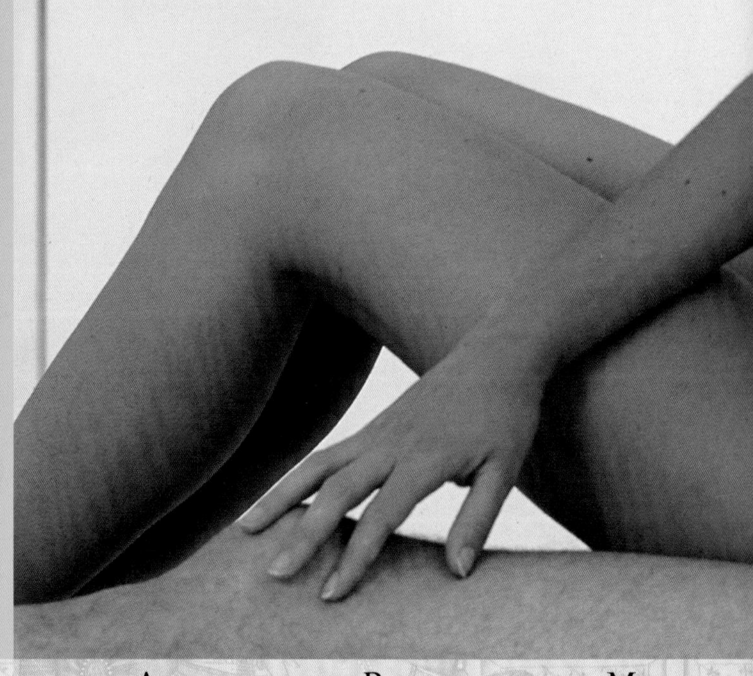

Pair of Tongs

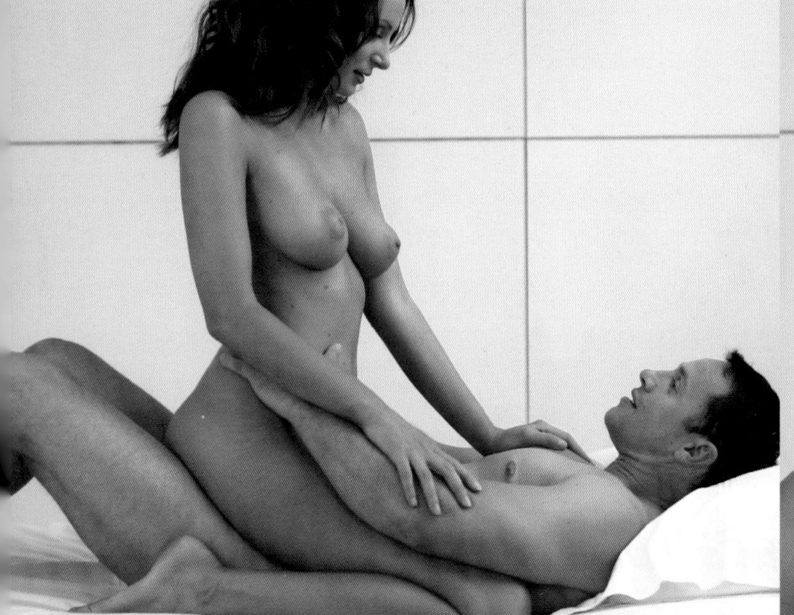

Acting the Part of the Man

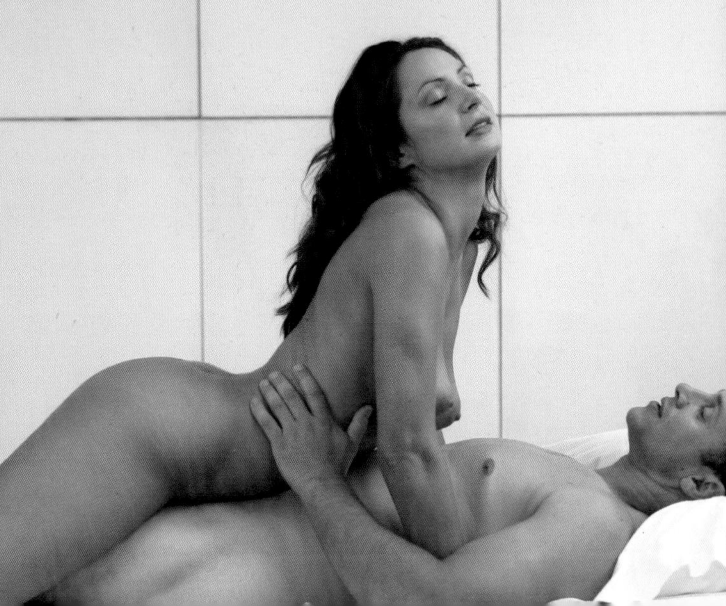

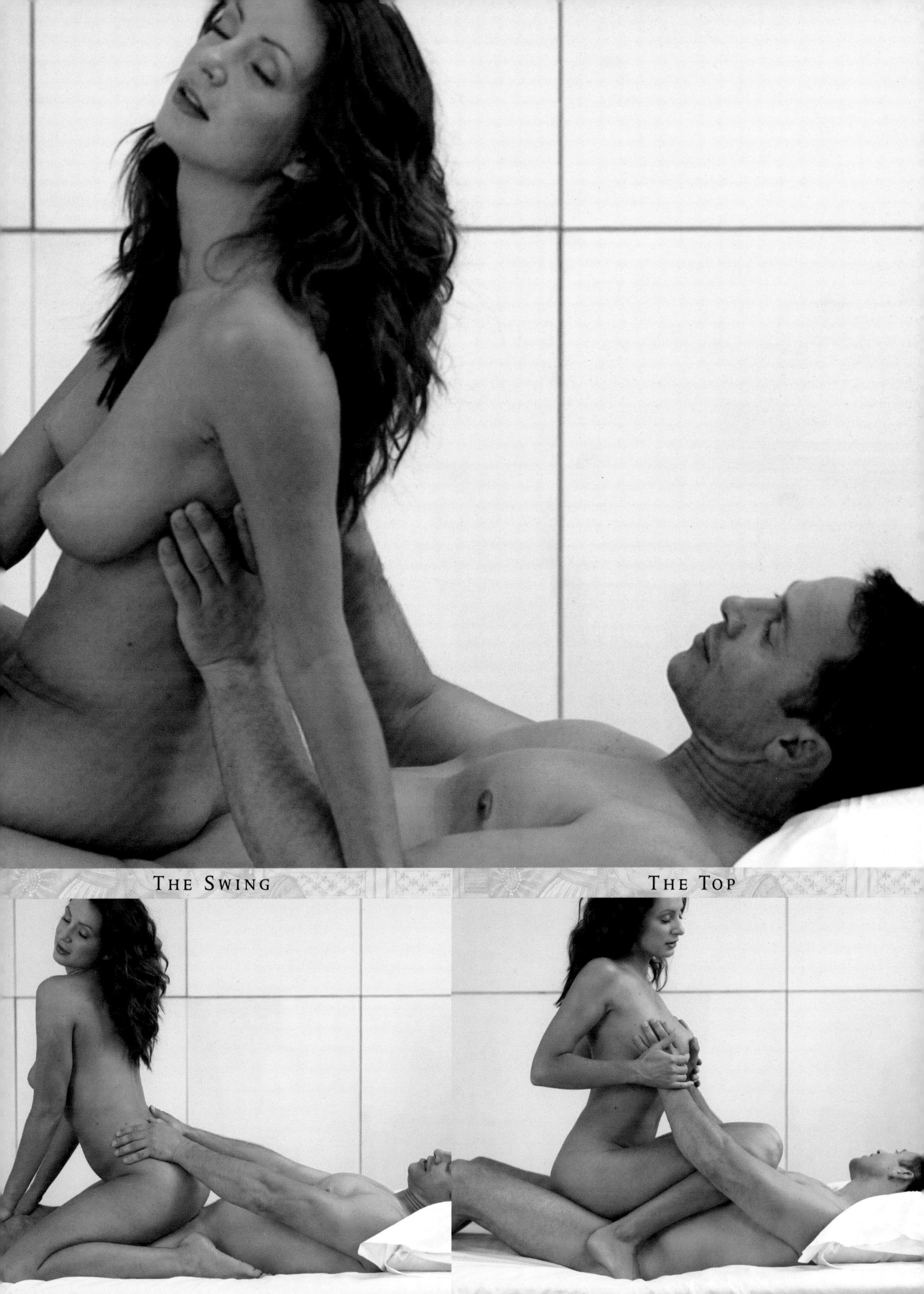

The Swing
The Top

Pair of Tongs

"When the woman holds the lingam in her yoni, draws it in, presses it, and keeps it thus in her for a long time, it is called the Pair of Tongs." The Pair of Tongs is a very sensual technique and, like the Mare's position (*see* pg.71), can be used in various postures. With her lover's penis inside her, the woman tightens her vagina. The sensations aroused as she repeatedly squeezes and releases is a real turn on for both him and her.

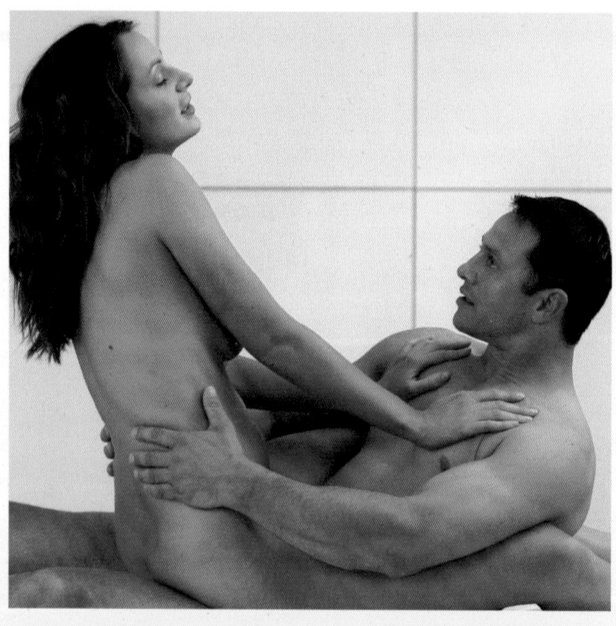

> SIT ASTRIDE HIS PRONE *and willing form (he might like to prop his head and shoulders up on a pillow) and bend your legs at the knee. Draw his penis deeply into your vagina, repeatedly squeezing it with your pelvic floor muscles (*see Kegel exercises, pg.158*). You can stimulate your clitoris to build up powerful sensations—and watch each other enjoying the shudders and spasms of pleasure that you're providing.*

∧ THE DOMINANT *positions described on the following pages link most naturally with sitting positions. From here you can push your lover down and if you like he can sit up again later for another long cuddle in a seated position.*

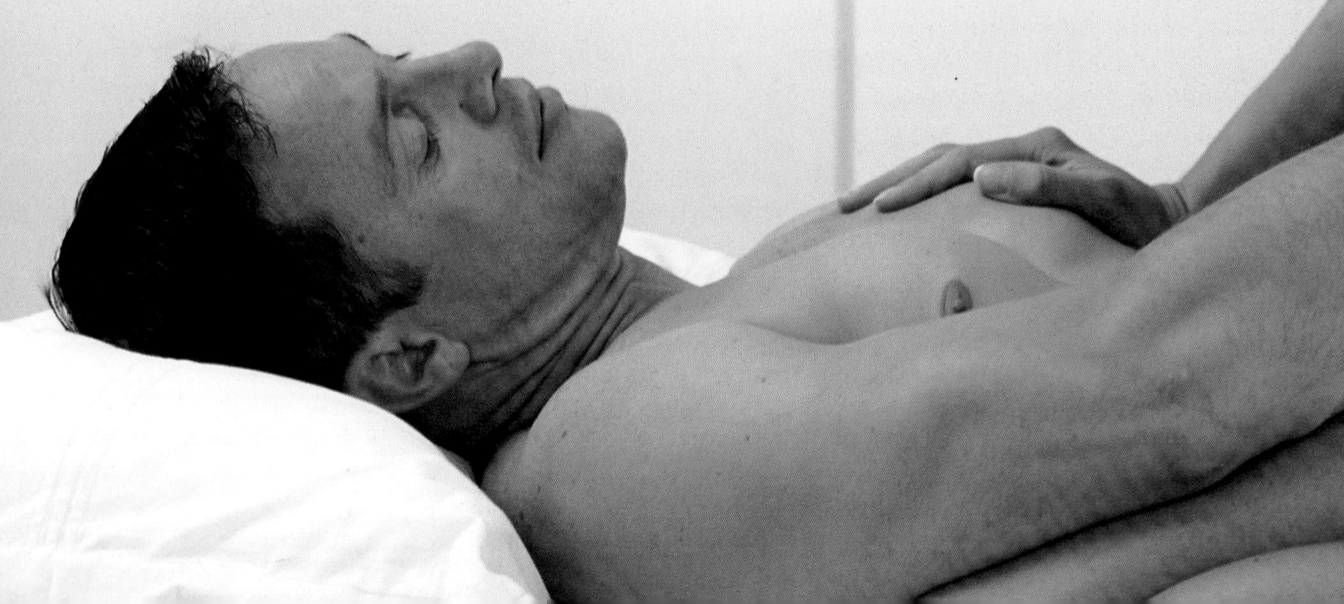

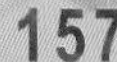

It's incredibly **liberating** and erotic to be able to "play the man" and see his pleasure at your prowess. It's also a chance to show off your vagina's special abilities as you **vary** depth, pace, and style of penetration. While this is going on, you can rub his chest and nipples, or reach behind to **fondle** his testicles. And meanwhile he's free to touch you, too.

What works for her?

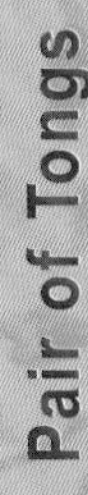

What works for him? ♂

You can ***abandon*** yourself to her wanton desire and focus entirely on your own ***pleasure***. This position is also an excellent way to overcome premature ejaculation, as the movements are ***gentle***, squeezing the penis rather than creating the friction that comes with thrusting.

Kegel exercises

These exercises (named after the gynecologist who popularized them) are simple movements that you can do to strengthen your pelvic floor and vaginal muscles. First, identify the muscles: When you next go to the lavatory, stop the flow of urine—the muscles you use to do this are those you want to strengthen. The first exercise consists of contracting these muscles for three seconds, then releasing them slowly for three seconds. You can also try doing this exercise more quickly. The second exercise consists of pretending that there is an elevator in your vagina and that you are pulling it up three floors in three stages. Hold it at the top, then let it go, again in three stages. Repeat these exercises several times a day. Practise them anywhere—at home, at work, on the train—at any time!

> THESE WOMAN-ON-TOP *positions also follow naturally from the supine, woman-on-top Inverted embrace (see pg.72). Alternatively, of course, you may decide to start your lovemaking in this way. However you get there, this is your chance to educate him in the delights that your body can offer his—delights he might be quite unaware of. He may take awhile to accept your new role, but be assertive; many men find they relish relinquishing control and abandoning themselves to pleasure. Completely seduce him by purposefully holding eye contact while you squeeze his penis in your vagina and simultaneously stroke his testicles.*

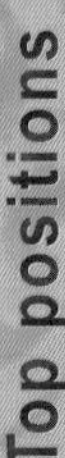

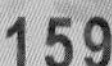

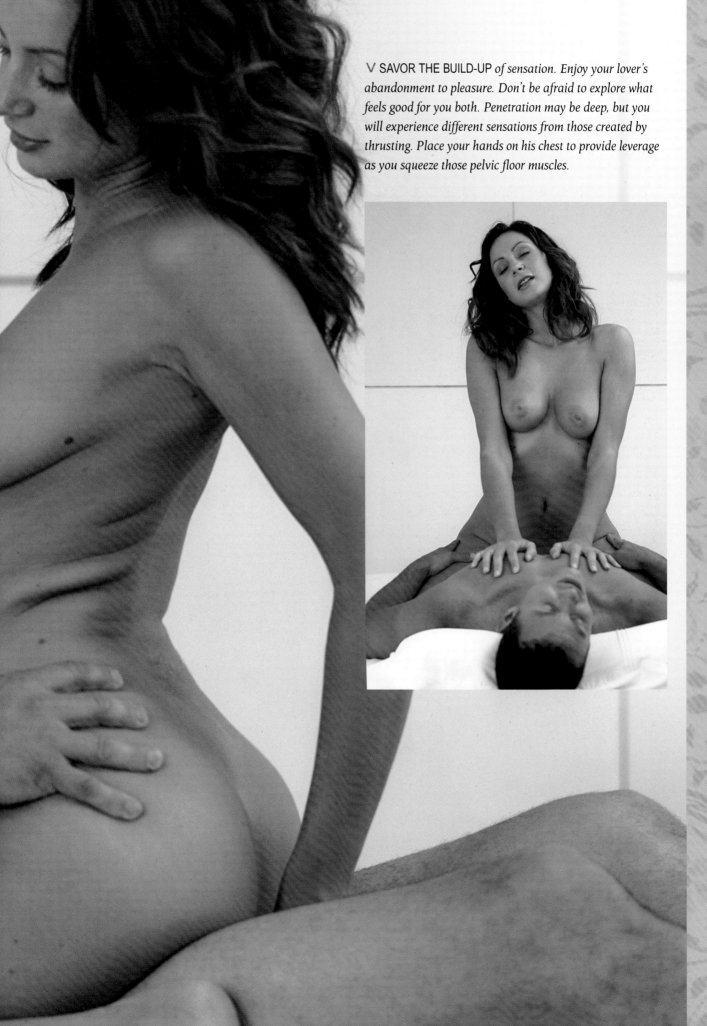

V SAVOR THE BUILD-UP *of sensation. Enjoy your lover's abandonment to pleasure. Don't be afraid to explore what feels good for you both. Penetration may be deep, but you will experience different sensations from those created by thrusting. Place your hands on his chest to provide leverage as you squeeze those pelvic floor muscles.*

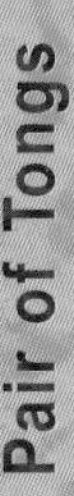

Acting the Part of the Man

Vatsyayana knew about the sexy side of role reversal: "When a woman sees that her lover is fatigued by constant congress, without having his desire satisfied, she should, with his permission, lay him down upon his back, and give him assistance by acting his part. She may also do this to satisfy the curiosity of her lover, or her own desire of novelty."

V CHANGE THE DYNAMIC *between you by making it obvious that you wish him to surrender himself to your sensuous attentions. Enjoy the feeling of mastery and the pleasure of his trust (and if he's tired, this is a great way of persuading him to play).*

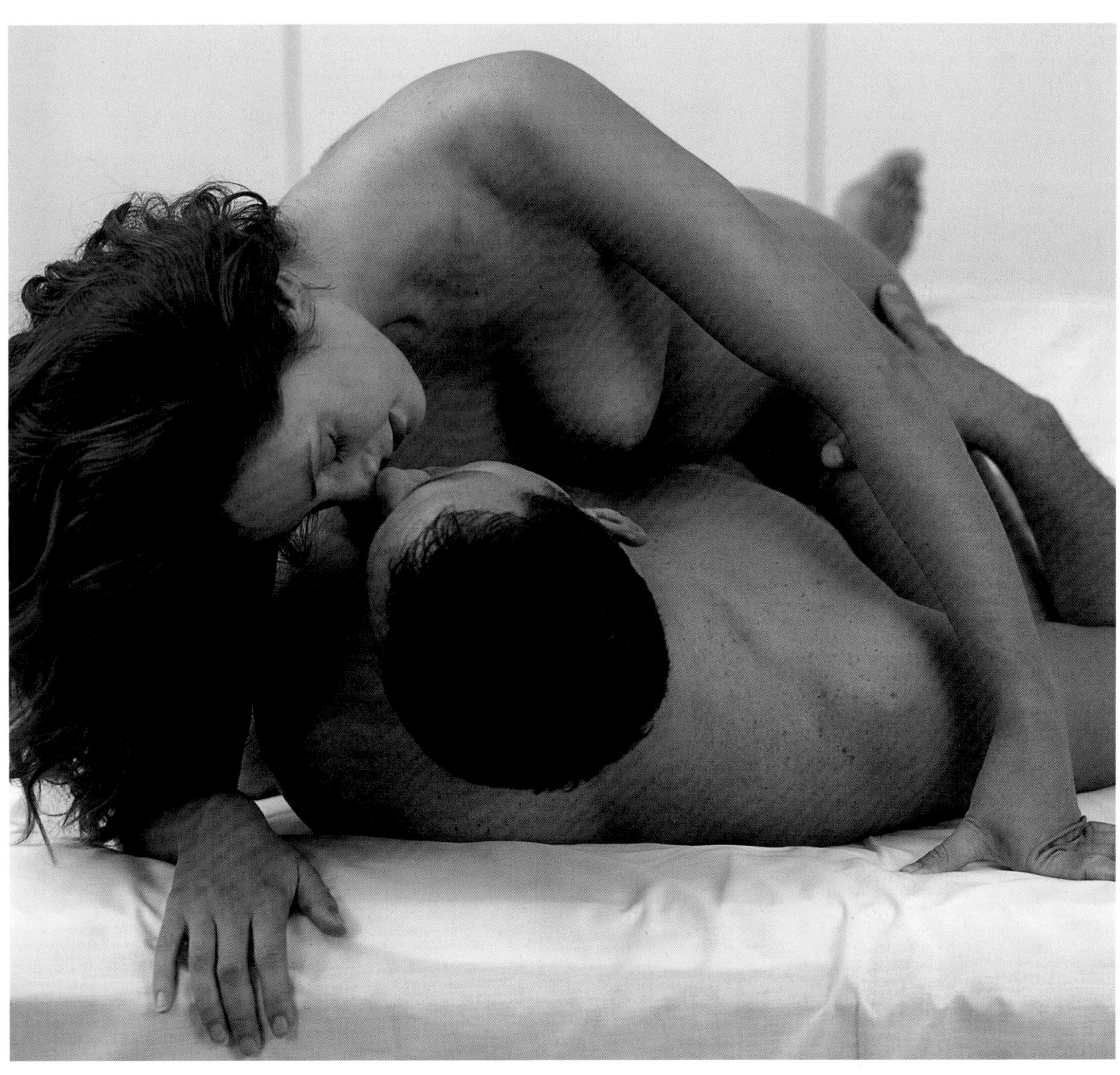

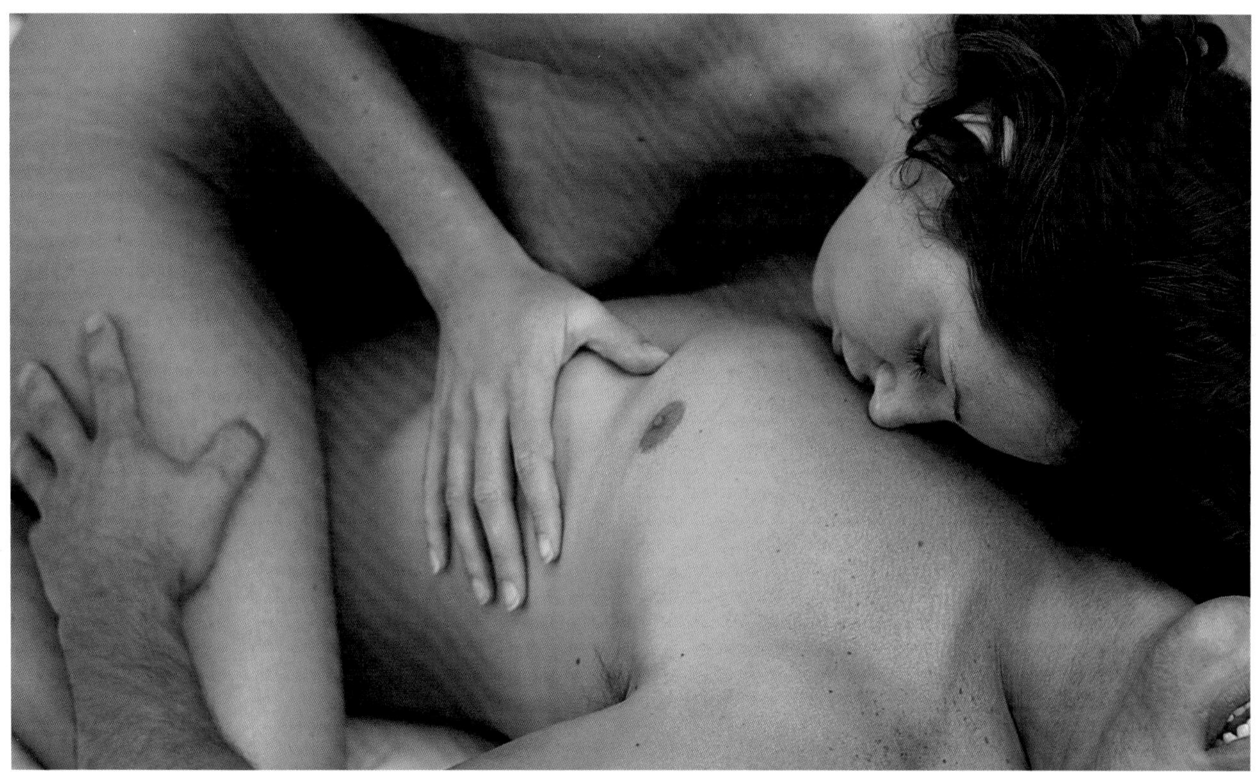

Role reversal

The Kama Sutra's description of the woman-on-top reads: "She acts the part of the man from the beginning. At such a time, with flowers in her hair hanging loose, and her smiles broken by hard breathings, she should press upon her lover's bosom with her own breasts, and lowering her head frequently, should do in return the same actions which he used to do before."

∧ USE YOUR TIME *on top to get to know him a little better, especially those scrumptious male nipples and pectorals. Knead, lick, tweak, and kiss. These bits become sensitive when he's aroused, so put them on your sexual agenda.*

∨ MANY MEN *love feeling their lover's body cover theirs—it's sensual and comforting. Some men who identify wholly with being the active partner may feel uncomfortable allowing you control, so build trust and introduce him gently to the concept of accepting pleasure.*

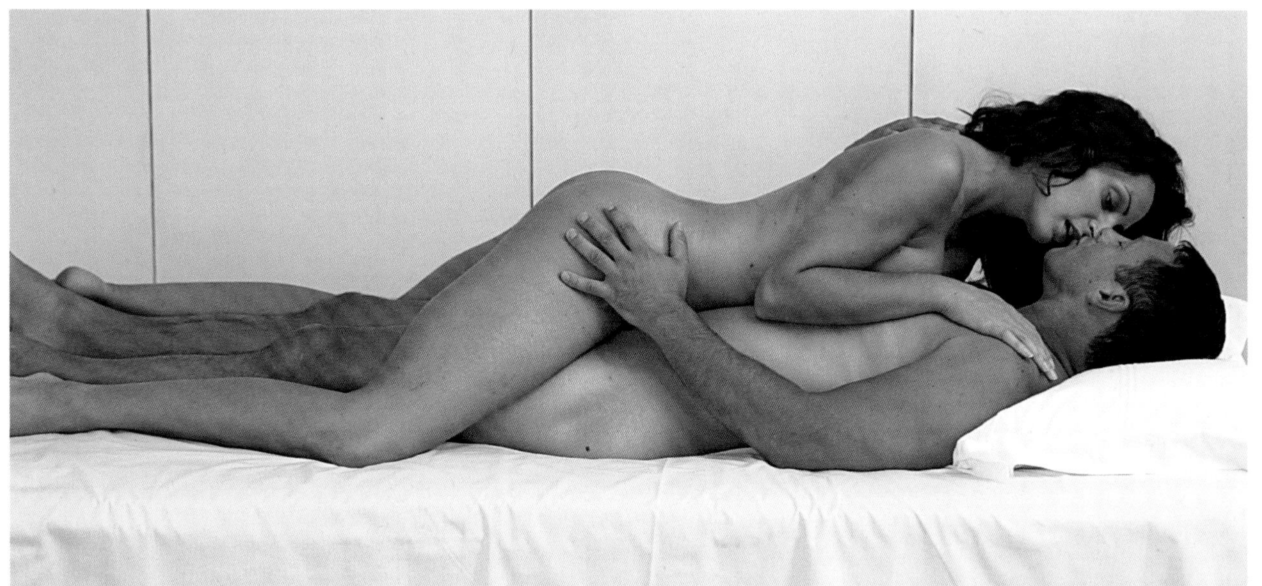

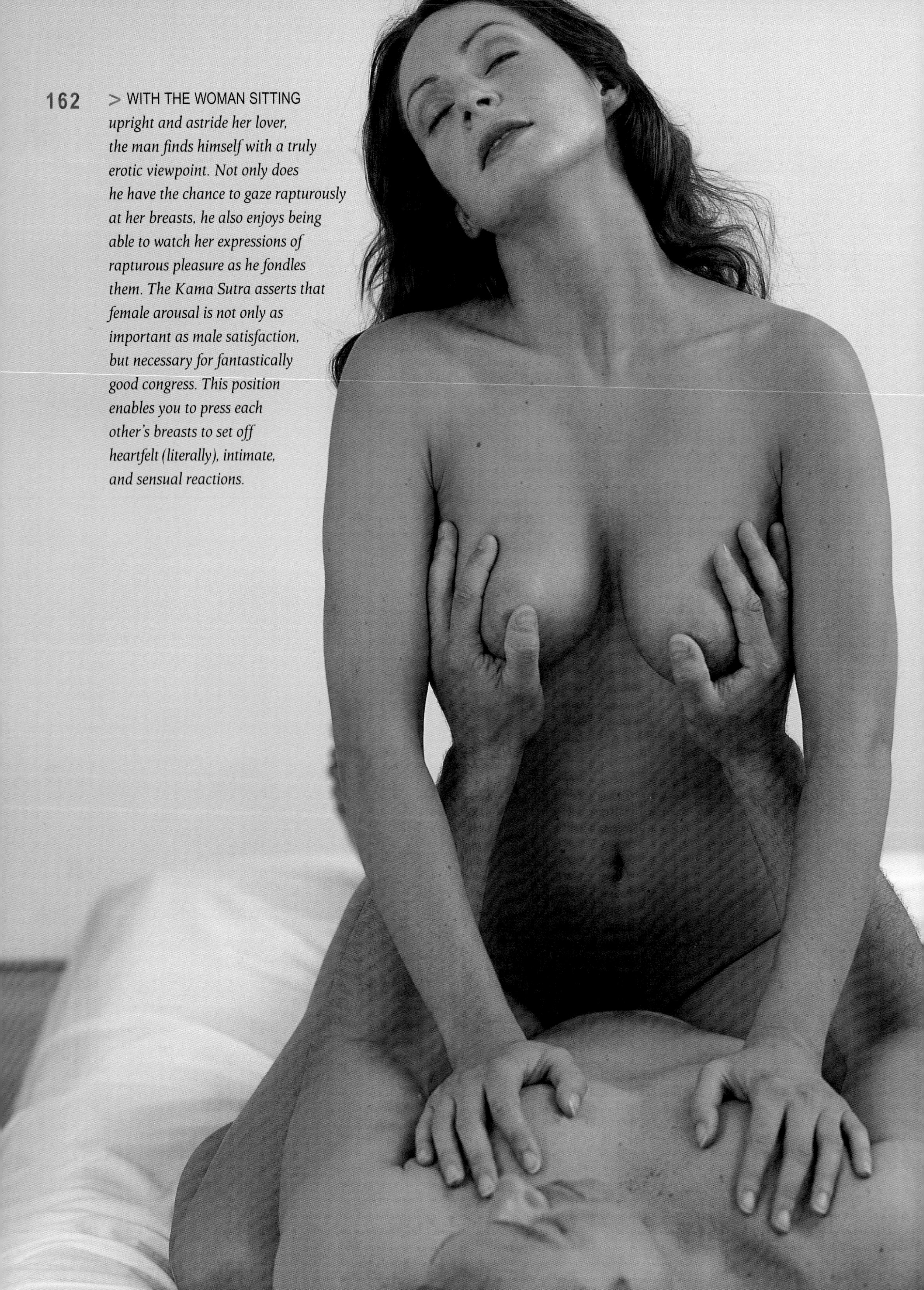

> WITH THE WOMAN SITTING *upright and astride her lover, the man finds himself with a truly erotic viewpoint. Not only does he have the chance to gaze rapturously at her breasts, he also enjoys being able to watch her expressions of rapturous pleasure as he fondles them. The Kama Sutra asserts that female arousal is not only as important as male satisfaction, but necessary for fantastically good congress. This position enables you to press each other's breasts to set off heartfelt (literally), intimate, and sensual reactions.*

Acts to be done by the man

"Whatever is done by a man for giving pleasure to a woman is called the work of a man," and when the woman acts the part of man, Vatsyayana suggests, she can choose from nine "acts to be done by the man." These include: churning [when the lingam is held with the hand and turned around in the yoni]; giving a blow [when the lingam is removed and then forcibly strikes the yoni]; the blow of the boar or of a bull [when one part, or both sides, of the yoni is rubbed]; and the sporting of a sparrow [rapid, shallow thrusting]. Vatsyayana encourages the woman to replicate the "male" actions that she most enjoys, but you should always feel free to experiment with your own variations to teach him a few new tricks!

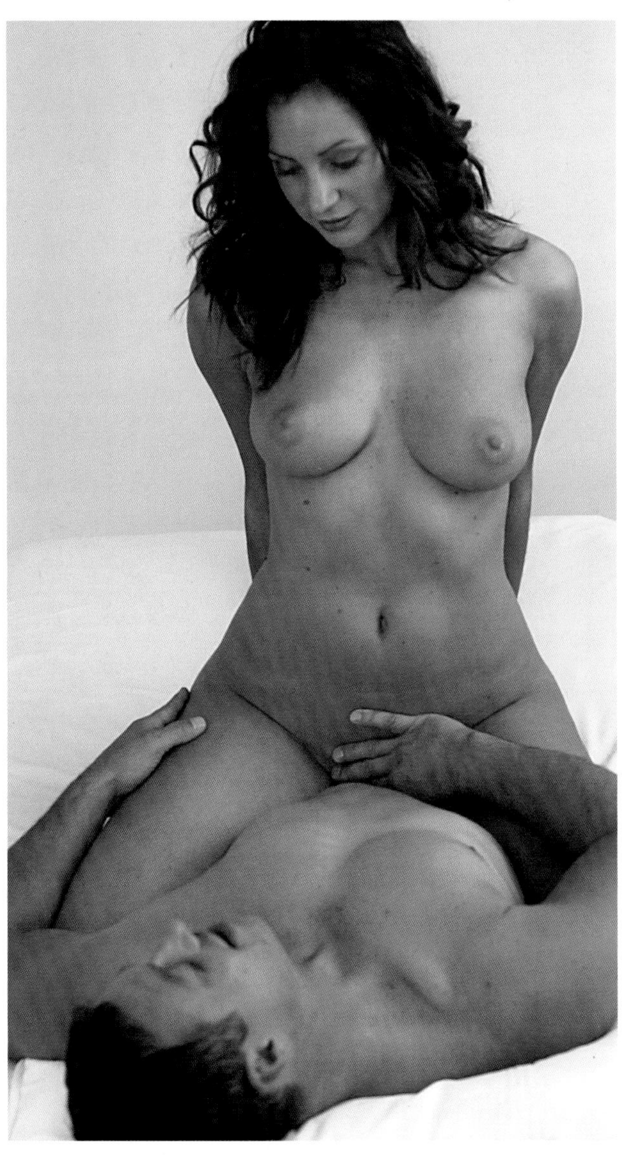

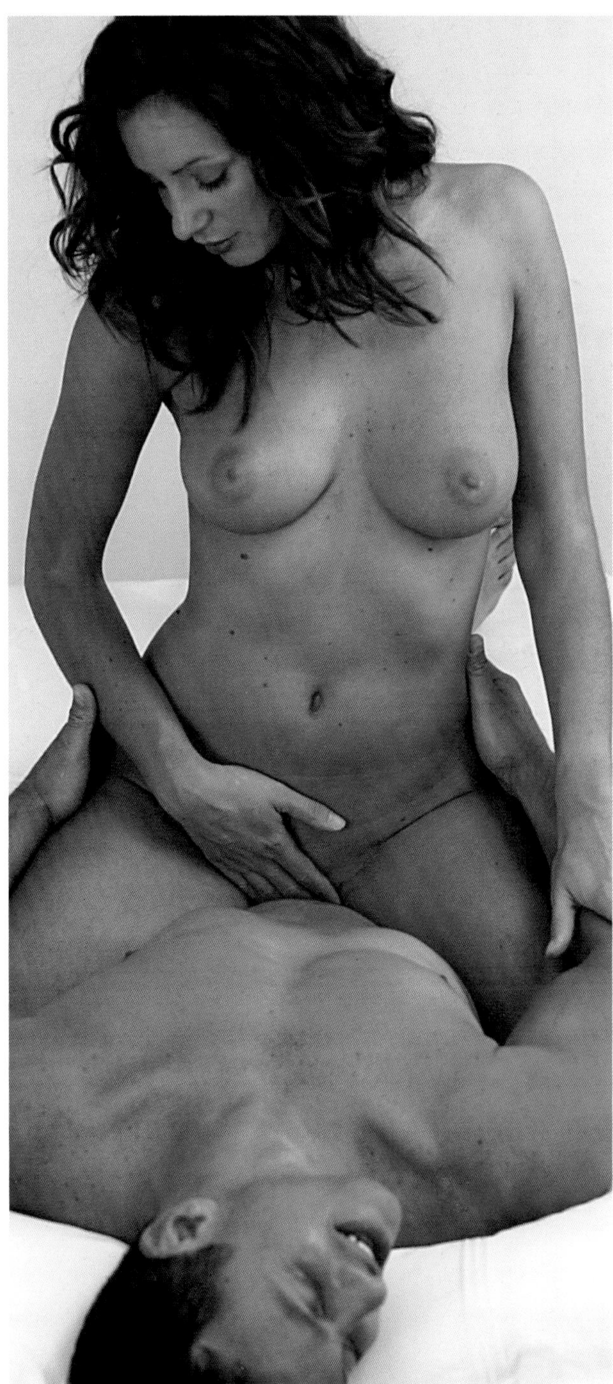

∧ AS YOU SQUEEZE *and grind your hips onto his penis, create further spasms and flutters by stimulating your clitoris. Play the "you can't touch me" game, where he just has to submit to your will and is allowed to touch you only when you say so.*

< THIS POSITION IS PERFECT *for hands-on help to heighten arousal. Keep eye contact while you fondle his testicles and he touches your clitoris. This is a slow burner, so keep communicating the different kinds of pleasure you're giving each other and wait for the fireworks.*

The Swing

"When . . . a man lifts up the middle part of his body, and the woman turns round her middle part, it is called The Swing." The man is supposed to arch his back while the woman twists around on top, swinging her pelvis back and forth. An interesting extension of the Top (*see* pg.166) perhaps, but he'd need a seriously strong back to sustain this position. Like The Top, it comes with a health warning!

V UNLESS YOU ARE WINNING *gold medals for being exceptionally strong and flexible, the original version of this position, as depicted in the painting opposite, is not practical. A safer option is for the man to prop himself up on his arms so he can move his lower back, and for her to keep her weight off him by balancing on her toes as she moves.*

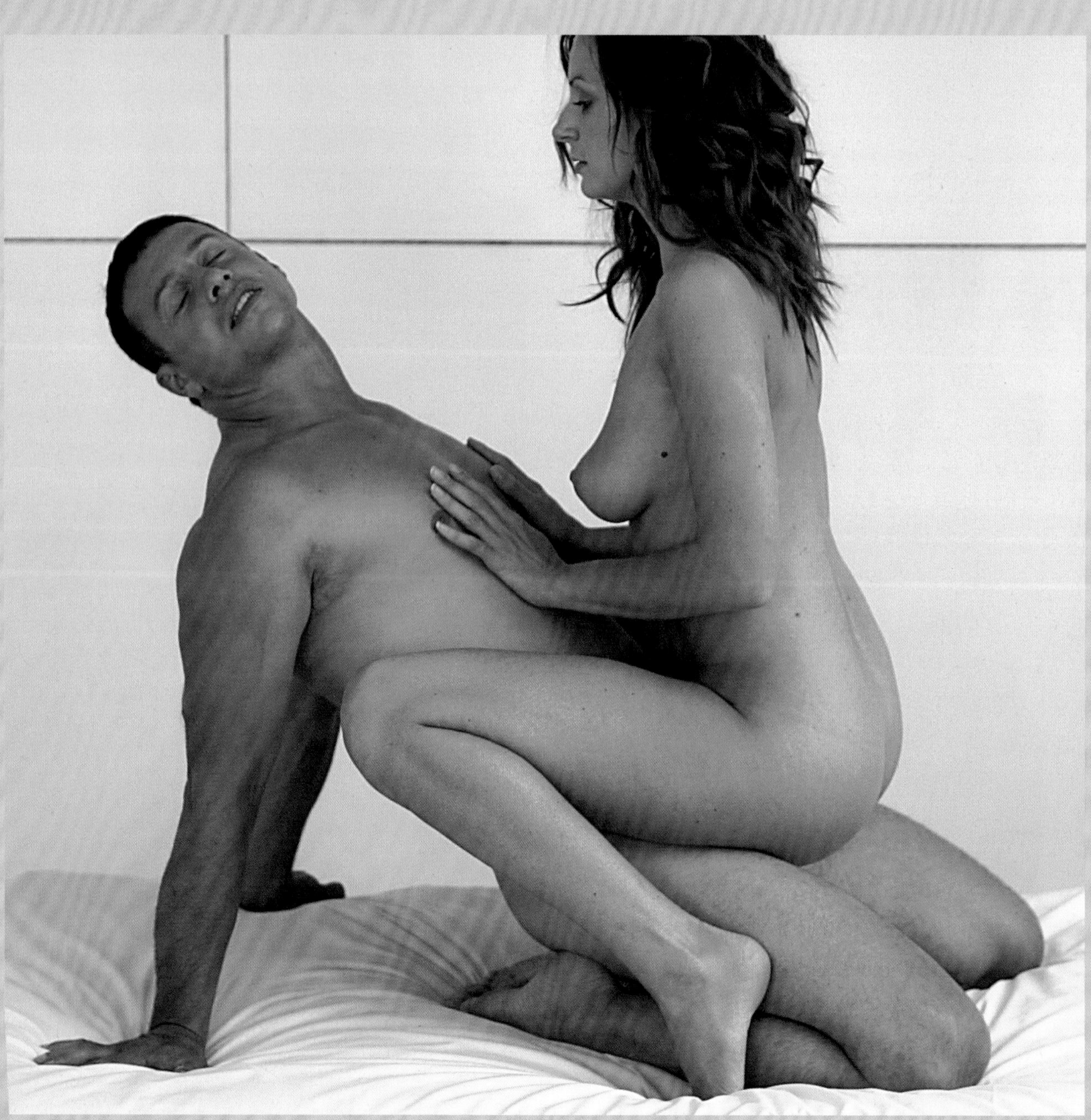

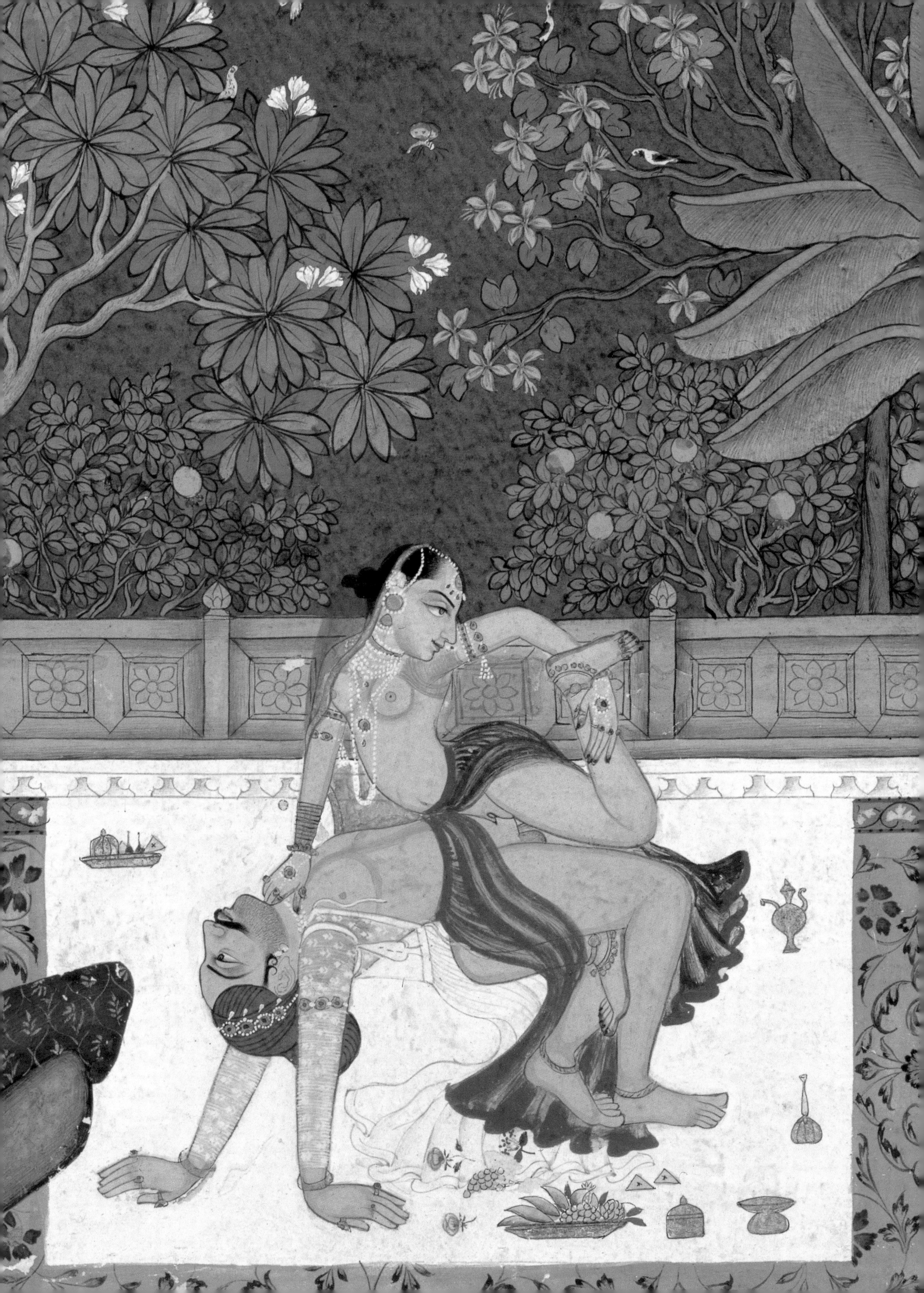

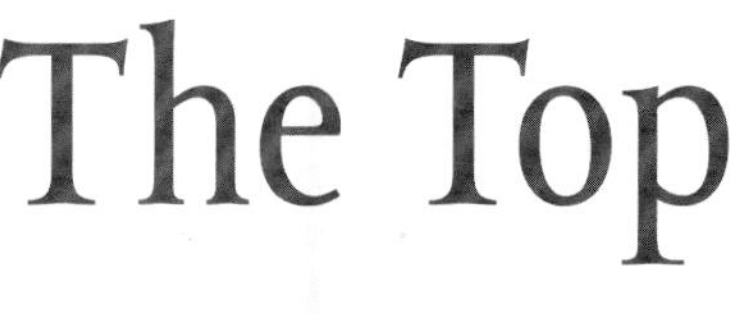

The Top

Theoretically this position offers a revolving 360-degree view of her body and some interesting penetration angles. In fact, the full sequence is more or less impossible to achieve without the penis slipping out at some point. Treat it like a woman-on-top variation of the Turning position (*see* pg.90)—that is, as something of an experiment. He must have complete trust that she will not injure his penis, because it isn't multi-hinged! So take it really slowly.

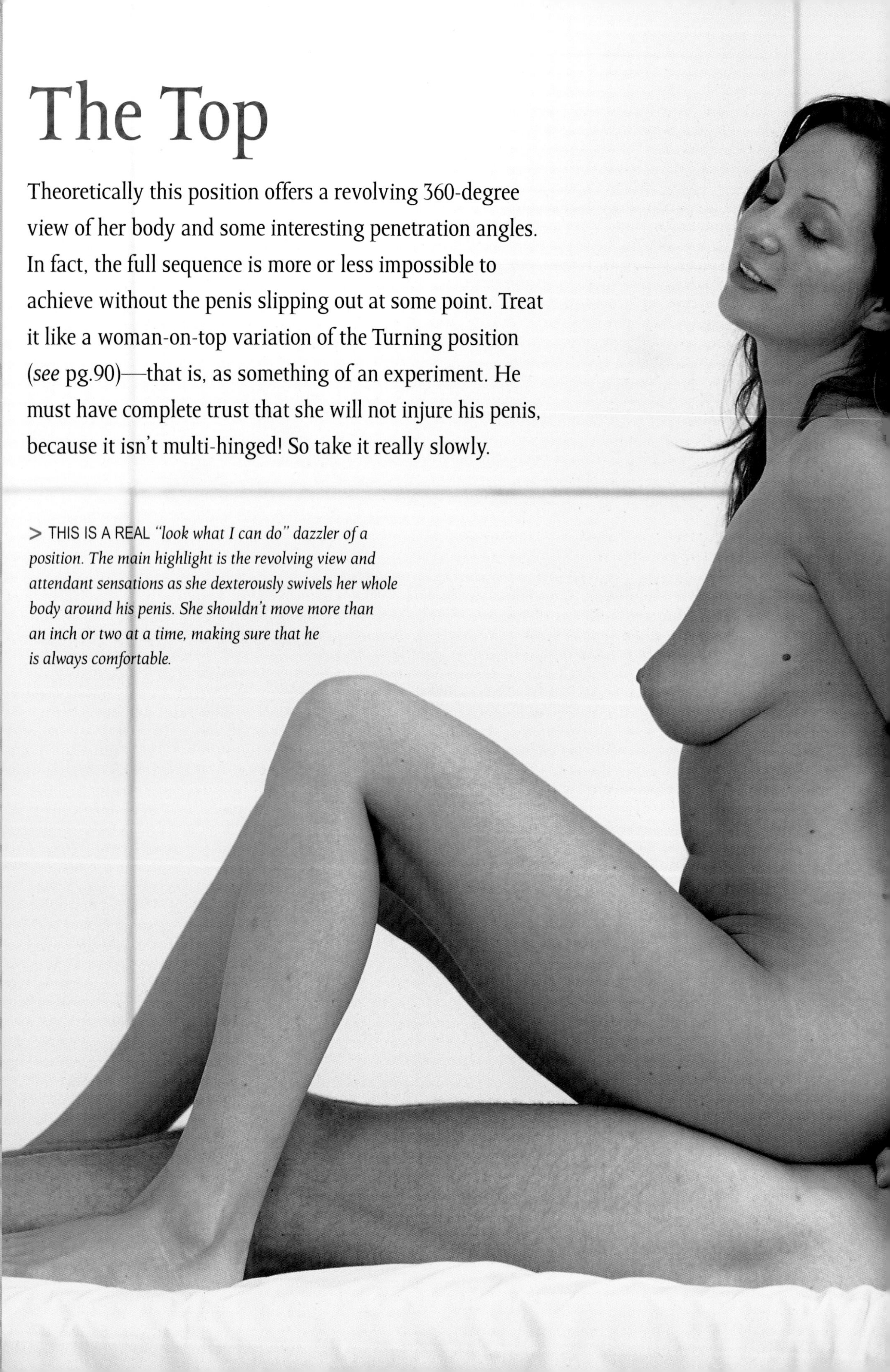

> THIS IS A REAL *"look what I can do" dazzler of a position. The main highlight is the revolving view and attendant sensations as she dexterously swivels her whole body around his penis. She shouldn't move more than an inch or two at a time, making sure that he is always comfortable.*

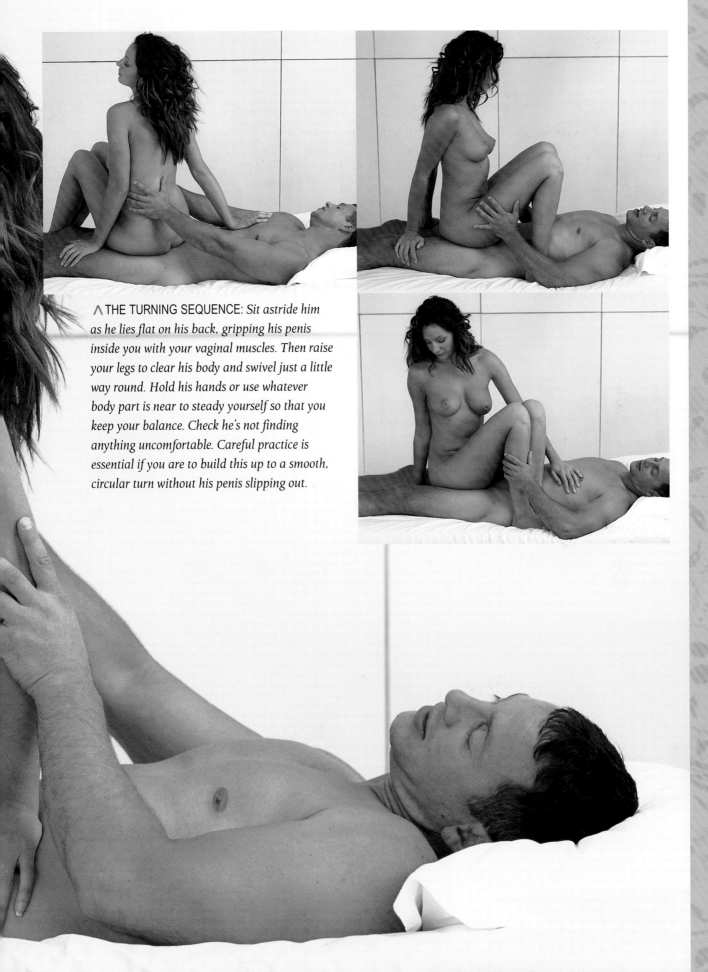

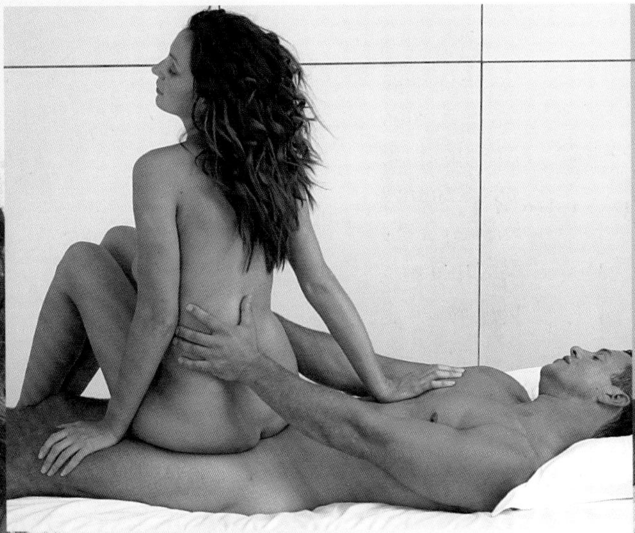

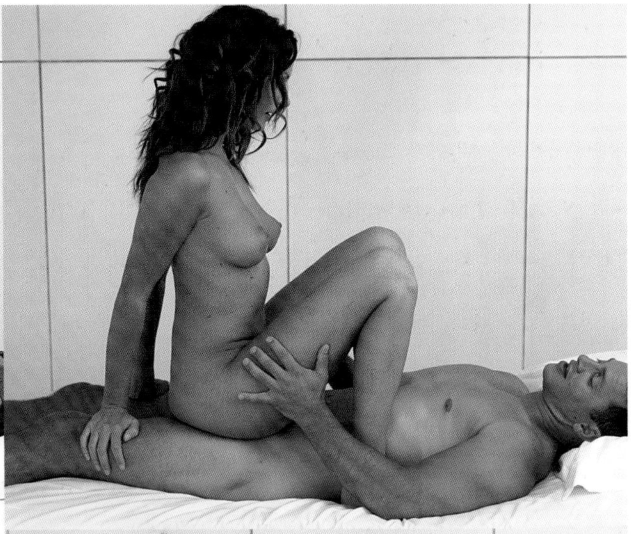

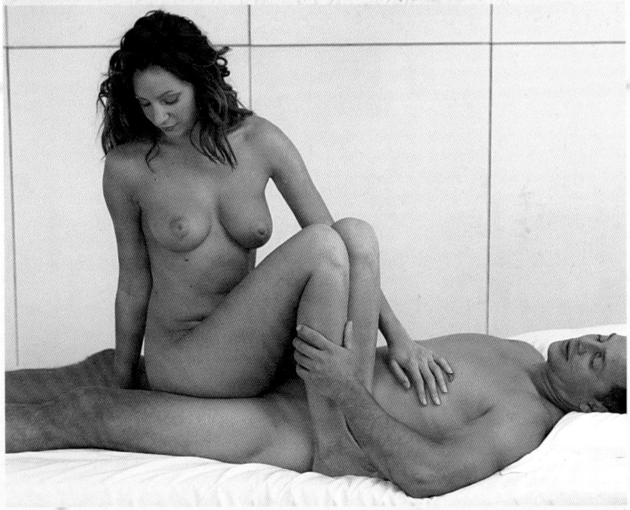

∧ THE TURNING SEQUENCE: *Sit astride him as he lies flat on his back, gripping his penis inside you with your vaginal muscles. Then raise your legs to clear his body and swivel just a little way round. Hold his hands or use whatever body part is near to steady yourself so that you keep your balance. Check he's not finding anything uncomfortable. Careful practice is essential if you are to build this up to a smooth, circular turn without his penis slipping out.*

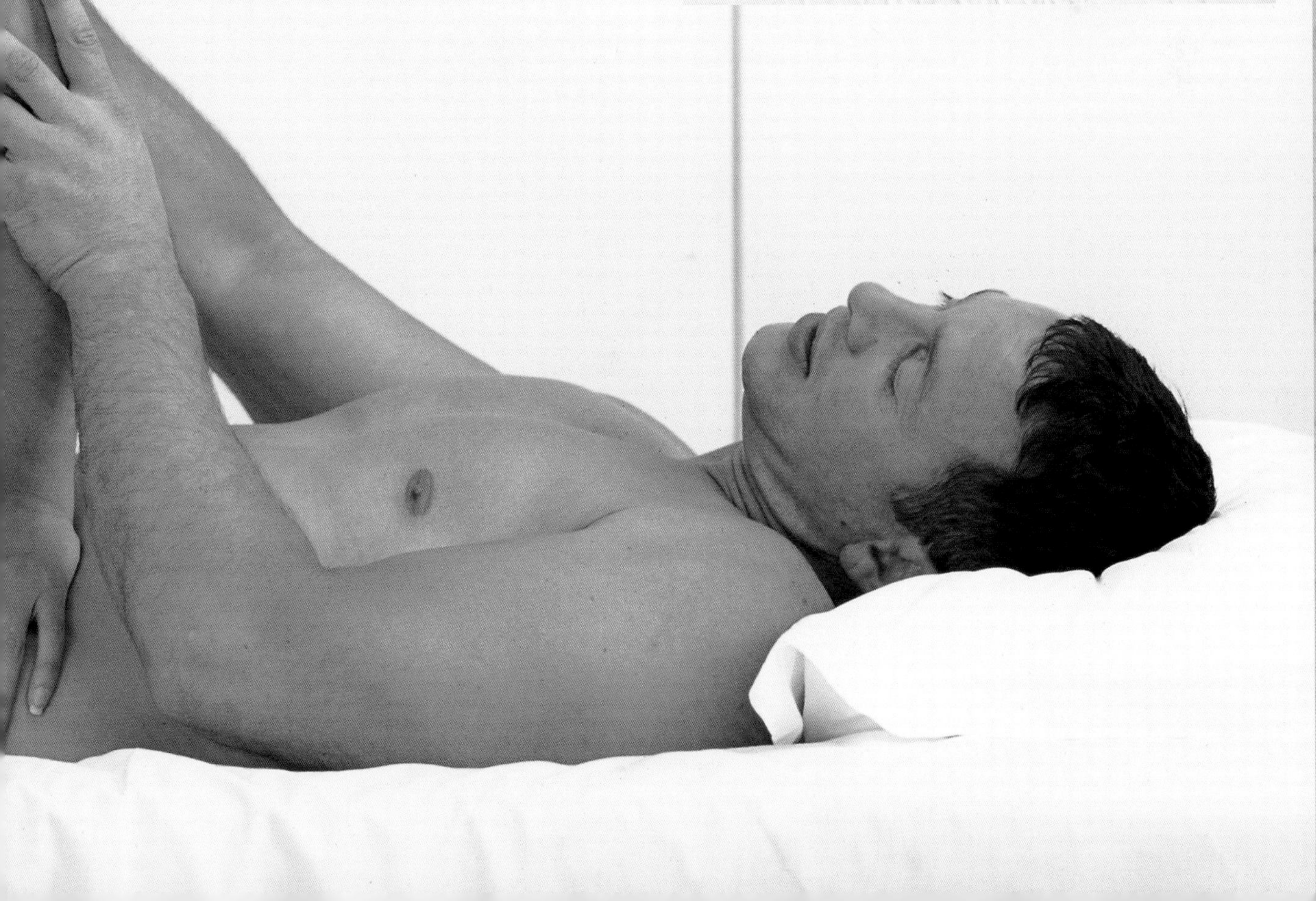

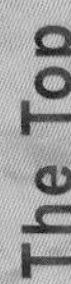

> EVEN WHEN YOU HAVE YOUR BACK *to your lover in the Top position, you can still enjoy a cuddle. You should receive maximum penetration at this angle, so ask him not to thrust, because this can jar the cervix. You can "act the part of the man" in this position, using your pelvic floor muscles to full effect while he holds you and surrenders to the blissful pleasure you're giving him. As for him, he gets an erotic view of—and access to—your buttocks.*

V TURN AWAY *from him to turn him (and yourself) on. Use this position to tease him slowly, control the pace, vary the movements of your pelvis, and contract your vaginal muscles around his penis. You have a not-to-be-missed opportunity to fondle his testicles. Hold them firmly as you gently rotate, bringing him to the point of orgasm. Meanwhile you enjoy the sensation of him touching your butt.*

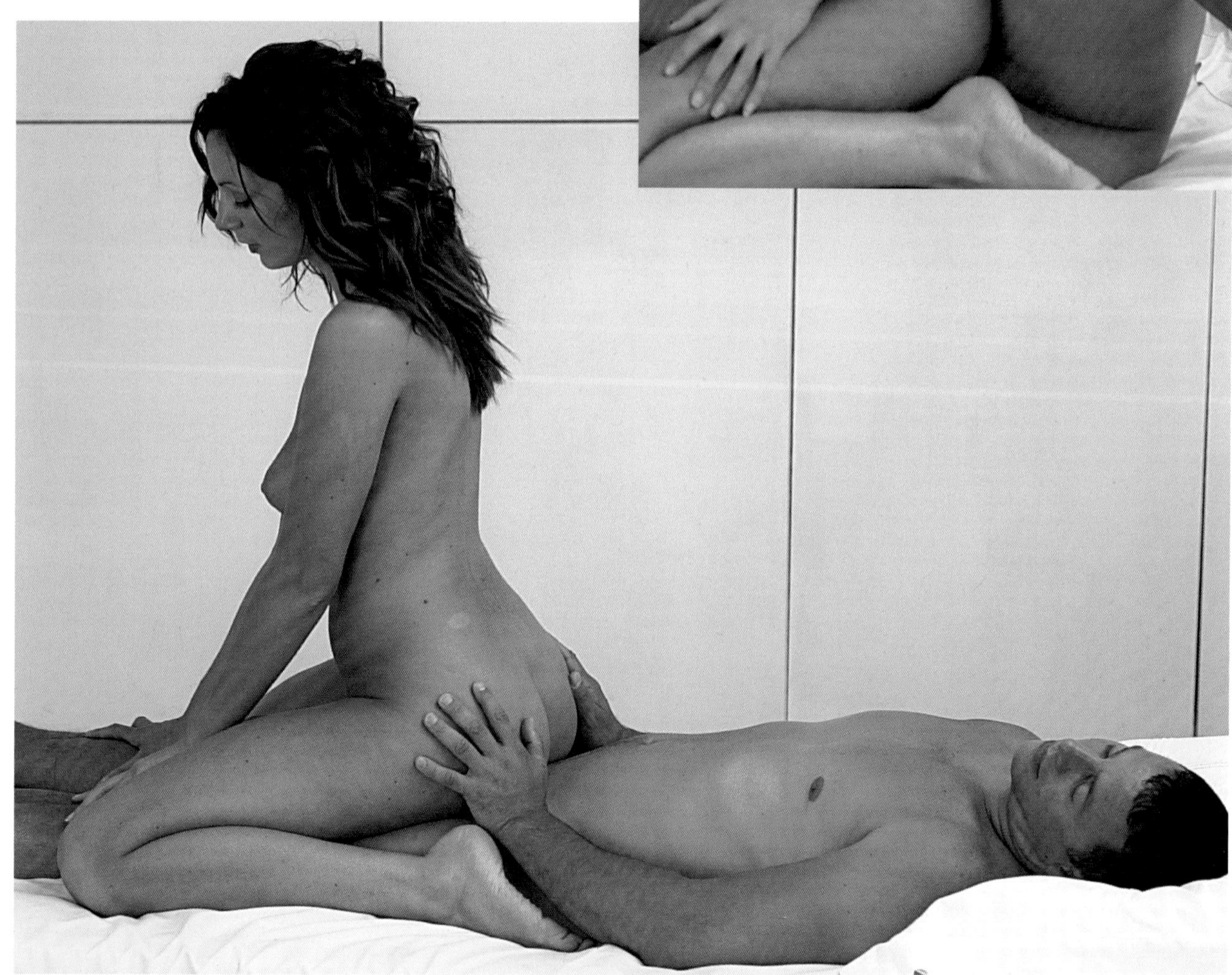

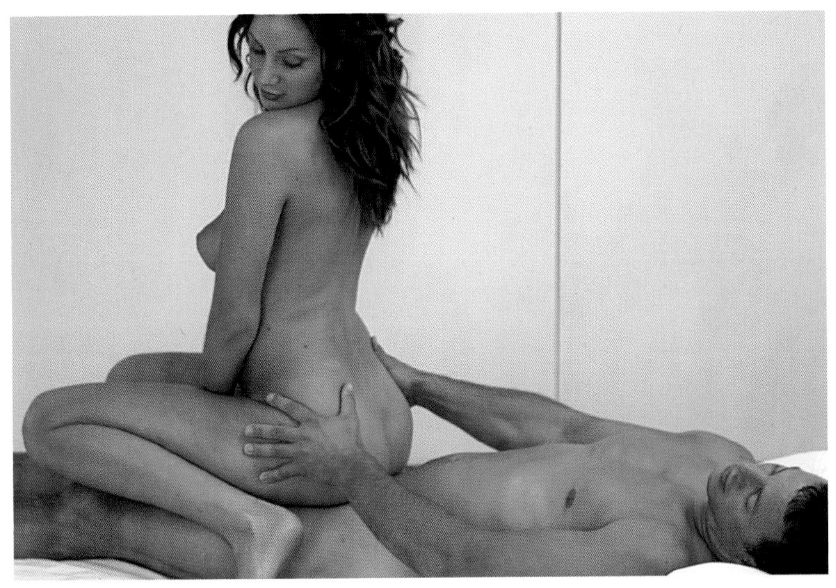

< THIS POSITION *offers the charms of rear-entry sex without engendering any possible feelings of female submissiveness. In this delicious role reversal, she has free reign to pleasure him as she sees fit. Another excellent feature of this position is the angle of penetration for its potential G-spot activation. In addition, your hands are free to tease and excite yourself or your lover to fever pitch. And it will give him a real thrill to watch your buttocks as you fuse together.*

V BE VERY CAREFUL *when you try this. Open his legs and place your feet between his thighs to allow deeper penetration. Lean forward to grasp his ankles for greater leverage. It's good for preventing premature ejaculation because it generates less intense sensations than when he thrusts freely.*

> DESPITE THE FACT *that these positions lack eye contact, they can be a source of deep, intimate sexual understanding. You can connect on a fundamental level with your lover by focusing on other senses, especially touch, and on the emotions aroused by your lovemaking.*

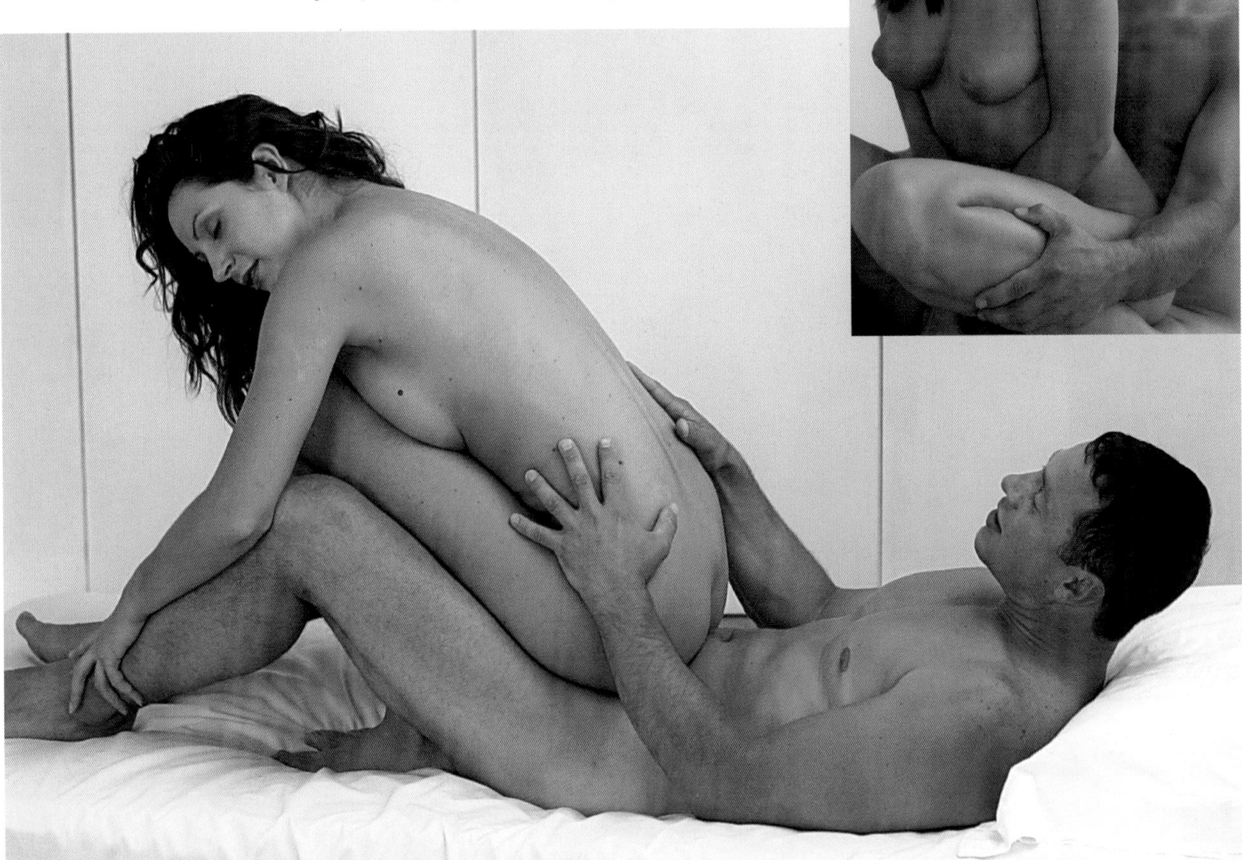

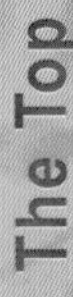

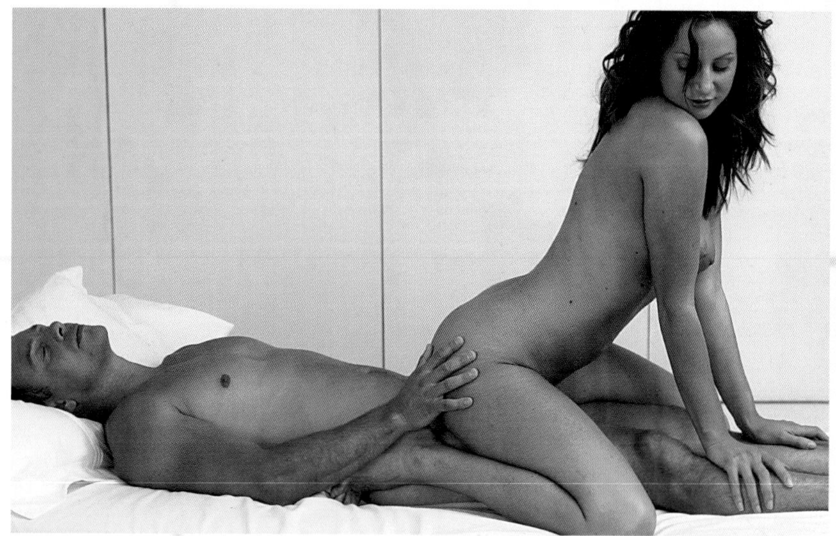

< BY TURNING AWAY *from him, you can give your rapt attention to the physical pleasure you're experiencing—or perhaps conjure up imaginary lovers. He can let himself go because he's not wholly responsible for your enjoyment. If you feel exposed on top, try blindfolding him. It'll heighten his other senses and free you to complete abandonment, knowing you are not being watched.*

> INTENSIFY YOUR *levels of intimacy and get all the skin-on-skin contact you can by lying back against him. This leaves your hands free to touch yourself, and it also permits his hands to rove all over your arched form. He will adore being covered by your body and feeling you move against him. The extra contact communicates every spasm of pleasure. Could anything be better?*

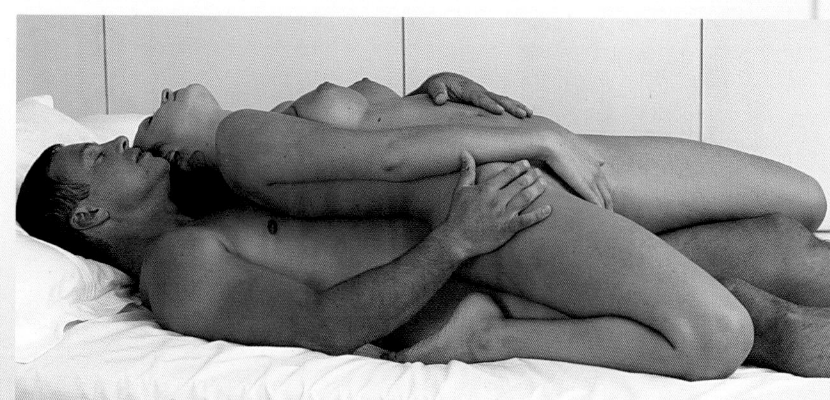

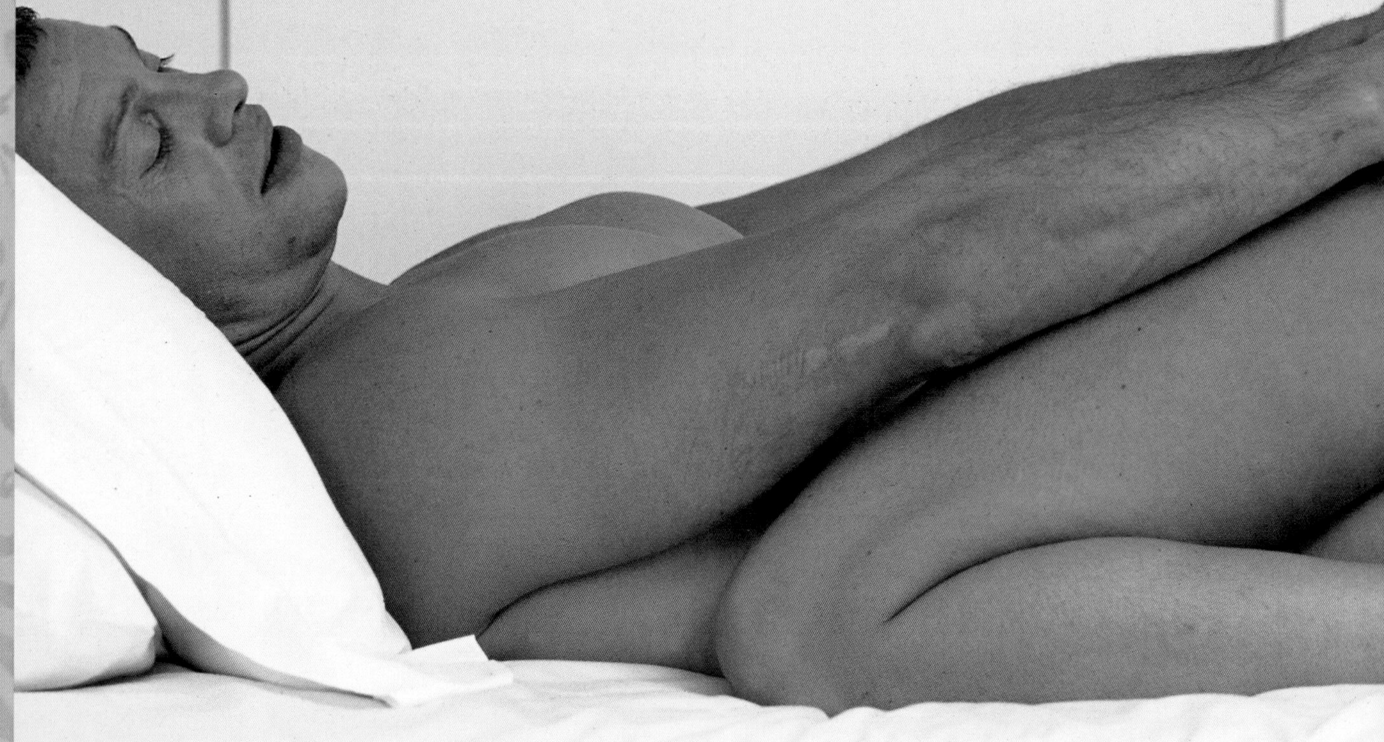

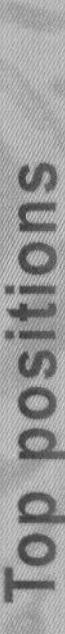

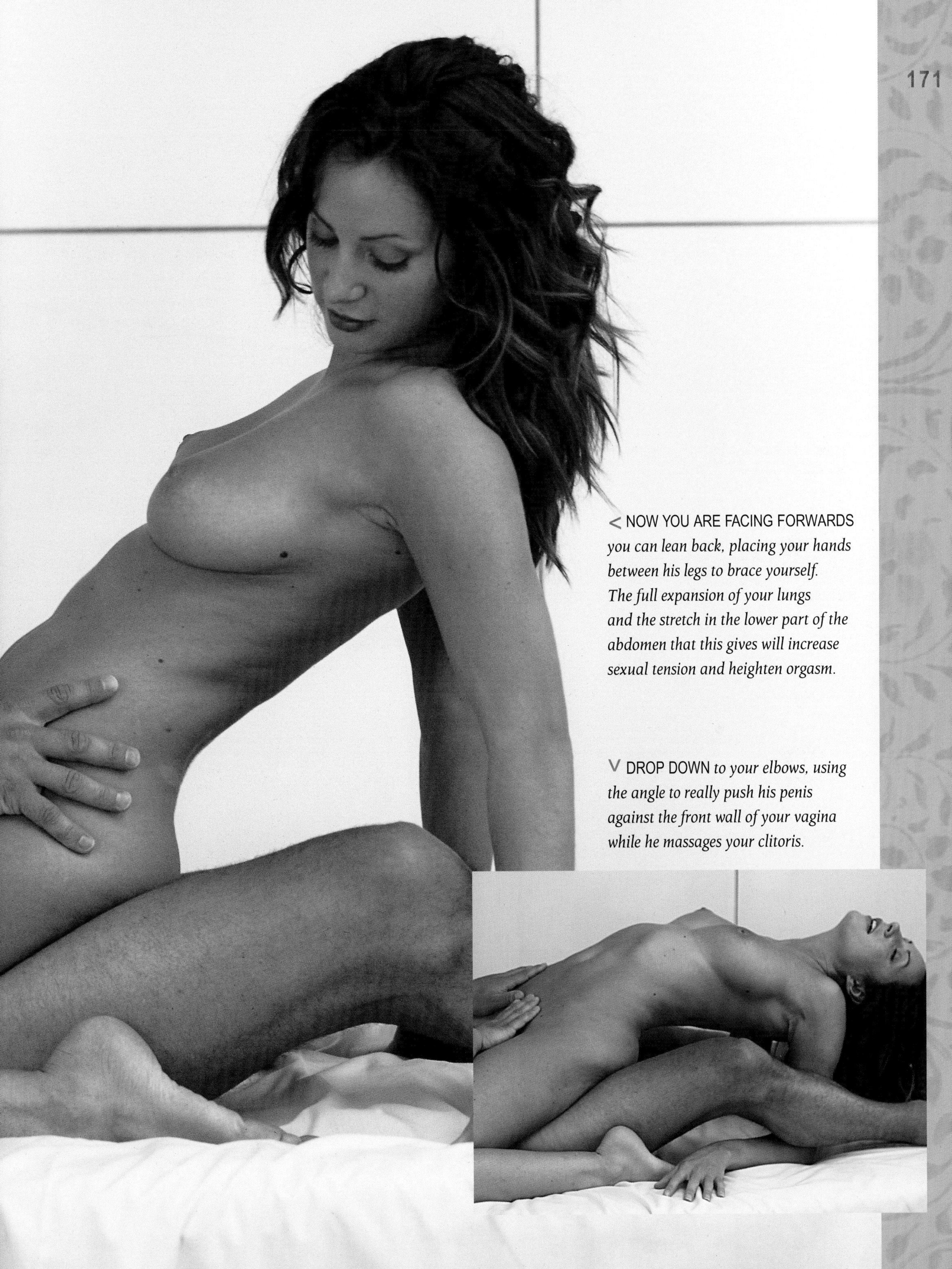

< NOW YOU ARE FACING FORWARDS *you can lean back, placing your hands between his legs to brace yourself. The full expansion of your lungs and the stretch in the lower part of the abdomen that this gives will increase sexual tension and heighten orgasm.*

V DROP DOWN *to your elbows, using the angle to really push his penis against the front wall of your vagina while he massages your clitoris.*

Kali energy

The Kama Sutra is informed by ancient Indian beliefs about the ultimate power of women. The mother goddess Kali was worshipped as the mysterious source of fertility and life. She could be both terrifying and nurturing—as well as incredibly sexy. All women have "Kali energy" inside, and this can be released at the height of sex. Passionate lovers can harness this energy to liberate their lovemaking, lifting it from the routine to the joyful, enriching and sublime experience it should be.

> THE WOMAN *in this painting is definitely delighting in her Kali energy, flinging herself passionately on top of her lover: "She acts the part of the man from the beginning . . . with flowers in her hair hanging loose."*

V DON'T BE SURPRISED *if, once he's realized the delights of the woman-on-top positions, your womanhood drives him wild. He'll soon be worshipping you as his very own sexy goddess.*

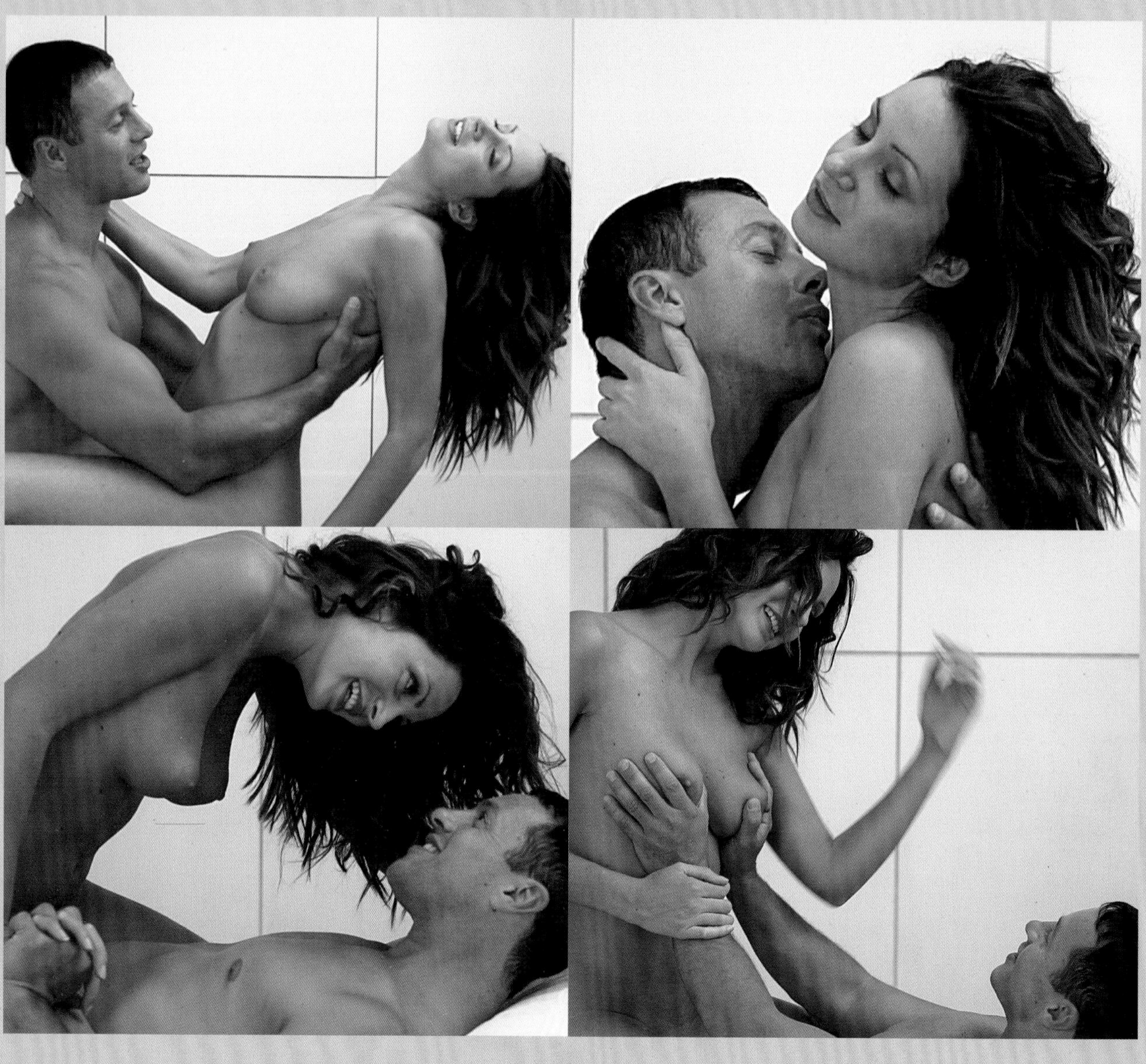

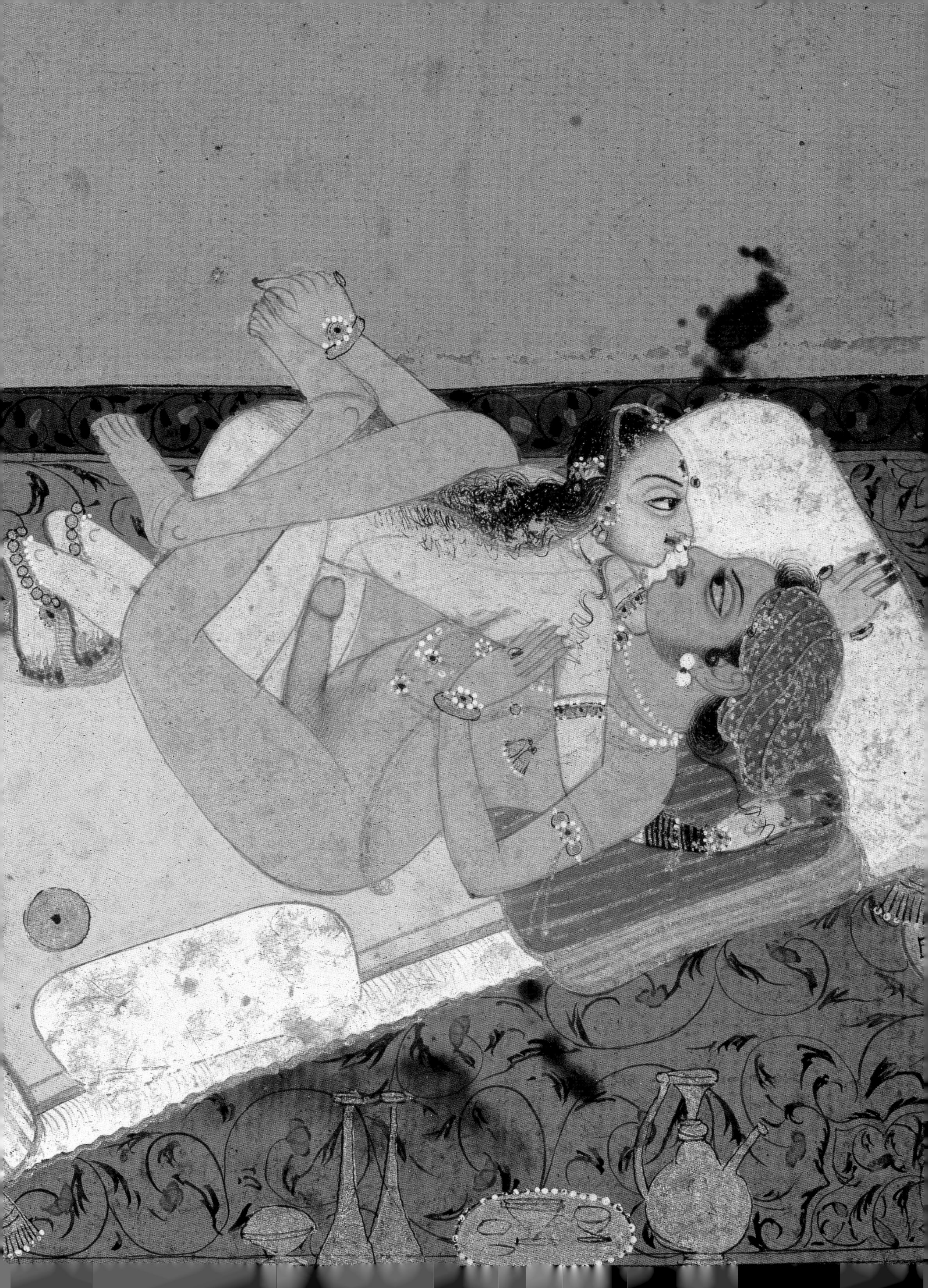

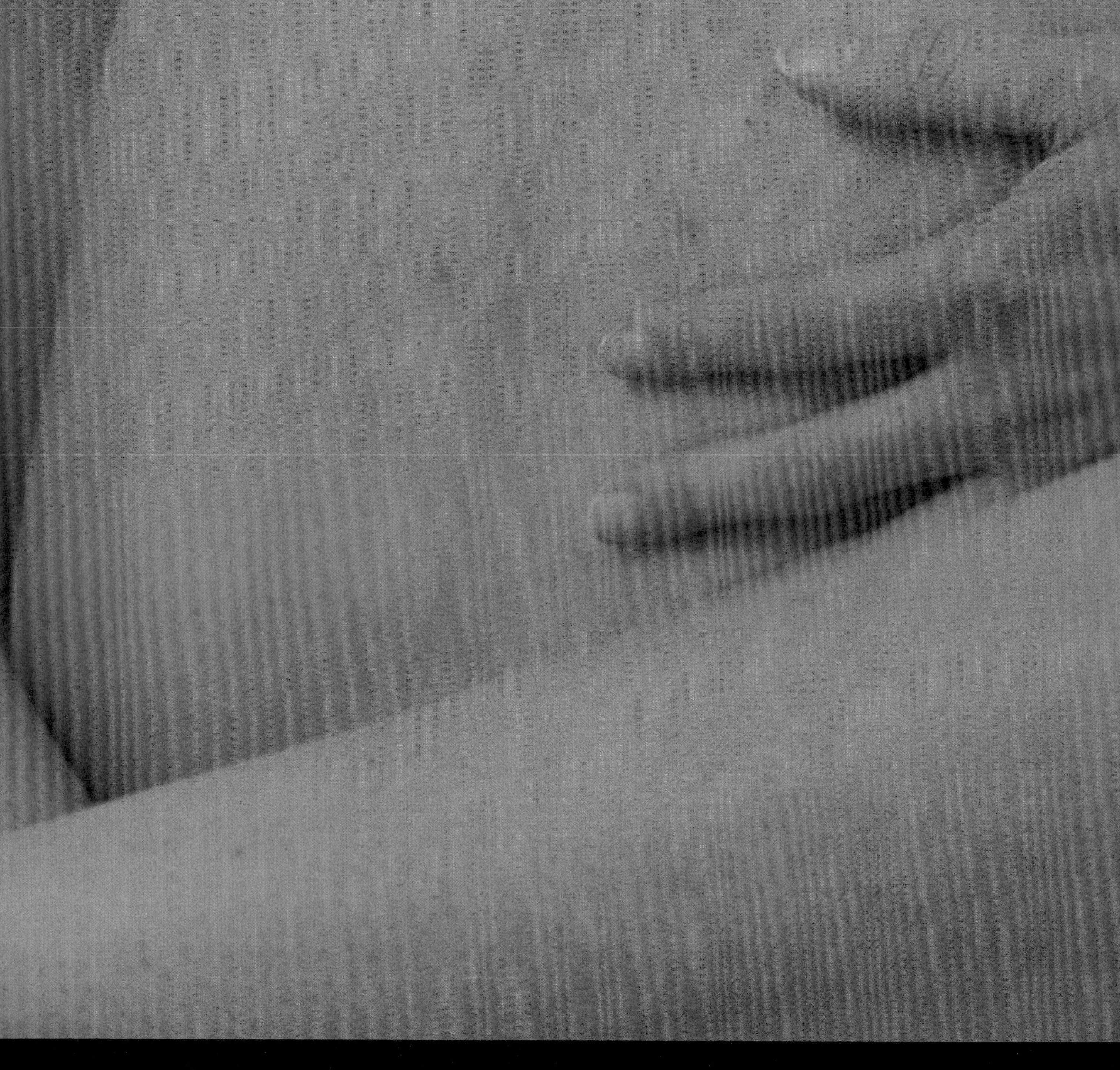

"The husband in this favorite position
sits cross-legged on the
bed or carpet, and takes his wife
upon his lap . . ."

ANANGA RANGA

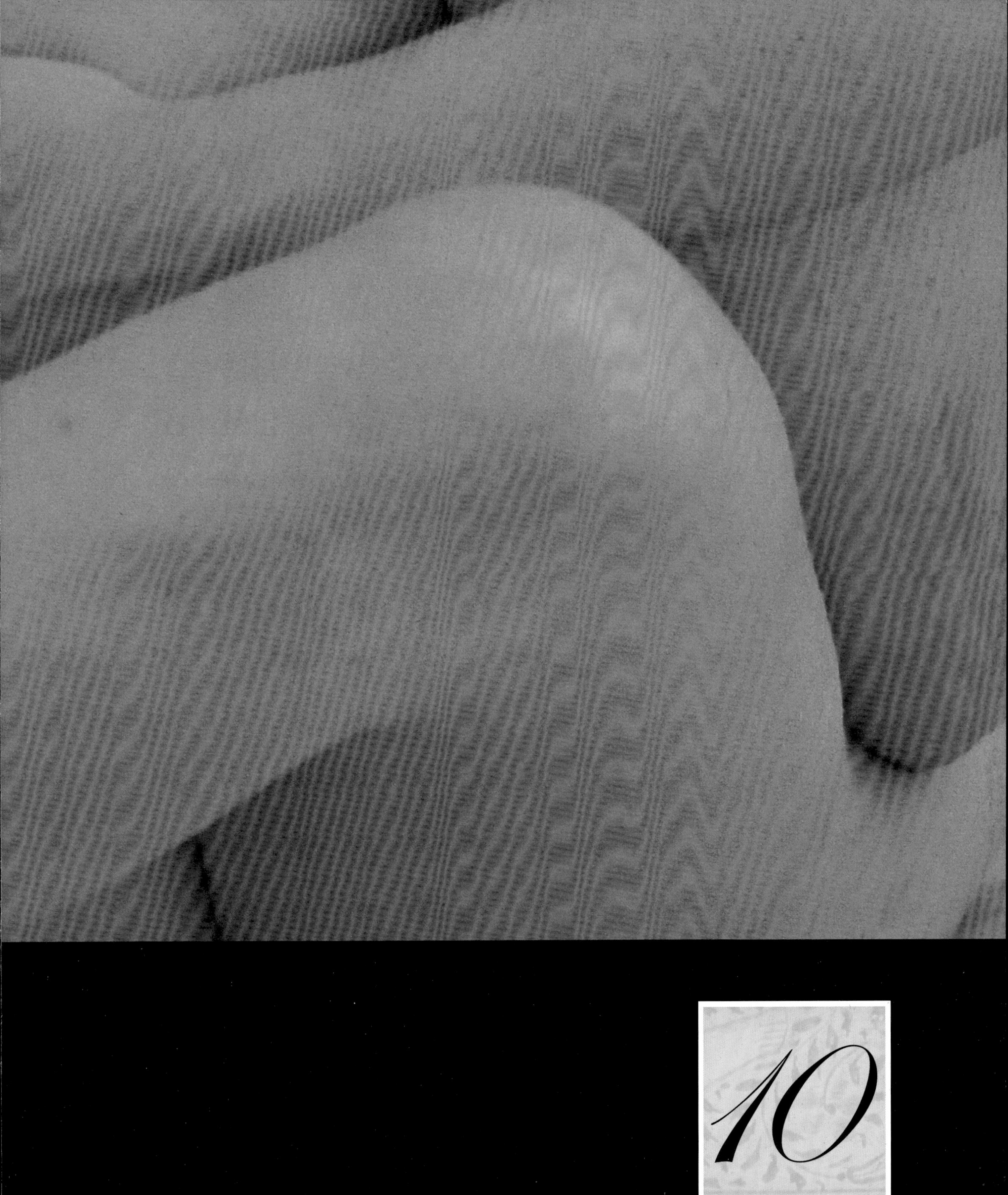
10

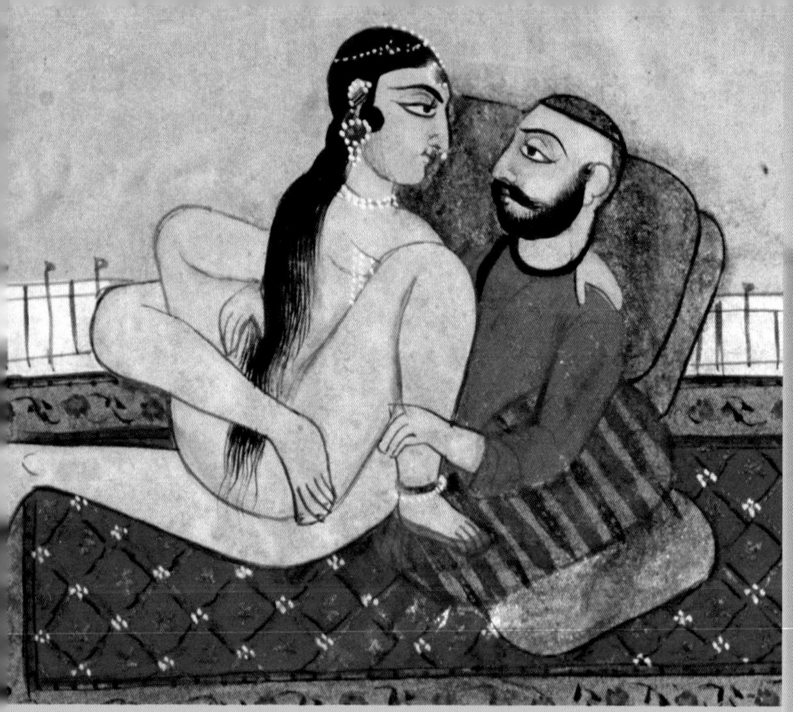

SITTING POSITIONS CAN BE the most tender and loving of all positions. It is an especially sensual and relaxed form of sex in which, although the female is usually the more active partner, the overriding feeling is of equality and intimacy. The relatively subtle movements necessitated by many of these positions can build up a potent sexual charge. Sitting positions are often used in tantric sex rituals.

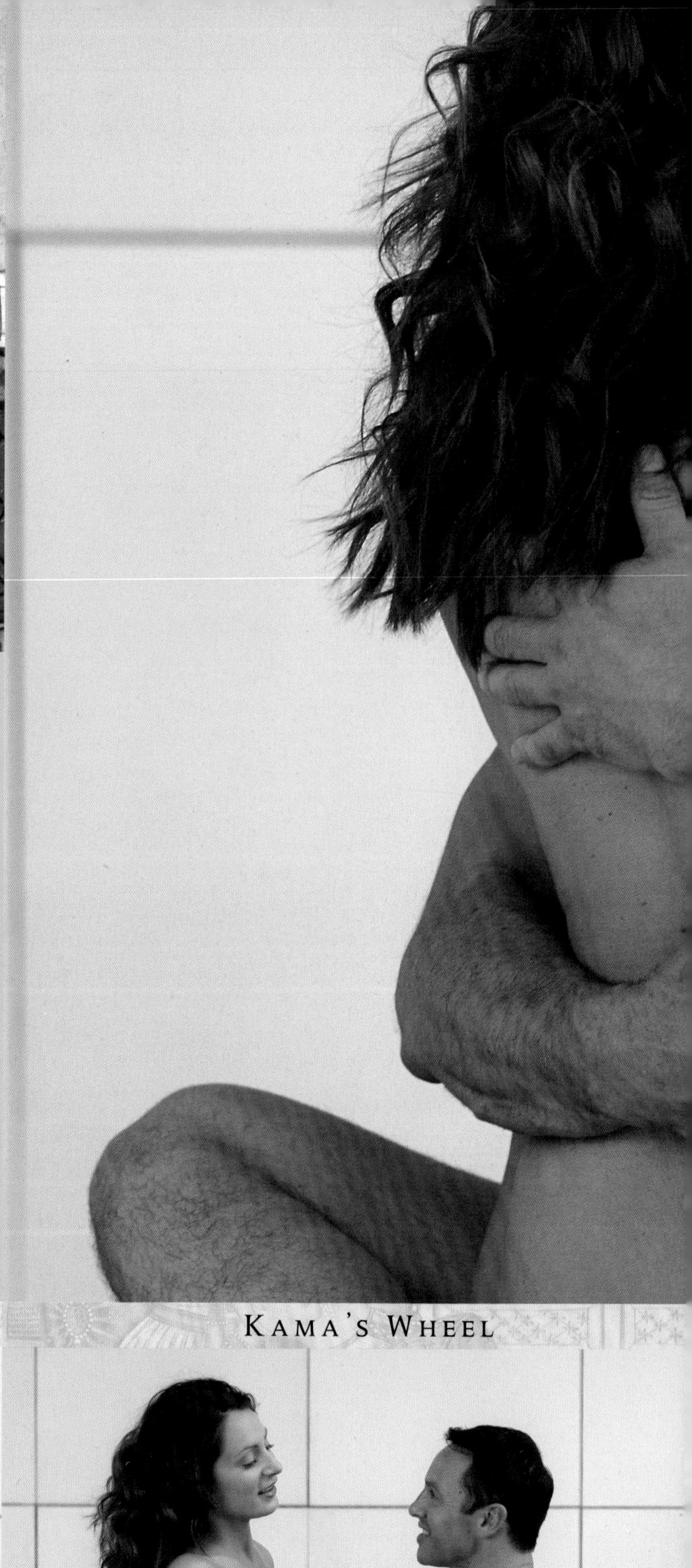

Lotus position

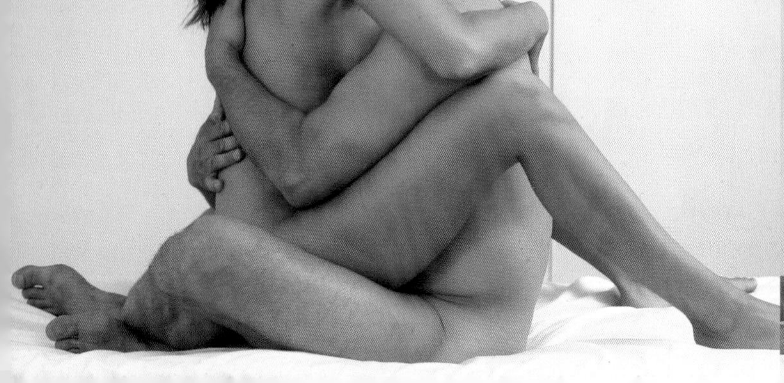

Kama's Wheel

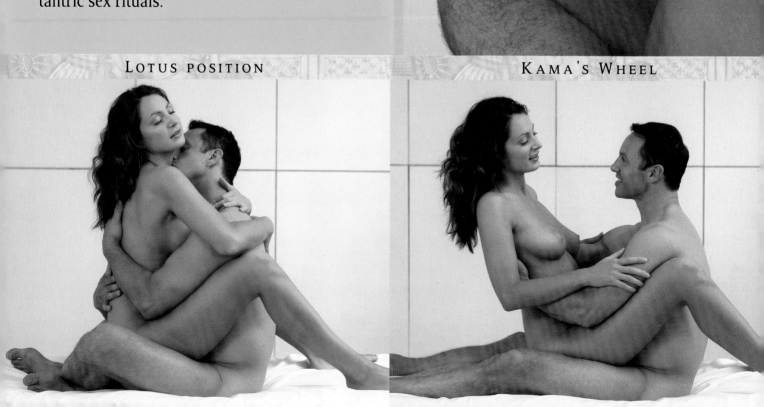

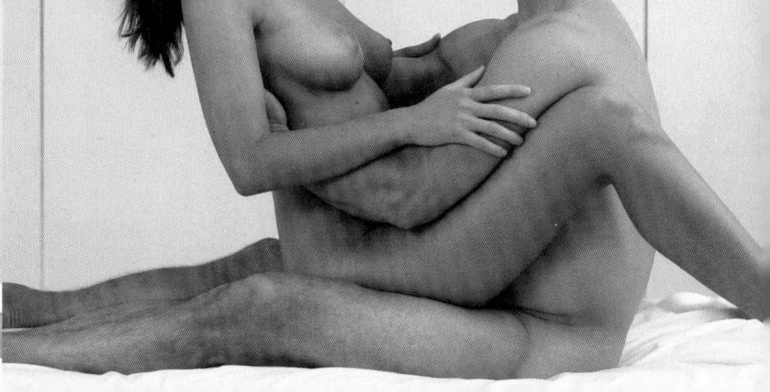

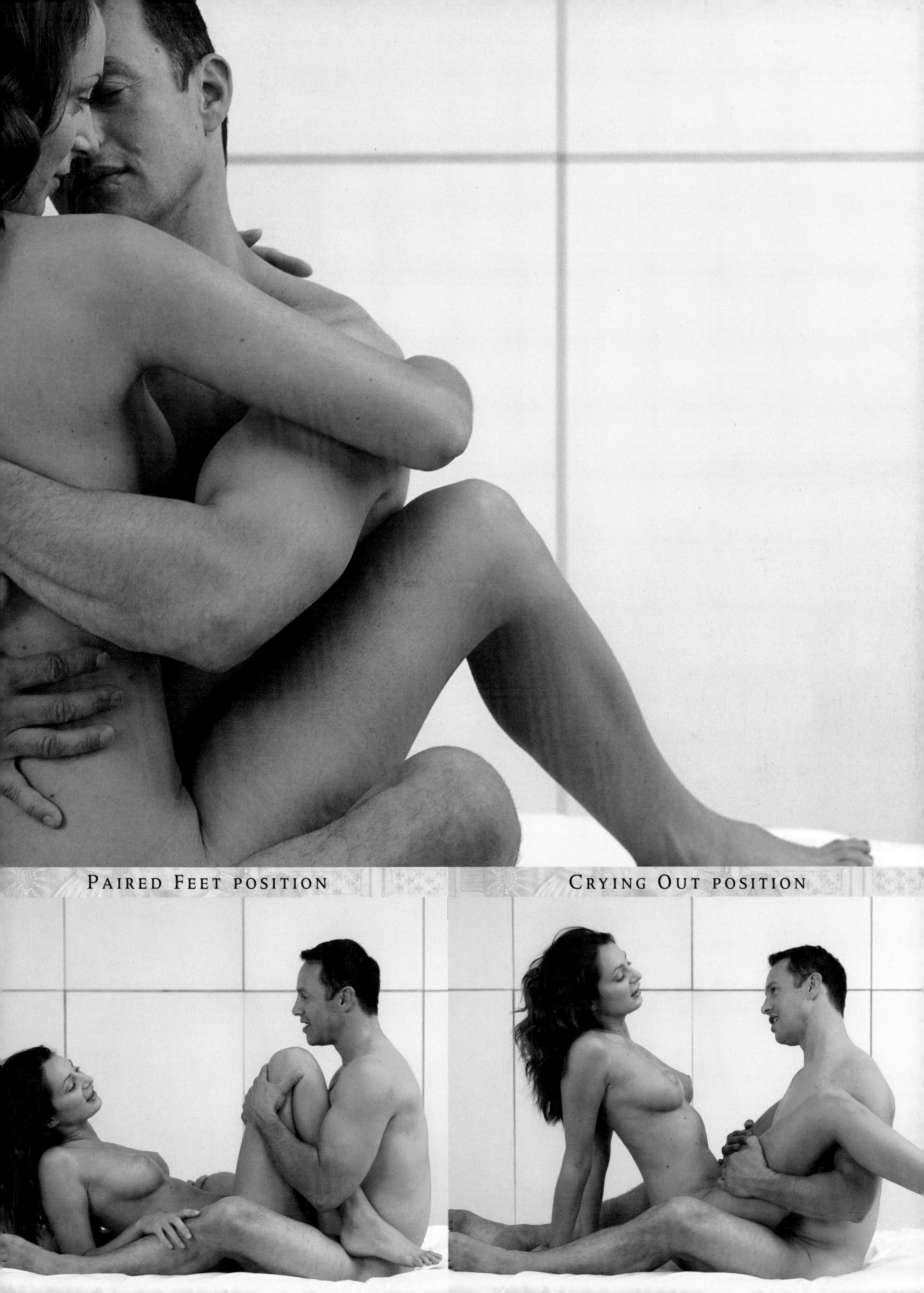

Paired Feet position

Crying Out position

Lotus position

The Lotus position, which is described as a "favorite" position in the Ananga Ranga, is actually the ancient tantric Buddhist position known as *yab-yum* (mother-father). It is a position that is revered by tantric practitioners as the sexual position of the highest form of union, in which it is possible to experience cosmic bliss. In Hindu mythology, Shiva and his wife Parvati (Kali) remained joined in this position for a thousand years.

V IN THIS SENSUOUS *lovemaking position, the man "sits cross-legged upon the bed or carpet, and takes his wife upon his lap." The woman sits astride him with her legs entwined around his waist. It doesn't stimulate the body as directly as other, more traditional postures, yet it is very arousing. Its eroticism lies in its intimacy, especially when your bodies are pressed tightly together.*

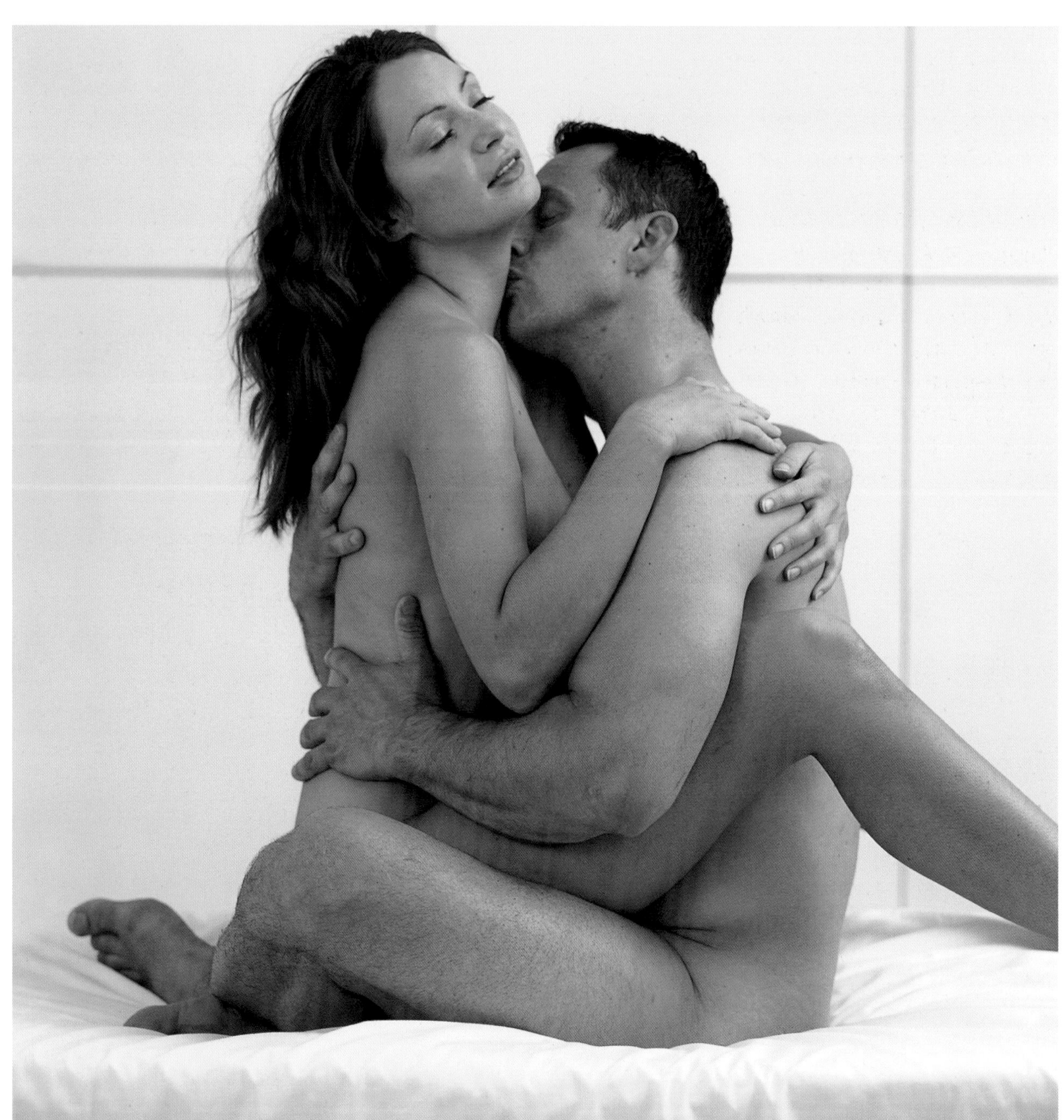

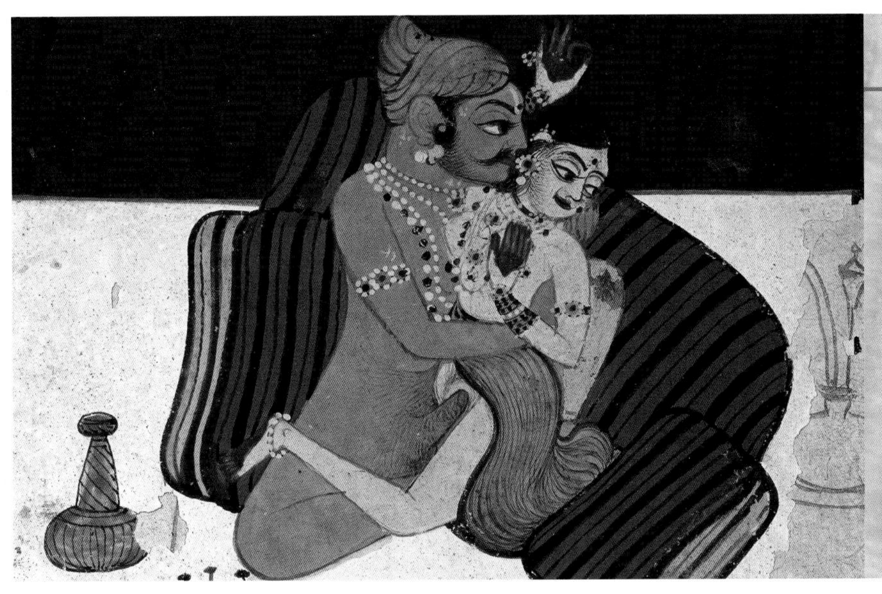

Teasing

Back support is definitely needed if you want to enjoy this position for any length of time. Here, the man has provided a number of large cushions for his partner's comfort. However, the woman is still wearing her skirt and seems to be resisting her lover's kisses. Perhaps this is an example of the playful teasing and counter-teasing that Vatsyayana recommends.

> THE ANANGA RANGA *describes a variation of the Lotus position in which the woman "slightly raises one leg." This subtly alters the tension between your vagina and his penis.*

V BY LEANING *backward you can change the angle of entry in your vagina and expose your breasts for your lover to kiss. Support your weight on one hand and, in the unlikely event that he doesn't take the hint, use your other hand to draw him toward you, urging him to lick and suck your breasts, telling him how good it feels.*

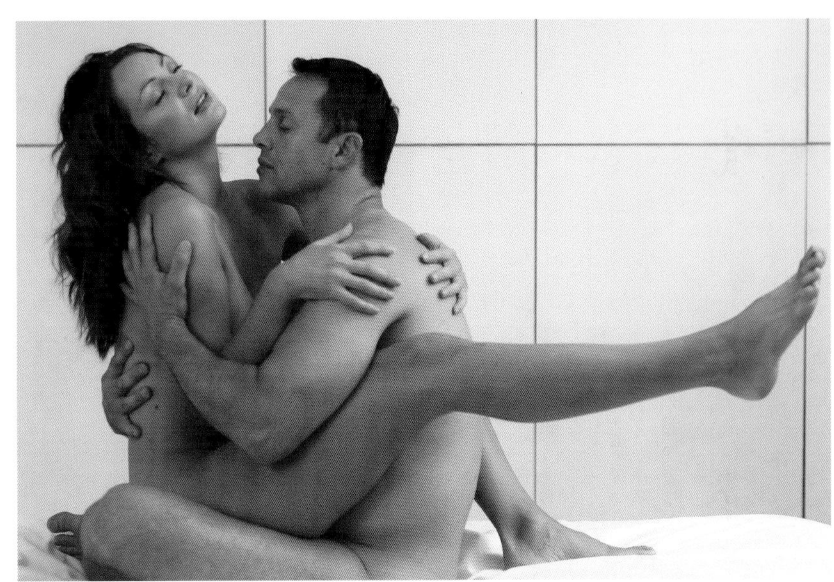

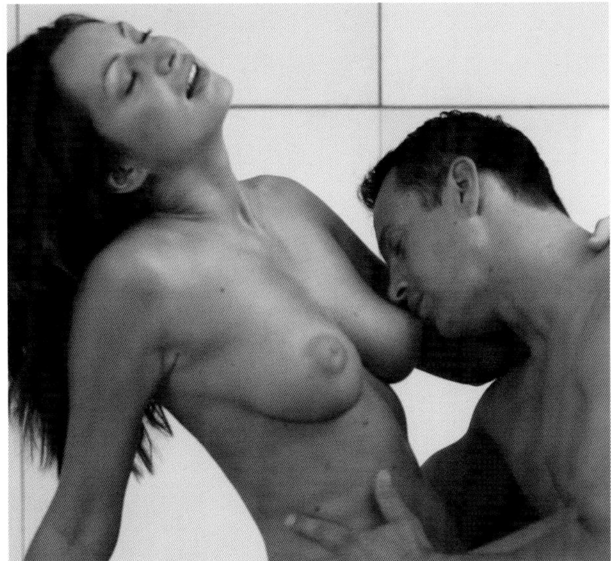

What works for him? ♂

Although sitting positions are popular for their ability to induce a meditative sexual mood during extended tantric sex rituals, they are also ideal for **impromptu** lovemaking sessions when time is short. They can be enjoyed with one or both partners more or less **fully clothed**. The fact that she is doing most of the work (and knowing that she is loving every minute of it) can be a major turn on. Open your legs wider and she will be able to sink **deeper** onto your penis.

These positions provide a great deal of **intimacy** and eye contact, and endless opportunities for kissing and **cuddling**. There is little movement, but you set the pace. However, some sitting positions can be tiring for the woman, so it is important to have moments of **stillness**.

What works for her?

> THIS PICTURE *shows one of the "practically impossible" tantric sitting postures. You would need to be a yogi, a contortionist, or a cat to be able to adopt this position.*

V PULL YOURSELF *closer to your lover by twining your legs around his back. If you want to quicken the tempo, move into the squatting position and pick up the pace. Use your feet for leverage, effectively bouncing up and down in his lap. Remember that it is easy to slip back into the woman-on-top positions if you decide the meditative mood is not for you.*

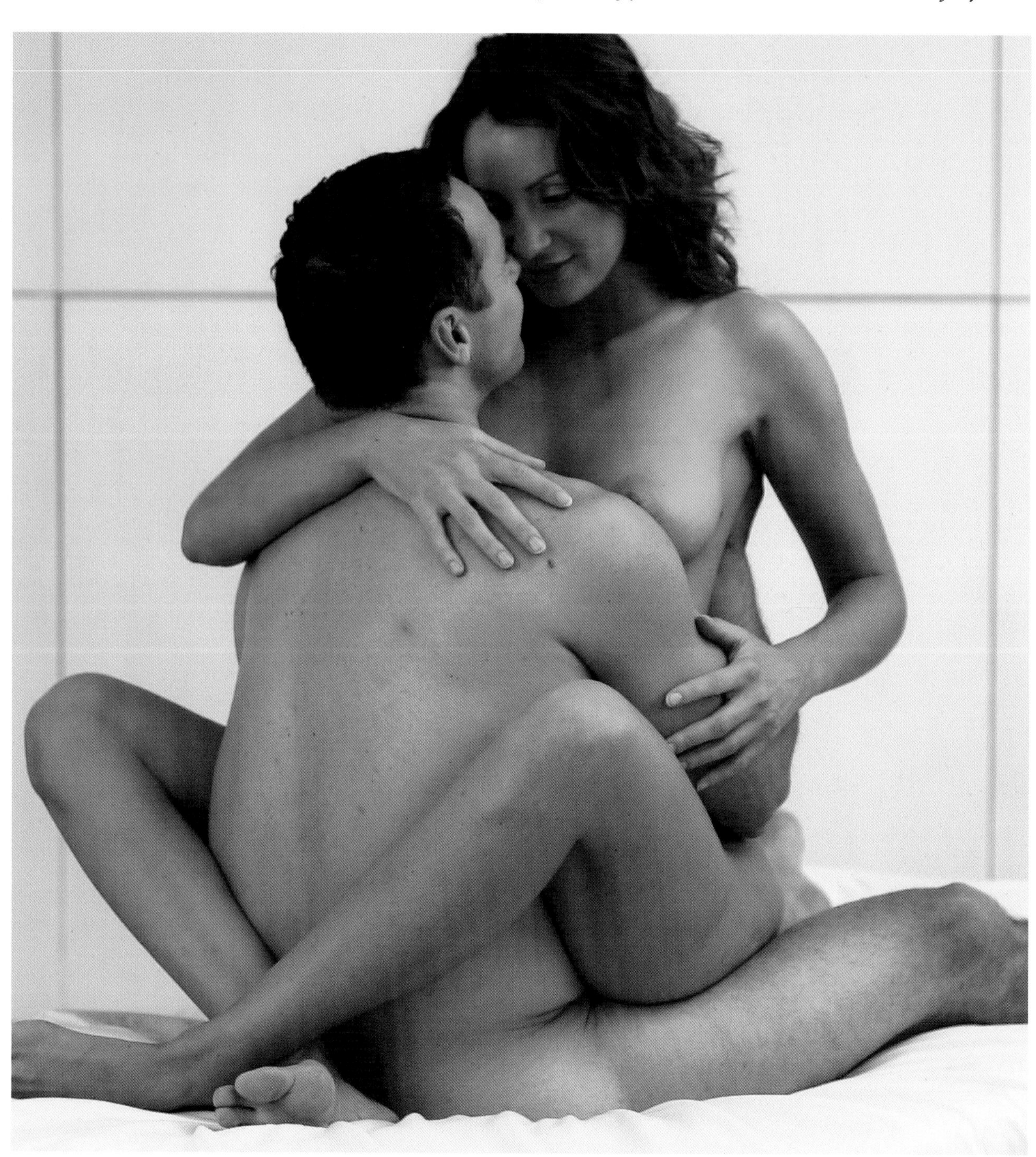

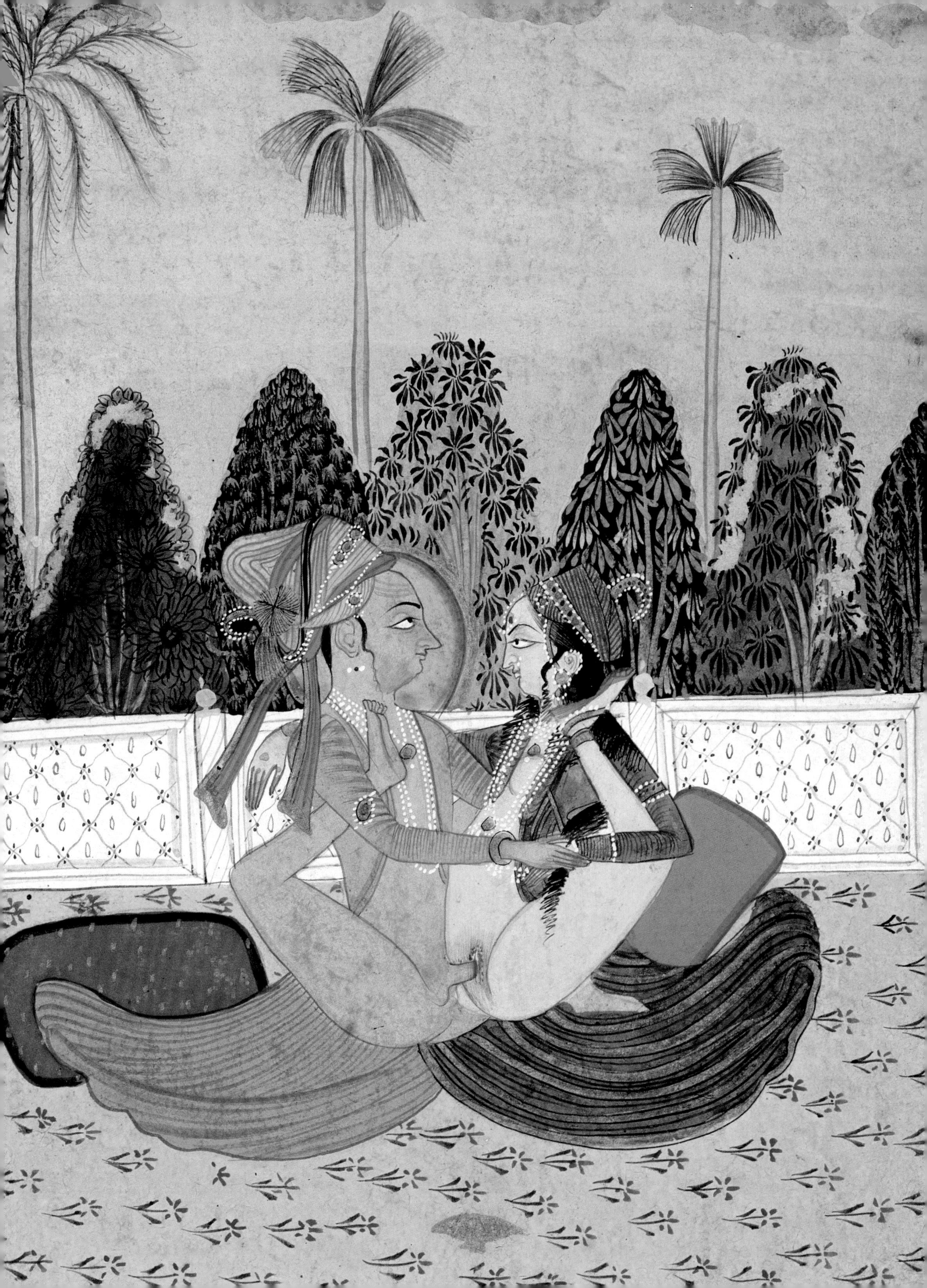

Kama's Wheel

Lovemaking in the sitting position can become very still and meditative, with the lovers simply holding each other closely, harmonizing their breathing, and allowing their bodies to sway and rock gently, without the usual thrusting associated with more active sexual positions. Kama's Wheel is also a position associated with meditative yogic and tantric rituals but here the partners lean away from each other. The man sits with his legs outstretched and his lover mirrors his position (thus creating the spokes of a wheel with their legs).

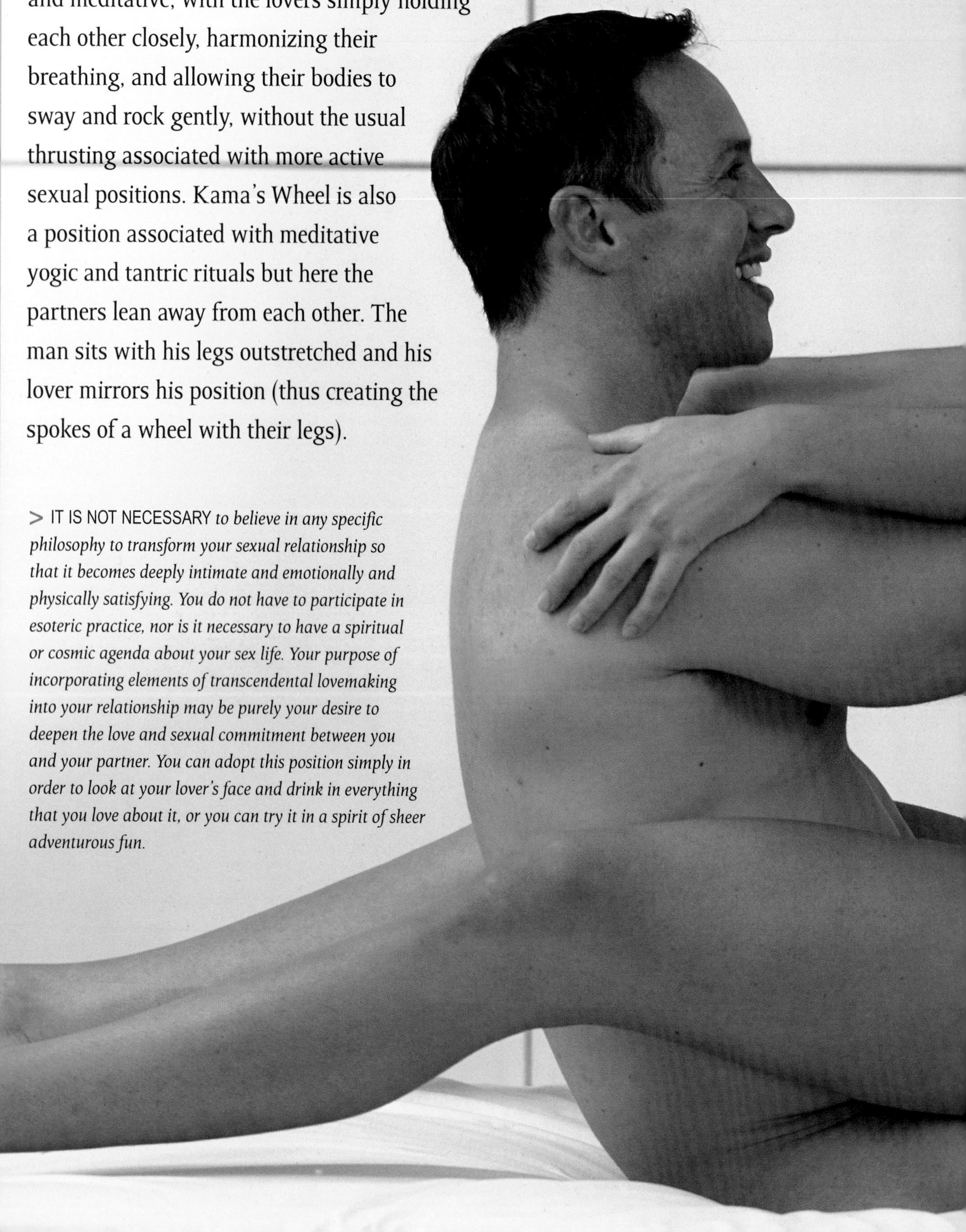

> IT IS NOT NECESSARY *to believe in any specific philosophy to transform your sexual relationship so that it becomes deeply intimate and emotionally and physically satisfying. You do not have to participate in esoteric practice, nor is it necessary to have a spiritual or cosmic agenda about your sex life. Your purpose of incorporating elements of transcendental lovemaking into your relationship may be purely your desire to deepen the love and sexual commitment between you and your partner. You can adopt this position simply in order to look at your lover's face and drink in everything that you love about it, or you can try it in a spirit of sheer adventurous fun.*

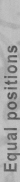

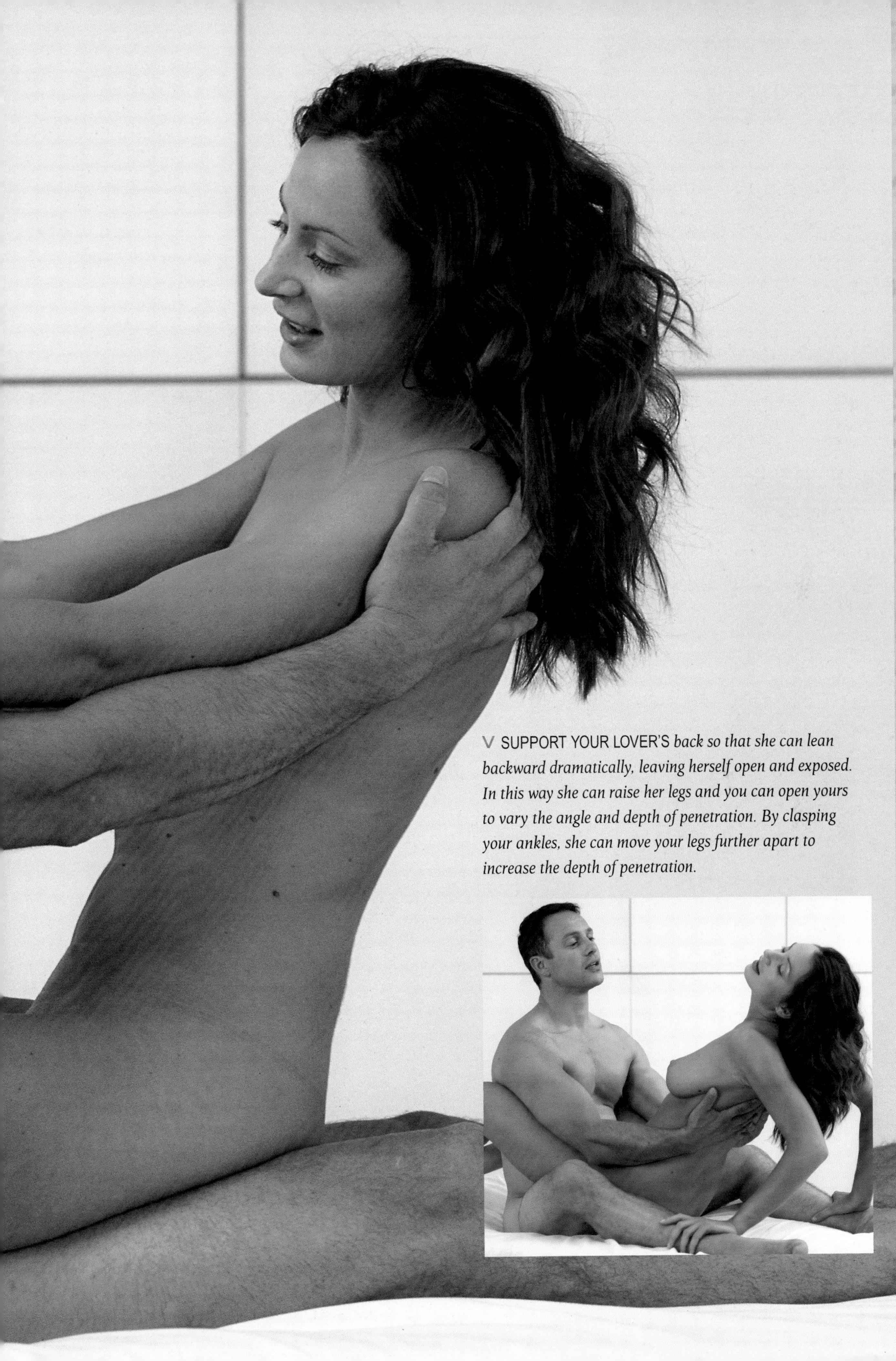

V SUPPORT YOUR LOVER'S *back so that she can lean backward dramatically, leaving herself open and exposed. In this way she can raise her legs and you can open yours to vary the angle and depth of penetration. By clasping your ankles, she can move your legs further apart to increase the depth of penetration.*

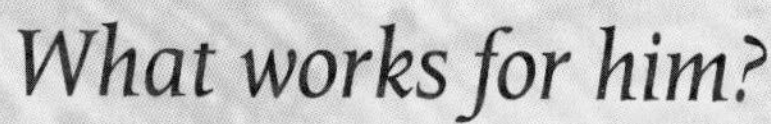

What works for him?

This is one of those positions that allows you both an exciting view of her vagina as it *slips* sensuously *up and down* the shaft of his penis. Look and learn as you begin to appreciate the eroticism of very *subtle* movements that are a million miles away from the masculine bump and grind. You will be very pleasantly surprised by the intensity of orgasm that can be reached.

> BY LEANING BACK *and holding on to your partner's ankles you can move into the Ananga Ranga position known as the Snake Trap. Use your pelvic floor muscles to grip your lover's penis and rock gently back and forth, tensing and relaxing your vagina. Rotate your hips slightly as you lower yourself onto the shaft of his penis, then slide back up to the tip without letting his penis slip out. Close your eyes—he can watch you without inhibition and you can focus on your own pleasure.*

Have you been practicing using those pelvic floor muscles? This is your opportunity to demonstrate just how good they can make you both feel. *Squeeze* your vagina around the tip of his penis and then make small circular movements to "milk" his penis. Listen to his *moans* of delight as the orgasmic tension inevitably *mounts*.

What works for her?

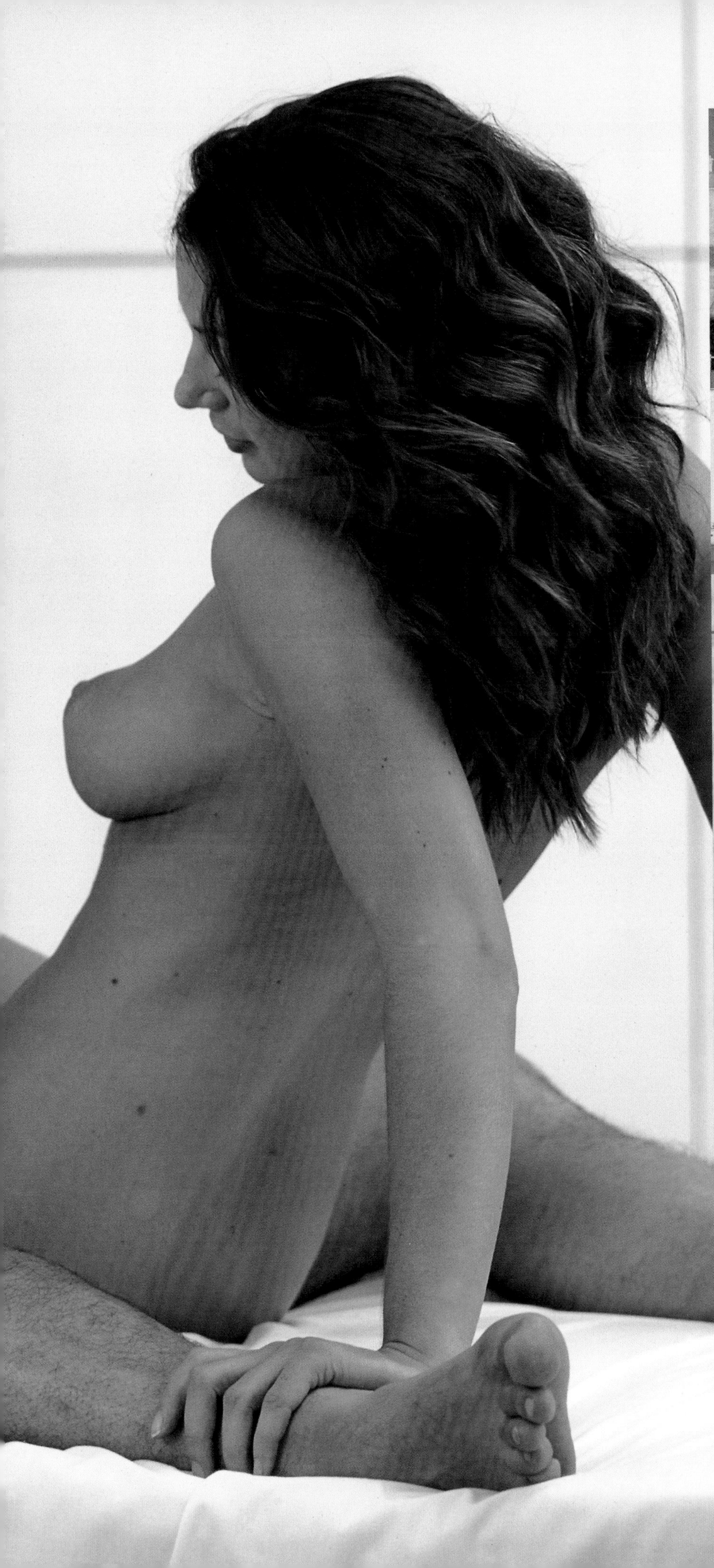

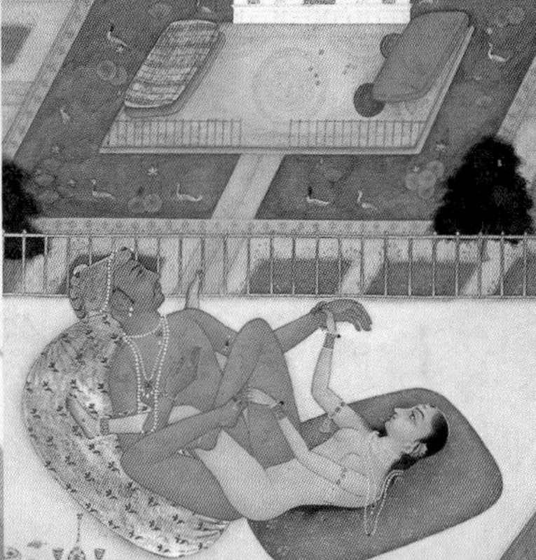

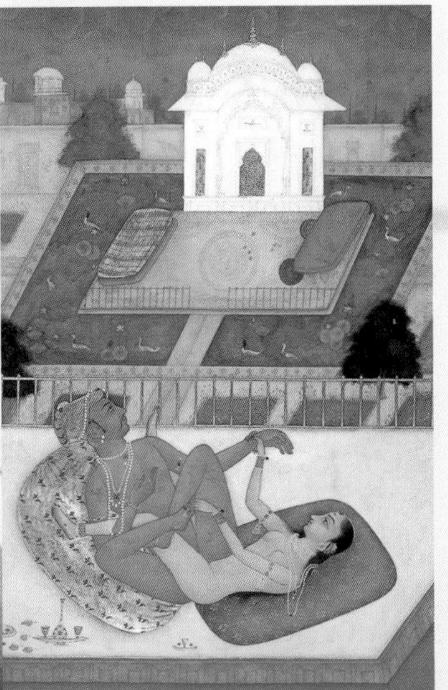

Spiritual energy

Here two lovers recline in a complex tantric posture, where the woman must use her vaginal muscles to maintain his erection. Sitting postures are employed in tantric sex rituals where the lovers can remain practically immobile for hours at a time, meditating and focusing on stimulating their subtle energy bodies rather than their physical bodies.

Upright seated positions encourage the release of *kundalini* energy, a spiritual energy that is usually represented in the form of a snake or serpent. The rising *kundalini* activates dormant power centers in the body, known as chakras. The crossed legs seal the flow of energy around the body.

As he becomes increasingly aroused, the man uses breathing techniques to control his semen and to retain and build on his orgasmic energy in order to transform or transcend his consciousness.

Paired Feet position

In this sensual position the woman leans back while drawing her legs up so that her shins are resting on her partner's chest. The man opens his legs wide apart, with her body between them, so that the woman can achieve full penetration. Then he presses her thighs together to intensify the sensations. Again, movement is very limited, so you may need a little help with stimulation. A bonus for him is the sexy view he gets of his lover's breasts.

V BY DRAWING *your knees up, your vaginal muscles naturally constrict around the penis giving you both intense pleasure. He can relax the pressure on your thighs occasionally and use his hands instead to stroke your thighs. If you need a little help to reach your orgasm, he can open your legs and gently massage your clitoris.*

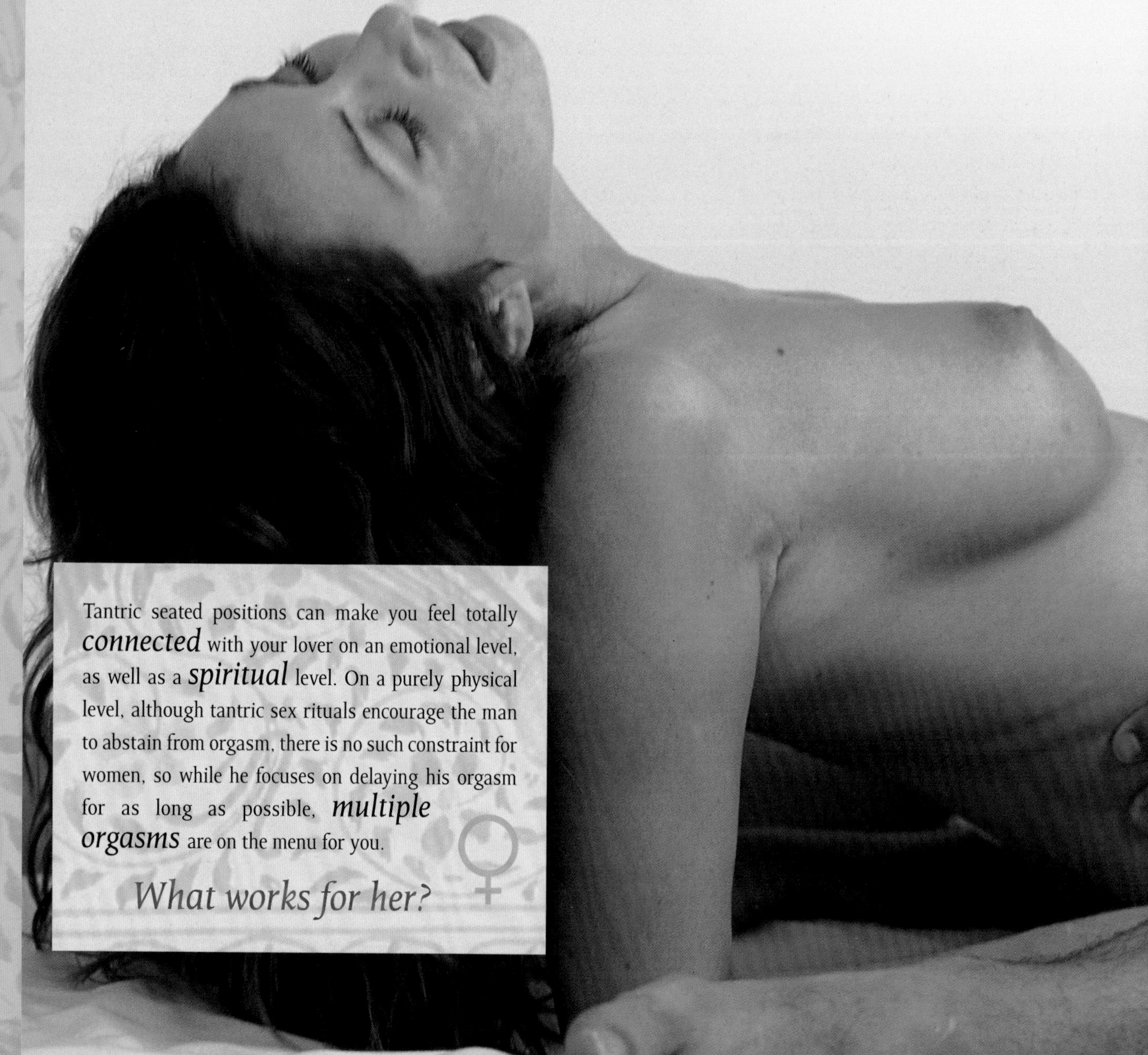

Tantric seated positions can make you feel totally *connected* with your lover on an emotional level, as well as a *spiritual* level. On a purely physical level, although tantric sex rituals encourage the man to abstain from orgasm, there is no such constraint for women, so while he focuses on delaying his orgasm for as long as possible, *multiple orgasms* are on the menu for you.

What works for her?

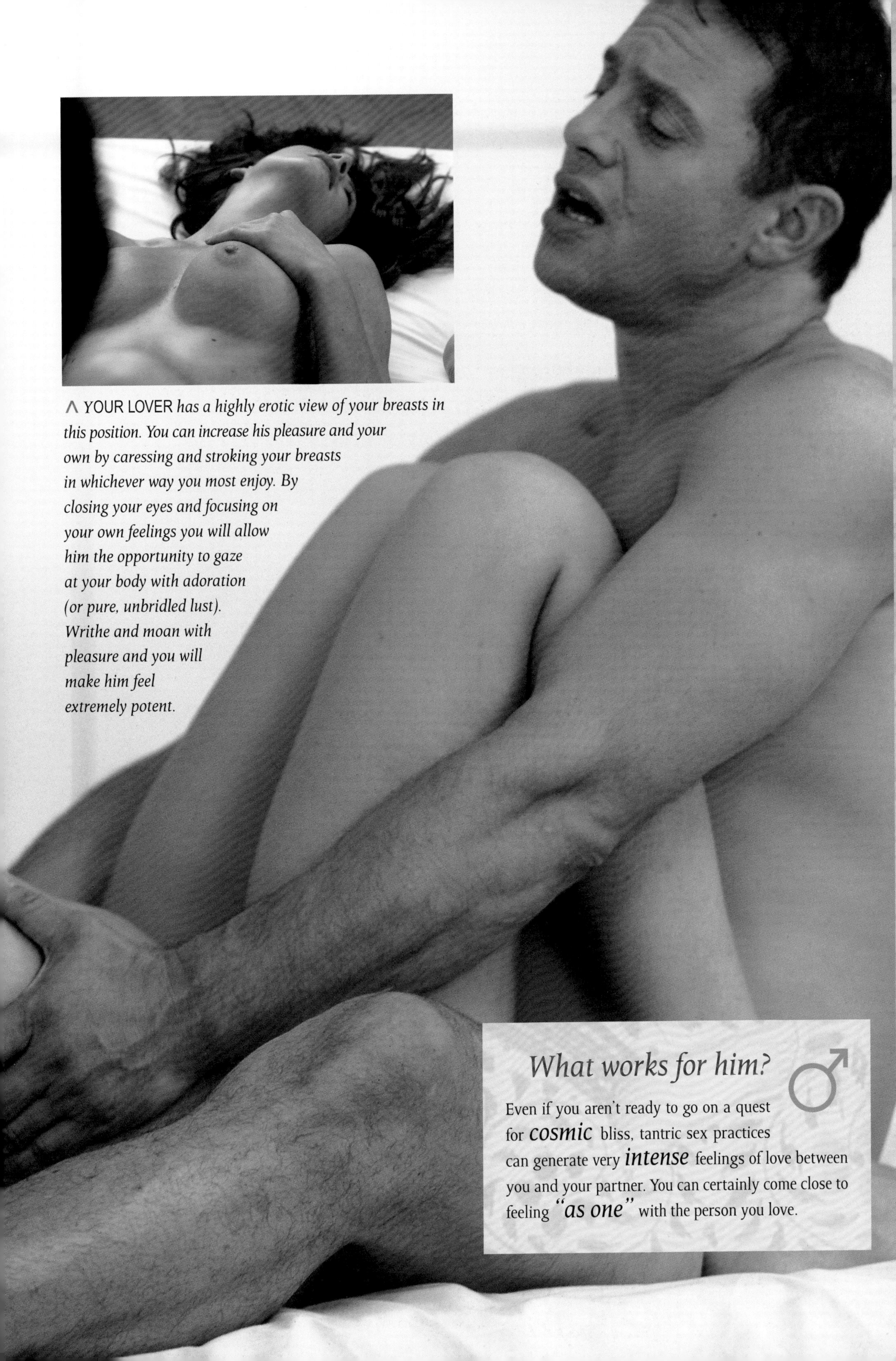

^ YOUR LOVER *has a highly erotic view of your breasts in this position. You can increase his pleasure and your own by caressing and stroking your breasts in whichever way you most enjoy. By closing your eyes and focusing on your own feelings you will allow him the opportunity to gaze at your body with adoration (or pure, unbridled lust). Writhe and moan with pleasure and you will make him feel extremely potent.*

What works for him? ♂

Even if you aren't ready to go on a quest for ***cosmic*** bliss, tantric sex practices can generate very ***intense*** feelings of love between you and your partner. You can certainly come close to feeling ***"as one"*** with the person you love.

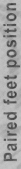

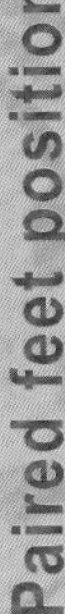

Crying Out position

According to the Ananga Ranga, this position is: "a form possible only to a very strong man with a very light woman; he raises her by passing both her legs over his arms at the elbow, and moves her about from left to right . . . until the supreme moment arrives." Penetration can be deep and the thrusting relatively vigorous, so it can indeed be a good position in which to reach the "supreme moment" of orgasm. It is also a simple step back from here into a long and loving post-coital cuddle in the Lotus position.

> THE SWORD AND DAGGER *in the foreground illustrate that this man is a warrior. The position in which he is depicted is further evidence that he is a man of great strength.*

V FROM THE PAIRED FEET *position he can slip his arms under your knees and put his hands on your waist to lift you. It may be a strain for him, so help him out by leaning back and taking some of your weight on your arms.*

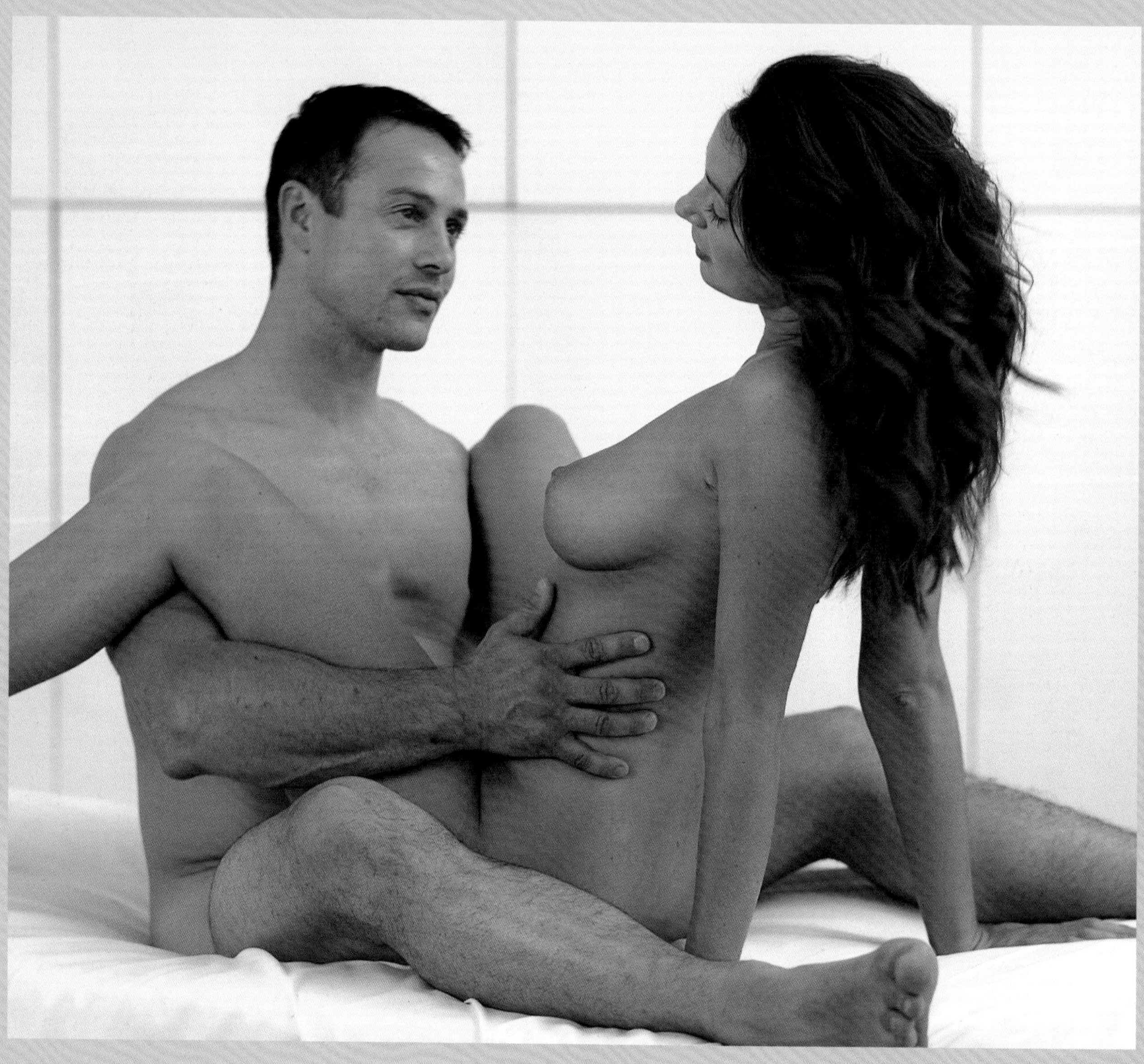

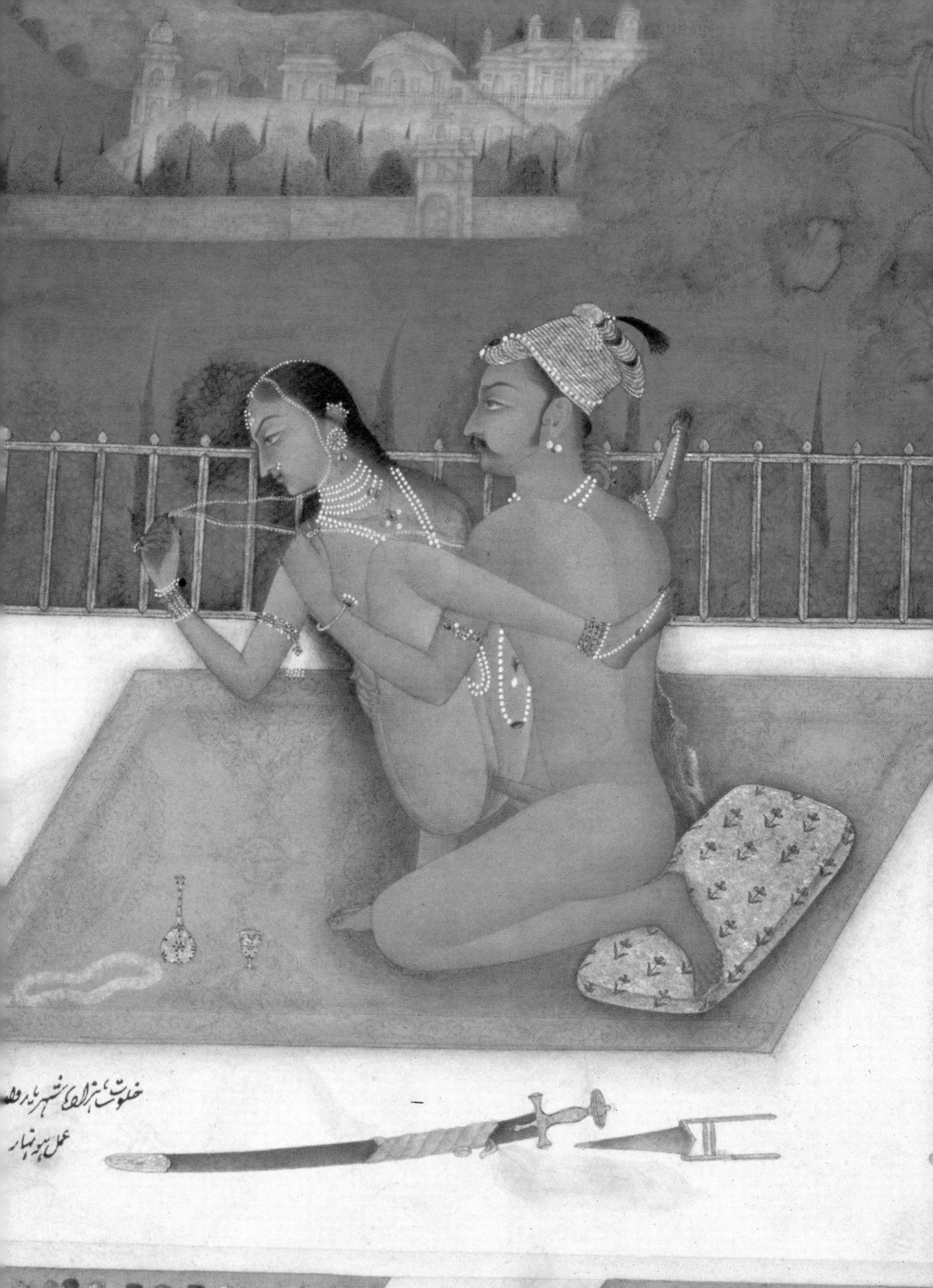

INDEX

ACKNOWLEDGMENTS

Studio Cactus are grateful to the following for their contributions to this project:
Picture research Jo Walton; design assistance Dawn Terrey and Laura Watson; proofreading Elizabeth Mallard-Shaw; Americanizing, Beth Adelman; indexing Jackie Brind; editorial assistance Aaron Brown. Our thanks also go to the models.

Picture Credits
All specially commissioned photography by Jeremy Hopley
Photographer's assistant: Clare Miller
Makeup artist: Sam Williams

AKG images/Jean-Louis Nou: 9, 18, 19 below
The Art Archive/JFB: 29 below, 66 above, 102 above, 118 above, 154 above, 176 above
Bridgeman Art Library
Archives Charmet/Private Collection: 15, 74 above, 82, 140 above
Ashmolean Museum, Oxford, UK: 20–21 Paris, France: 14
British Library, London, UK: 27
Fitzwilliam Museum, University of Cambridge, UK: 10, 23 above left, 23 above right, 23 center left, 55, 86, 91 above, 99, 127, 133, 136 below, 149, 185, 189
Lahore Museum, Lahore, Pakistan: 51
Lauros/Giraudon/Musée Guimet, Paris, France: 13 above
Ann and Bury Peerless Picture Library/Baroda Museum, Baroda, Gujarat, India: 12 above
Private Collection: 8, 11, 25, 30, 35, 38–39, 40, 43, 59, 60, 63, 144 above, 165, 173, 179 above, 181
Victoria and Albert Museum, London, UK: 4–5, 6–7, 13 below, 26 above, 32, 41, 44, 47